Mental Health Approaches to Intellectual/Developmental Disability: *A Resource for Trainers*

– SECOND EDITION –

Robert J. Fletcher, DSW, ACSW, LCSW, NADD-CC

Melissa Cheplic, MPH, NADD-CC

Daniel Baker, Ph.D., NADD-CC

Juanita St. Croix, BSc., NADD-CC

Jeanne M. Farr, M.A.

NADD
An association for persons with developmental disabilities and mental health needs.

321 Wall Street
Kingston, N.Y., 12401

Contributions to Module 11 were made by Carly Winnie.
Book design by Michael Frazier.

ISBN: 979-8-9853366-2-7
Library of Congress Control Number: 2022931462

Printed in the United States of America

TABLE OF CONTENTS

Introduction

Welcome to the second edition of *Mental Health Approaches to Intellectual/ Developmental Disability: A Resource for Trainers.* This is a landmark contribution to the field of support for persons with intellectual or developmental disabilities (IDD) and mental health concerns. This resource can be used by a myriad of different professionals and care providers for a variety of different purposes. *Mental Health Approaches to Intellectual/Developmental Disability: A Resource for Trainers* may be used to train others for professional development (train-the-trainer model); as a resource guide for individual study; or as a reference guide. Proper support of mental wellness among persons with IDD requires a significant body of information and knowledge, and the authors of this resource are happy to offer it as a means for educating professionals and care providers.

This resource is designed to be used with a variety of audiences, including Direct Support Professionals and the full spectrum of behavioral healthcare professionals. The resource is organized into modules, within which materials are presented in Microsoft PowerPoint slides and speaker notes. For professionals seeking more extensive information, references have been provided at the end of each module.

To access the digital version of the material in this book, please visit **thenadd.org/presentations**.

Using the Resource for Trainers to Train Others for Professional Development
Exercises and Case Studies are included to give attendees a chance to practice and interact with the materials being presented. Please read the chapter on Cultivating Training Mastery to learn about all aspects of developing and delivering a training workshop.

A workbook, *Trainee Workbook for Mental Health Approaches to Intellectual/ Developmental Disability, Second Edition*, is intended to be used by participants in your trainings. It contains the slides (without speaker notes) and space for the participant to write notes. The workbook contains pre- and post-tests for each module to measure and assist in learning. These tests are also included in the appendix of the resource for trainers.

Using the Resource for Trainers for Individual Study

When used for individual study, we encourage reviewing and reading the entire resource for trainers.

Using the Resource for Trainers as a Reference Guide

The organization of this resource is in a module format, so if you have specific interest in any area, you can review that topic specifically.

About the Authors

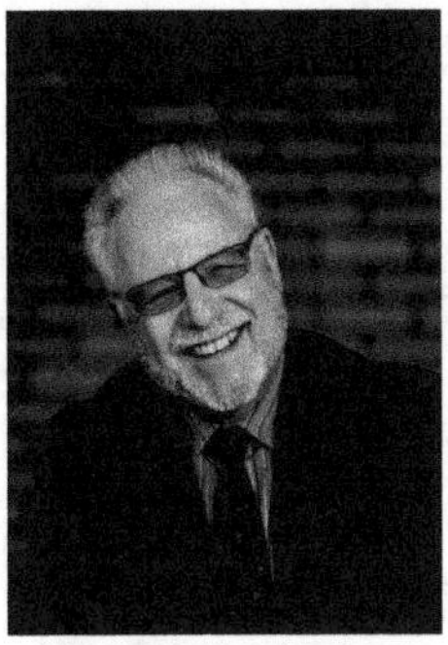

Robert J. Fletcher, DSW, ACSW, LCSW, NADD-CC

Dr. Rob Fletcher is the founder and Chief Executive Officer Emeritus of NADD. He has dedicated his professional career to improving the lives of individuals who have a dual diagnosis of mental illness (MI) and an intellectual disability (ID). Dr. Fletcher has authored articles, book chapters, and books in areas concerning clinical, programmatic, policy, and research in the field of dual diagnosis. He is the Chief Editor of both the textbook and clinical guide of the *Diagnostic Manual – Intellectual Disabilities (DM-ID and DM-ID-2)*. Additionally, Dr. Fletcher has provided consultation services and lectures worldwide on various topics related to mental health aspects in persons with intellectual disabilities.

Rob earned a bachelor's degree from Marquette University, a master's of social work from Washington University and a doctorate in social work with honors from Hunter College School of Social Work-City University of New York.

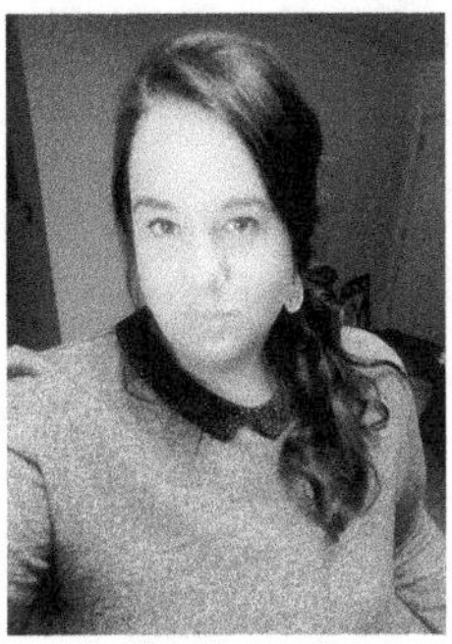

Melissa Cheplic, MPH, NADD-CC

Melissa Cheplic is a Senior Training and Consultation Specialist at The Boggs Center on Developmental Disabilities at Rutgers Medical School – New Jersey's University Center for Excellence in Development Disabilities. Melissa develops and delivers training and technical assistance to community provider and state agencies, building capacity in behavior and mental health and identifying strategies to coordinate behavior intervention with clinical supports for individuals with dual diagnosis. Melissa holds a master's degree from the Rutgers School of Public Health.

Melissa has designed and delivered nationally recognized curricula and presented at national conferences. She serves as the Chairperson of the NADD Direct Support Professional Certification Committee. In this role, she coauthored competency-based curriculum in dual diagnosis and was honored as NADD member of the year in 2015. Her work has been featured in the NADD Bulletin and other publications. Melissa currently co-chairs the NADD U.S. Policy Committee, collaborating with community and government partners on improving services for persons with IDD across systems.

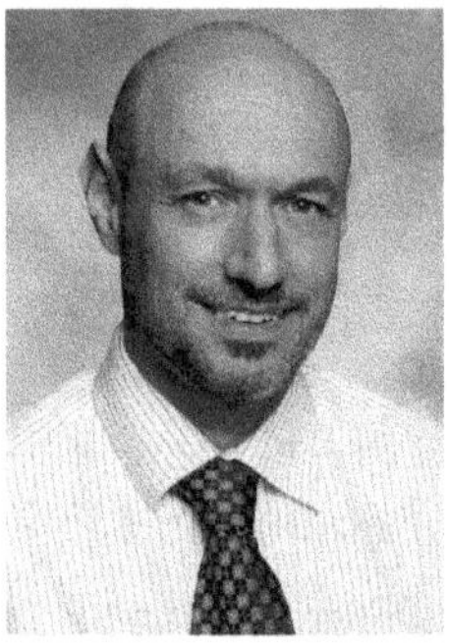

Daniel Baker, Ph.D., NADD-CC

Dr. Dan Baker is with the Minnesota Department of Human Services, where he serves as the Positive Supports Compliance Specialist with Quality Assurance and Disability Compliance Services. Dr. Baker also provides clinical supervision for the Successful Life Project. Dr. Baker is involved with the design, development and monitoring of treatment and intervention programs to align with the Positive Supports and a person-centered culture. Dr. Baker's clinical focus is on positive behavior support, models of community and educational support, transition services and mental health services for persons with disabilities.

Dan is well published in books and literary journals, primarily addressing strategies for teaching direct care staff to work with persons who present challenges. His contributions earned him the 2010 Clinical Practice Award from NADD. Dr. Baker is a reviewer for the journals *Intellectual and Developmental Disabilities, American Journal of Intellectual and Developmental Disabilities* and *Research in Developmental Disabilities*. Dr. Baker is very involved with NADD; he serves on the Board of Directors and co-edited the *NADD Bulletin* from 2006-11.

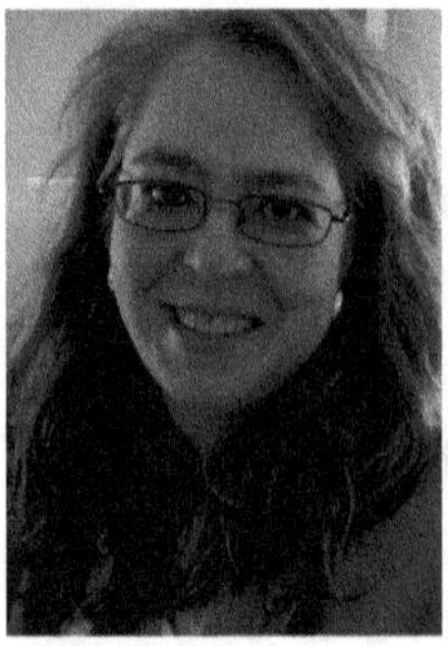

Juanita St. Croix, BSc, NADD-CC

Juanita St. Croix's home province is Newfoundland and Labrador in Canada. She credits the culture and spirit of community there with shaping her goals and her approach to working with people. Ms. St. Croix attended Western University in London, Ontario, where she stayed once her studies were complete. She has worked in human services for more than 30 years, primarily in developmental services with organizations providing services and supports for people with a dual diagnosis.

Juanita has been an active member of NADD since 2012 and has had her NADD-CC designation since 2019. Her current work involves building collaborations based on the needs of people who have a dual diagnosis and require services across multiple sectors. Her ongoing passion is building capacity to provide effective services and supports through developing resources, publications and research.

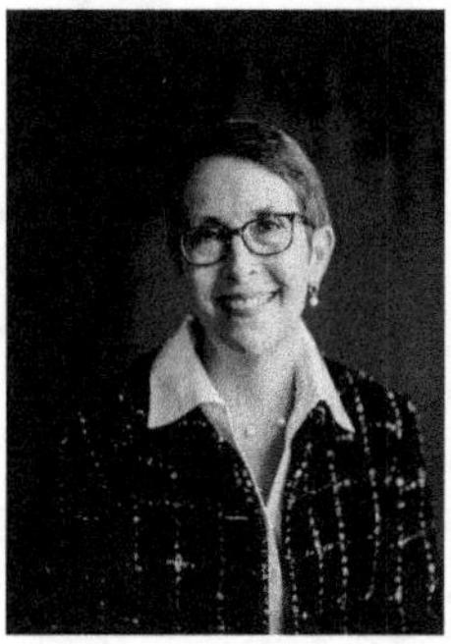

Jeanne M. Farr, M.A.

Jeanne M. Farr, Chief Executive Officer of NADD, has served in nonprofit executive leadership positions for more than 30 years and has won multiple awards honoring her exceptional professional contributions.

Jeanne serves on a variety of university and state advisory committees and nonprofit boards. She is Chair of the Board of the National Alliance for Direct Care Professionals and Chair of the Board of Ripple Effect Images. She serves on the advisory boards for the School of International Studies at University of the Pacific and the National Mental Health and Intellectual Disability Training Center. She is also a member of The Arc's Center for Future Planning Advisory Council.

Jeanne earned a master's degree in intercultural relations from University of the Pacific and has completed executive leadership programs at Harvard Business School, Columbia Business School and the Kellogg School of Management. She is the founder of Coexistence Collaborative, a social enterprise dedicated to fostering intercultural understanding and effectiveness focusing on organizational consultation, leadership, cross-cultural and diversity training and intercultural executive coaching.

Cultivating Training Mastery

Introduction

Teaching is more than imparting knowledge; it is inspiring change.
Learning is more than absorbing facts; it is acquiring understanding.
— William Arthur Ward, Writer/Educator

Being a trainer is a privilege and responsibility. People take precious time out of their lives, dedicate fiscal resources and depend upon you to make valuable use of their time and investment. This book is designed to support you as a trainer. Whether you are a seasoned trainer or new to this professional endeavor, this chapter is intended to be a resource and expand your capacity as a trainer. This text and the accompanying workbook are equally applicable whether you are training a group on the content in this book or training professionals to teach this material. The various modules in the book can be taught independent of one another. You can create a training with just one or any grouping of modules that are relevant for your needs. To access digital files you can use in your training, visit **thenadd.org/presentations**. The digital files correspond directly to the PowerPoint slides in this book. Being a good or excellent trainer is a skill that incorporates many qualities. While good content is essential, it is only one piece of the complex tapestry of skill, preparation, intercultural sensitivity and self-awareness that together make a trainer not just competent but confident and inspiring.

In this chapter, we will cover the characteristics that excellent trainers work to embody; the strategies and importance of training design; essential considerations that require focus before, during and after a training; and best practices in developing and delivering virtual training.

Training the modules contained in this book, in their entirety, will take several days. When planning your training, covering three modules in one day is a good estimate to use.

There will be different approaches to training this material and different types of training professionals using this book. We invite you to take these ideas and work with them in whatever way makes sense for you and your role and goals as a trainer.

General Characteristics of Excellent Trainers

... as important as methods may be, the most practical thing we can achieve in any kind of work is insight into what is happening inside us as we do it.
– Parker Palmer, Author/Educator/Activist

In this chapter, we are going to provide information to support you in becoming the best trainer that you are uniquely qualified to become. We all bring our cultural background, history, experience, sensitivity and relationship to the material into the training environment. This chapter will support you in harnessing your strengths and using your vulnerabilities, so you are able to be an authentic, engaging and compelling instructor.

Developing an understanding of culture and cultivating emotional intelligence will give you the awareness and skill to effectively train and navigate unexpected responses from your audience during the training session. When we use the term "culture," we are referring to the shared, learned, symbolic system of values, beliefs and attitudes that shapes and influences perception and behavior. When we refer to "emotional intelligence," we are using the following definition, developed by Lee Gardenswartz, Jorge Cherbosque and Anita Rowe from the Emotional Intelligence and Diversity Institute (https://www.eidi-results.org/): "Emotional Intelligence is the ability to feel, understand, manage, articulate, and effectively apply the power of emotions as a source of human energy."

We are all complex cultural beings, influenced by many things, including our ethnicity; gender identity; sexual orientation; age; abilities/disabilities; current and family of origin socioeconomic status; religion; where we were raised; our professional background and that of our parents; our education and the educational background of our family, etc. Understanding how these factors influence our worldview is key to self-awareness. Effective trainers know themselves and have explored the ways in which their cultural background and attitudes toward others (that we are often unaware of) influence how they come across as trainers and how they react under stress. They know their strengths as trainers as well as their vulnerabilities, triggers and emotional responses to things that irritate them in a training environment. They bring not only an awareness of themselves but also know how to remain balanced and manage their emotions and physical reactions to stressors (mistakes, technological issues, disruptive participants, etc.) that may arise during training sessions.

The best trainers are continuous learners and keep up to date with the current research on adult learning and the current best practices in the field of study they are training. They know how to engage their audience and can effectively adapt the material to the specific group being trained. They are flexible and patient and know how to deal with disruptions gently (participants multitasking, one person dominating a conversation, etc.). They are excellent communicators and role models in how to actively listen and respect the perspectives of others. They are knowledgeable and have experience relating to the material they are training. They are clear and consistent in their delivery of the material and they utilize their body language consciously (gesture with hands and arms, move around the space effectively, visually connect with all participants, etc.).

The best trainers have systems in place, such as checklists, to ensure that the only uncertainty going into the training is what the audience or environment may produce. And finally, excellent trainers are constantly learning from feedback, evaluating their sessions and improving their skills.

Preparation for the Training

If you can't explain it simply, you don't understand it well enough.
– Albert Einstein, Mathematician/Physicist

While the basic training content is provided in this text, there are a number of important training design elements to consider and incorporate into your training.

First and foremost, you need to know and understand the material you are teaching. You will get many questions during your training session. You will need to thoroughly understand the terminology and be prepared to talk in depth and with familiarity about the content you are teaching. You can review the references outlined in the appendix or contact NADD if you would like to have a conversation with an expert on the information covered in this book. We want to support you in being a confident and knowledgeable trainer in any way we can.

As you design the training, it is critical to understand the needs and makeup of the audience and the training goals of the organization or individual hiring you to train. At the early stage of training design, you will want to identify someone with influence and knowledge who can be a cultural informant. By that, we mean a person who will clearly articulate the goals of the training and tell you honestly about the makeup of the participants. Considerations include, but are not limited to, the specific training need you have been hired to address; the professional makeup of the group (e.g., are there supervisors and direct reports together?); interpersonal dynamics that may influence participant engagement; the ethnicity and age of participants; the geographic location of the training; the motivation of the participants (e.g., are the participants there because they are excited by the content or are they being forced to attend the training?); etc. These factors will greatly influence the types and content of examples you use in your training. What is appropriate and humorous in one region is not necessarily so in another region or country.

Once you know the material, understand the needs being addressed, have clarity about the overarching training goals and understand the characteristics of the group you will be training, then you will be prepared to incorporate effective storytelling and relevant examples throughout your session. As you are envisioning your training session, please consider the following:

- Always start each day with a clear outline or agenda for the day. Start and end each day with an exercise that brings people together. The outline needs to spell out the breaks, lunch and ending times. How you choose your opening and closing exercises will be influenced by time, the size of the group and the training goals. Know what you are trying to achieve with your opening and closing exercises. Are you trying to help the group focus, to leave their regular lives outside of the training session and begin to form a cohesive unit, or are you trying to foster deeper team building? You could use simple questions, such as "one thing no one in this room knows about me is..."; "one thing I want to take back into my work after this training is..."; or "one thing I learned today is...". There are many creative tools to use for icebreakers or meeting closing exercises. Please keep in mind that not everyone is comfortable with public participation. Make sure you have icebreaker or closing activities that allow for feedback via Post-it notes or in pairs or small groups.

- For this unique group at this particular time, what stories can be woven into the material? Emotionally compelling stories that the participants can relate to will be the most memorable and will keep them paying attention. Ideally, you will have personal examples that directly relate to the participants' work or lives. Of course, those examples must be within clear professional boundaries and not convey too much personal information.

- While the book content provides learning objectives, make sure to link those learning objectives to the organization's (or individual's) identified training needs and goals. Every topical area needs to lead to the next. It must all be connected and coherent.

- Use the pre- and post-tests included in the workbook.

- If you are training virtually, email the participants instructions on how to access the platform and include screenshots so they may familiarize themselves with the platform before the training session.

- Social interaction fosters emotional connectivity. Incorporate as many interactive exercises as you can manage effectively, grouping people differently with each exercise and being cognizant of the hierarchical relationships in the room. Make sure the exercises are concretely linked to the learning objectives. Ensure that the training methods attract the engagement of all types of learners and are inclusive of different learning styles. Involve people in the process of learning and sharing so that the collective experience of the group enhances the learning for everyone involved. Remember to keep people moving around and interacting as much as you can.

- Make sure that the examples, images and vignettes are relevant, and that your language is culturally appropriate for each unique group.
- Create the ideal physical environment for your training. Have the chairs and tables organized for maximum group work. Ensure the lighting is as soft and inviting as the space will allow. Try to manage the room temperature effectively, and always have good treats and beverages available throughout the session.
- Be sure to incorporate frequent breaks into the schedule and regular shifts in training methodology (dyad work to group work to individual work to triad work, etc.).
- If possible, provide a gift or tool to the group, such as a notebook to record observations or some other item that will remind the participants of the training in the future.
- If you have handouts, ensure they are attractive and professional.
- Develop a backup plan for presenting your training should technology not work correctly.
- Use the training checklist we have provided in the appendix or create your own checklist. If you are not bringing these materials yourself, make sure you have arranged for all the audiovisual equipment (computer, projector, adapter, flash drive with your presentation, microphone, etc.), meeting supplies (flip chart, Post-it notes, pens, Sharpies, icebreaker materials, etc.) and training materials (handouts, workbooks, etc.) to be waiting for you when you arrive.

Once the training is designed and planned out, create a script or outline for yourself. Incorporate speaker notes to guide you in each section. Begin each section by briefly summarizing the previous content and outlining the next section. After you have completed your preparation, review your work with someone who can give you clarifying feedback. Once finalized, allow yourself time to practice so that when you enter the training session, you are prepared, confident and excited to share the important information you are teaching.

Plan what you will do the morning of the training, so you can be at your best during your session. Spend time quietly, have a brief workout or do whatever self-care supports your preparation to be on stage for the day. Ensure that your attire is both professional and comfortable, in alignment with and slightly more professional than your audience. Have healthy snacks and water within easy reach so you can maintain your energy level throughout the session.

Not every person who trains is comfortable being a trainer. Sometimes it is part of one's job and a professional challenge. If you are one of those people, determine what you can do to ease your nervousness before the training, as well as during the training should something throw you off balance and generate stress. Plan ahead and expect the unexpected. Know exactly what you will do to manage your emotions should an unexpected variable throw you off course.

During the Training

One important key to success is self-confidence.
An important key to self-confidence is preparation.
–Arthur Ashe, Tennis Professional

Following are 10 time-tested strategies to ensure your training is successful.

1. One of the most effective things you can do to start your training with confidence and clarity is to arrive at the training location very early. This will give you time to make sure everything is working and the environment is as exactly as you had planned (AV and safe electrical cord placement, lighting, temperature, training materials placed where you want them, general room setup, etc.).

2. We are relational beings and respond to personal attention. To set the

tone and create an informal and welcoming environment, greet and spend time with participants as they arrive. Ask them about themselves and what excites them about their work. Modeling this as people enter the room provides a natural segue for you to ask people to share their own experience throughout the day.

3. When you first address the group, tell them about yourself, ideally including a relevant short story and elements of your background that relate to the material you are training. This will help participants get to know you and understand why you are qualified to train them.

4. Then, co-create a set of ground rules to make expectations clear regarding things like being on time, respecting other opinions, texting, taking phone calls or doing other work while in the training. Calling these things out and having the group develop the set of behavioral standards for your collective time together supports a healthy, safe and predictable training environment with clear boundaries. Be sure to model the established ground rules. For virtual training, include expectations regarding screen presence. A consideration would be whether or not participants need to have their screen on in order to receive credit for the training.

5. Be prepared to positively address disengaged or disruptive behavior. Here are examples for you to consider. If you notice pairs or small groups staying to themselves, not interacting or commenting during the session, you can rotate people around the room several times during the session to encourage engagement across groups. If you find people multitasking, you may want to encourage full engagement by thanking everyone who is fully present and by sharing how much everyone benefits from the collective wisdom in the group. If you find an individual is so talkative that there is no room for other viewpoints, you could say something like "in an effort to hear from everyone, please finish your thought and let's hear from another one of our colleagues" or "in an effort to honor our timeline today, let's move on." If there is a person raising issues or information that is outside the scope of the training, you could say: "Thank you for bringing that up. Let us have a side conversation at the break (or after the training)." If questions are raised that you do not know

the answer to, you can always say: "Thank you for asking. Please email me and I will be happy to send you the latest information on that."

6. Create a "parking lot" or place you can capture questions and issues that need to be addressed. Be sure to allow time at the end of the day to discuss each item on the list.

7. Always scan the room for engagement. Ask for feedback if you sense things are not working well. Change your approach if how you are teaching a segment is not being received as you had hoped.

8. Always stay within the agreed timeline. Start when you say you will start, and end the day on time or a little early.

9. Personally connect in some way with each person in the room, so everyone feels seen, heard and valued.

10. Let the group know you will seek their feedback at the end of each day, so that you can learn from their experience and improve your capacity as a trainer. If you are training on behalf of NADD, there will be an evaluation tool to administer. If not, you can create your own. Be sure to allow time at the end of each day for people to complete the evaluations before they leave the room.

Before you end the session and invite people to complete their evaluations, thank them for their engagement, for dedicating the time to increase their skills and for the learning you gained by working with them. Give them specific information on how they can contact you or NADD for additional resources or learning opportunities.

After the Training

The key to learning is feedback.
It is nearly impossible to learn anything without it.
–Steven D. Levitt, Economist

After the training session, collect the evaluations and return the room to its original condition. You may want to ask for volunteers to help you.

When reviewing the evaluations, please don't be disturbed by negative comments. No training works well for everyone. There are always people who will say things that are difficult to read. Take all feedback and consider each comment for the lessons you may learn and incorporate into your next training. There are always opportunities for learning and improvement. If there are trends, those are worthy of deep consideration and learning. Isolated comments may not be particularly helpful. If you are doing a multi-day training, start each subsequent day with a very general summary of the trends of the feedback (not individual comments) and how you are addressing their insights.

Virtual Training

Technology will not replace great teachers, but technology in the hands of great teachers can be transformational.
–George Couros, Educator/Author

Training with a virtual platform can be very effective but is significantly different than training in person. Using a virtual platform requires different preparation as well as a different delivery methodology. When employing a virtual format, you gain enormous flexibility, but you lose the synergy of the group and elements of personal connection. This is a significant shift. When you are conducting an in-person training, you have a wealth of information with which to gauge how your material is being received (body language, group interaction, etc.). Without in-person feedback, an online trainer must devote significant energy to reading the reactions of the participants remotely. This takes practice and a very different type of focus and engagement. Since training on virtual platforms is increasingly common, we offer these basic considerations and best practices when planning and conducting your trainings in a virtual format.

Most of the basic elements for developing mastery as a trainer covered in this chapter can be adapted for the preparation and delivery of virtual training. However, there are fundamental differences that will require a restructuring of your design and delivery. We invite you to consider and incorporate the following suggestions as you prepare and present your sessions in any online format:

- If possible, the training should be conducted on a virtual platform that allows for video participation if applicable, as well as break-out sessions, polling and extensive interaction opportunities. Regardless of the format for training delivery, one constant is that social interactivity fosters emotional connectivity. Personal engagement is essential in keeping participants engaged, connected and interested.

- As mentioned earlier, if you are training virtually, email the participants instructions on how to access the platform and include screenshots so they may familiarize themselves with the platform before the training session.

- Emotionally compelling stories, videos and pictures are even more important when training remotely.

- To keep participants focused, the training modules need to be broken down into small increments of about 20 minutes, with engaging activities between the 20-minute increments.

- Make use of the screenshare function to post handouts, graphics, videos and relevant information so you minimize words on the screen.

- To ensure participant learning, trainings will not be able to occur in a full eight-hour day as they would when training in person. Instead, it is ideal when possible that the content be broken out over multiple days, with no more than four full hours in a day, including breaks, or six hours including breaks and a lunch break.

- It is critical that you are trained and proficient with the virtual platform you are using.
- Before the day of your training, practice all aspects and phases of your training to make sure they work effectively (group video engagement, break-out sessions, screenshare, etc.).
- Be sure you present a professional and calming presence. Don't wear bright colors or extreme patterns. Wearing a pastel color with a gentle neutral background is important. Also wear a color that contrasts with your skin so your hands are distinguished from your clothing when you are gesturing and using your hands in communication.
- Be aware of your vocal tone, and also where your eyes are focused. Be a welcoming presence to those watching and listening.
- Add to your opening session a tutorial on the details of the virtual platform so participants know how to use the chat function, how to raise their hand to speak, why it is important to remain muted unless speaking, etc.
- To maintain a professional atmosphere, incorporate into the tutorial a description of virtual etiquette, including how to: position their camera, use the microphone, create the best lighting, ensure their environment is free of distractions, etc.
- Convert your evaluation process into polls, surveys or questions and allow for completion after each day of training, so you can learn from participant feedback before you next train.

Consideration about Training Timeframes and Final Thoughts

Generally speaking, modules that are trained virtually take less time than when in person, primarily because there is less back-and-forth engagement when conducting a training using a virtual platform. Other than that, there are no specific rules regarding training timeframes. Numbers of participants in a training and a person's training style also impact the time it takes to move through a module.

This material is very versatile and can be used in many ways both in person and virtually. The modules can be trained individually or in any grouping that matches specific training goals. Modules can be used as a tool in clinical supervision or with a person receiving services. They can be taught at staff meetings or in classroom settings as a half- or full-day training. You will take all these factors into consideration as you design your training.

We are delighted that you have chosen to train this material. If there is any way we can further support you or if you are interested in additional resources on any of the topics covered in this or the other chapters, please visit thenadd.org or contact us at info@thenadd.org.

Module I

Understanding Dual Diagnosis Basics

Slide 2

This module covers basic information about the nature of mental health disorders among persons with intellectual or developmental disabilities (IDD). The following content will be covered: definitions of IDD and mental illness (MI), prevalence, indicators, characteristics, vulnerability factors, and similarities and differences between MI and IDD.

Slide 3

Learning Objectives

- Define "dual diagnosis."
- Describe vulnerability risk factors.
- Articulate the similarities and differences between MI and IDD.

Slide 4

- **Coexistence of two disabilities: Intellectual/Developmental Disability (IDD) and Mental Illness (MI)**
- **Both IDD and mental health disorders should be assessed and diagnosed.**
- **All needed treatments and supports should be available, effective and accessible.**

It is only within the past 40 years or so that professionals have recognized that it is possible for individuals to have both intellectual/developmental disability and mental illness.

Trained professionals are needed to conduct mental health assessment in people with IDD.

Services available for people with MI should also be available for people who have IDD/MI. Availability is not enough; we need staff who have a level of competency in dual diagnosis. The services need to be conducted by professionals who are trained in dual diagnosis. This helps to achieve effectiveness.

Slide 5

Terminology

The DSM-5 was published in May 2013 with many changes in diagnostic criteria and terminology.

One of these is the change from the term "mental retardation" from DSM-IV to the term "intellectual disability" or "intellectual developmental disorder." This change better reflects terminology changes by medical, educational and service professionals and advocacy groups.

DSM 5, 2013

Terminology in the DSM-5 is also reflective of new federal statute in the US – Pub.L. 111-256, Rosa's Law. This law replaces the term "mental retardation" with "intellectual disability."

Intellectual developmental disorder is a disorder with onset during the developmental period that includes both intellectual and adaptive functioning deficits in conceptual, social and practical domains. The three following criteria must be met:

1. Deficits in intellectual functions, such as reasoning and problem-solving, planning, abstract thinking, judgment, academic learning and learning from experience, confirmed by both clinical assessment and individualized, standardized intelligence testing.

2. Deficits in adaptive functioning that result in failure to meet developmental and sociocultural standards for personal independence and social responsibility. Without ongoing support, the adaptive

deficits limit functioning in one or more activities of daily life, such as communication, social participation and independent living, across multiple environments, such as home, school, work and community.

3. Onset of intellectual and adaptive deficits during the developmental period. (American Psychiatric Association, 2013)

Together, these revisions bring the DSM into alignment with terminology used by the World Health Organization's International Classification of Diseases and other professional disciplines and organizations, such as the American Association on Intellectual and Developmental Disabilities and the U.S. Department of Education (American Psychiatric Association, 2013).

Slide 6

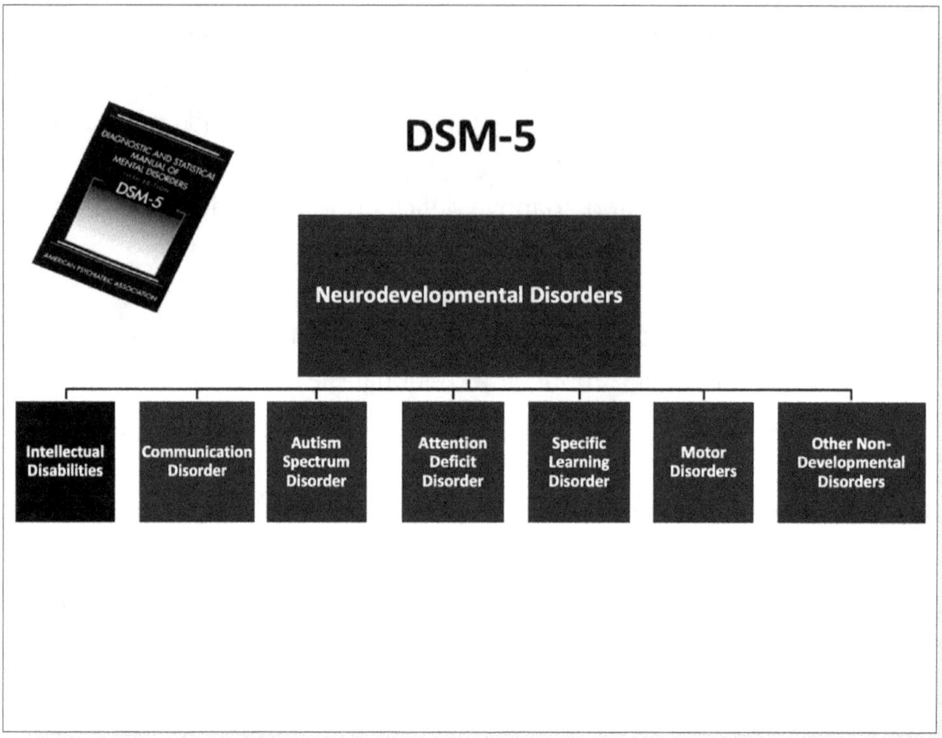

Neurodevelopmental disorders are deficiencies in growth and development of the brain or central nervous system. Included within the category of Neurodevelopmental Disorders in the DSM-5 is Intellectual Disability.

The DSM-5 includes in Neurodevelopmental Disorders:

- Intellectual Disability (Intellectual/Developmental Disorder)
- Communication Disorder
- Attention Deficit Disorder
- Autism Spectrum Disorder
- Specific Learning Disorder
- Motor Disorders
- Other Non-Developmental Disorders

Slide 7

Intellectual/Developmental Disorder

The following three diagnostic criteria must be met:

1. Deficits in intellectual functioning, such as reasoning, problem-solving and planning, abstract thinking, academic learning and learning from experience, confirmed by both clinical assessment and individualized standardized testing.
2. Deficits in adaptive functioning that result in failure to meet developmental and sociocultural standards for personal independence and social responsibility. Without ongoing support, the adaptive deficits limit functioning in one or more activities of daily life, such as communication, social participation and independent living, across multiple environments, such as home, school, work and community.
3. Onset of intellectual and adaptive deficits during the developmental period.

DSM 5, 2013

The criteria are based on adaptive functioning and not IQ scores, because adaptive functioning determines the level of supports required. IQ scores alone do not give much information about the supports needed. Those are generally based on adaptive function and patterns of behavior.

Slide 8

Disorder Characteristics: Three Domains

Intellectual/Developmental Disorder involves impairments of general mental abilities that impact adaptive functioning in three domains or areas. These domains determine how well an individual copes with everyday tasks:

- **The Conceptual Domain** includes skills in language, reading, writing, math, reasoning, knowledge and memory.
- **The Social Domain** refers to empathy, social judgment, interpersonal communication skills, the ability to make and maintain friendships and similar capacities.
- **The Practical Domain** centers on self-management in areas such as personal care, job responsibilities, money management, recreation and organizing school and work tasks.

DSM 5, 2013

Adaptive functioning refers to a person's capacity to gain personal independence, based on the person's ability to learn and apply conceptual, social and practical skills in their everyday life. As noted in the slide, adaptive functioning abilities are determined on the basis of the three domains: conceptual, social and practical. Formal assessment will examine the level of functioning in each of the three domains.

Slide 9

- Self-care
- Language and communication
- Community use
- Independent living skills

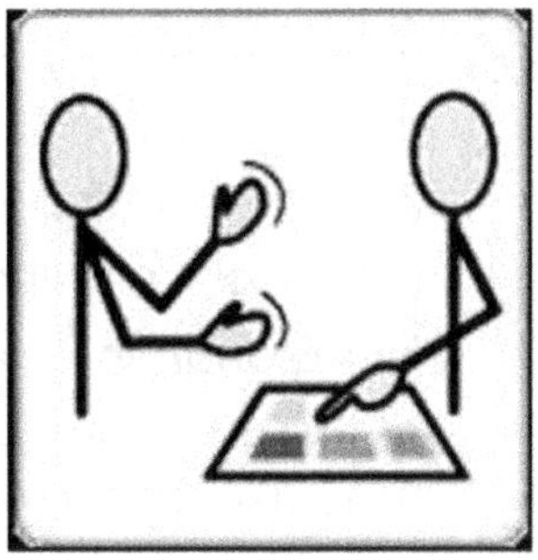

DM-ID, 2007

Deficits in adaptive behavior are one of the criteria to meet the definition of IDD. Deficits in adaptive behavior are also one of the three criteria to be eligible for services in the IDD system.

While change in terminology is reflected in federal statute, the federal Developmental Disabilities Act, 2000 (P.L. 106–402), still uses the term "developmental disability" and has not been formally updated.

Federal Definition of Developmental Disabilities

According to the Developmental Disabilities Act, section 102(8), "the term 'developmental disability' means a severe, chronic disability of an individual five years of age or older that:

1. Is attributable to a mental or physical impairment or combination of mental and physical impairments;

2. Is manifested before the individual attains age 22;

3. Is likely to continue indefinitely;

4. Results in substantial functional limitations in three or more of the following areas of major life activity;
   (i) Self-care;
   (ii) Receptive and expressive language;
   (iii) Learning;
   (iv) Mobility;
   (v) Self-direction;
   (vi) Capacity for independent living; and
   (vii) Economic self-sufficiency.

5. Reflects the individual's need for a combination and sequence of special, interdisciplinary or generic services, supports or other assistance that is of lifelong or extended duration and is individually planned and coordinated, except that such term, when applied to infants and young children means individuals from birth to age five, inclusive, who have substantial developmental delay or specific congenital or acquired conditions with a high probability of resulting in developmental disabilities if services are not provided."

Slide 10

- **Socialization skills**
- **Health and safety**
- **Work**
- **Self-direction**

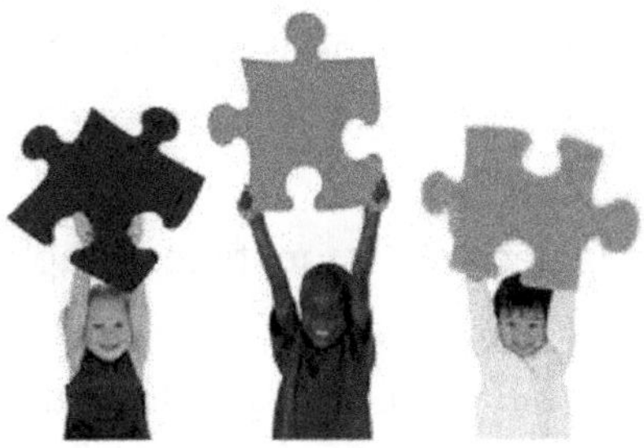

DM-ID, 2007

There is a clear trend for agencies to require identifiable and substantial deficits in adaptive behavior as one of the three criteria to meet eligibility for services. Assessment of functioning must consider typical behavior as opposed to optimal behavior.

There are several methods of adaptive function assessments including traditional, norm-referenced rating scales and alternative methods. Considerations of best practice guidelines and benefits and limitations of each method should be considered before choosing the most appropriate/effective method for the particular assessment need.

Two of the more frequently used assessments for adaptive behavior are:

1. *The Vineland Adaptive Behavior Scales (VABS)*, third edition (Vineland-30) by Sara S. Sparrow, Domenic V. Cicchetti & Celine A. Saulnier, 2016. This tool measures adaptive behavior from birth to adulthood.

2. The *Adaptive Behavior Assessment System*, second edition (ABAS-II; Harrison & Oakland, 2000), which uses a behavior-rating format to assess adaptive behavior and related skills for individuals five through 89 years of age.

Slide 11

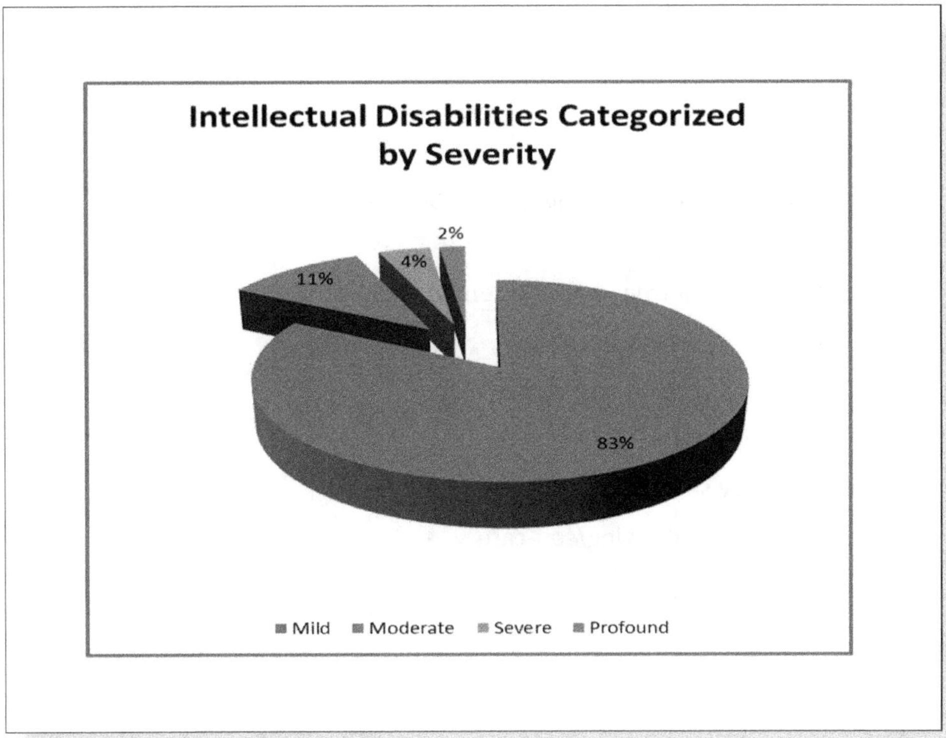

As 80-85 percent of people with IDD fall in the mild range, it is likely that the people you will come in contact with will have a certain degree of expressive and receptive language skills. The way in which we interact with persons in the mild range is not significantly different than the way we would interact with someone who does not have IDD.

Individuals with mild IDD can often acquire academic skills and can become fairly self-sufficient. Individuals with moderate IDD can carry out work and self-care tasks with moderate supervision and are able to live and function successfully within the community, typically in a supervised environment. Individuals with severe IDD may master very basic self-care skills and some communication skills. Individuals with profound IDD may be able to develop limited self-care skills and some may learn to use communication devices with appropriate support and training. They generally need a high level of structure and supervision.

Slide 12

Mild: 80-85 percent of people with IDD:

- **Slower-than-normal development in all areas**
- **Unusual physiology is rare**
- **Typical skill repertoire includes:**
  - **Practical skills**
  - **Literacy skills**
  - **Tasks of daily living/self-care**
  - **Social skills**

DSM 5, 2013

Note that as the person experiences greater levels of IDD, skill deficits become more significant, so instruction and supports become of paramount importance. Also as severity of IDD increases, the need for more precise/ systematic means of instruction grows.

Slide 13

Moderate: 10-12 percent of people with IDD:

- Noticeable delays, particularly with speech and communication
- May have unusual physiology
- Typical skills repertoire includes:
    - Simple communication skills
    - Simple health and safety skills
    - Some tasks of daily living/self-care
    - Independence in the community in familiar places

DSM 5, 2013

Slide 14

Severe: 3-4 percent of people with IDD:

- Significant delays in some areas
- Delayed motor development
- Limited expressive communication skills
- Typical skills repertoire includes:
    - Daily routines and repetitive activities
    - Less complex tasks of daily living/self-care
    - Social skills with support and supervision

DSM 5, 2013

Slide 15

Profound: 1-2 percent of people with IDD:

- Significant delays in all areas
- Congenital abnormalities present
- Require specialized/attendant care
- May respond to regular physical and social activity
- Need intensive support and supervision to do self-care and activities of daily living

DSM 5, 2013

Slide 16

Exercise and Discussion

- What do you know about each of the severity levels of IDD (mild, moderate, severe, profound)?
- What is your personal experience with someone who has a disability?

Slide 17

People occasionally experience mental health problems that may:

- **Change the way they think and understand the world around them**
- **Change the way they relate with others**
- **Change the emotions and feelings they have**

These changes can have a short-term impact on the way they deal with day-to-day life.

However, if the impact is very great (ongoing problems with repeated relapse episodes), then we consider the possibility of mental illness.

From time to time, we all experience situations in our lives that contribute to increased stress and anxiety. These are usually externally driven. That is to say, impacts from environmental/social situations can cause a great deal of stress in our lives. These stressors can contribute to short-term anxiety and worry. For example, moving from one home to another can be an extremely stressful situation, but that stress will last for only a limited time.

However, when the impact of the stressful situation continues for a long period of time, i.e., over three months, and the severity of the stress interferes with day-to-day functioning, then we are looking at more than just a mental health problem. If the stressful situation goes on for a period of time and has frequent and intense episodes, then we may be looking at mental illness rather than just a mental health problem.

Slide 18

- MI is a psychiatric condition that disrupts a person's thinking, feeling, mood or ability to relate to others and can impair daily functioning.
- MI can affect people of any age, race, religion, income or level of intelligence.
- The DSM-5 or the DM-ID provide diagnostic criteria for mental disorders.

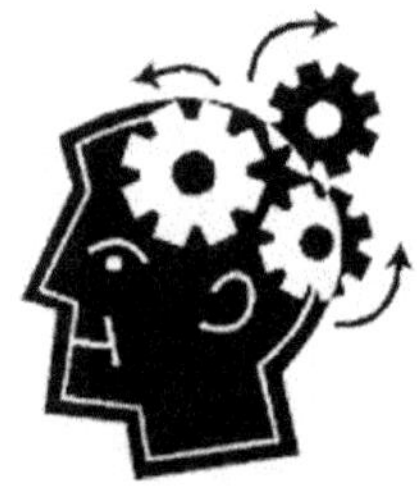

"A mental disorder (mental illness) is a syndrome characterized by clinically significant disturbance in an individual's cognition, emotion regulation or behavior that reflects dysfunction in the psychological, biological, or developmental processes underlying mental functioning. Mental disorders are usually associated with significant distress or disability in social, occupational, or other important activities" (American Psychiatric Association, 2013).

A mental illness is a psychological or behavioral pattern generally associated with subjective stress. A mental illness may consist of a combination of affective, behavioral, cognitive and perceptual components.

Onset of mental illness generally occurs at late adolescence or early adulthood. However, all ages are susceptible.

Slide 19

Mental illness is a biological process that affects the brain. Some refer to it as a brain disorder.

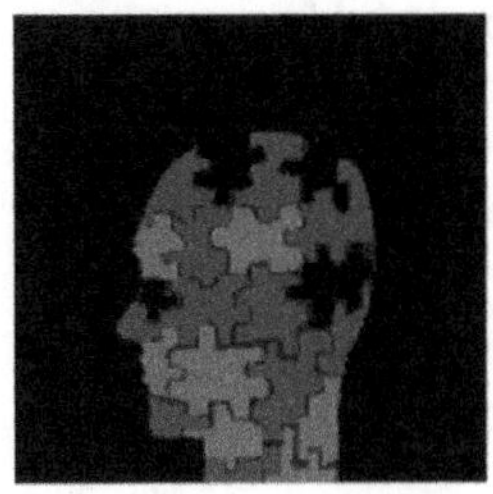

Emerging research indicates that most psychiatric disorders are biologically driven. We are finding that brain abnormalities are the cause of many serious mental illnesses.

Mental disorders can arise from a combination of sources. In many cases, there is no single accepted or consistent cause currently established.

For people who have IDD, current thinking is that there are likely to be bio-psycho-social influences that contribute to the development of mental illness.

Slide 20

Mental illnesses (mental disorders) can also be defined as a variety of psychiatric conditions that may be a result of vulnerabilities in:

- Environment
- Biology
- Psycho-social factors

DSM 5, 2013

Environmental factors can include:

- poverty
- interrupted nurturing in adolescence/childhood
- substance abuse
- work/school problems
- abuse
- rejection by others
- stressful relationships
- low social supports
- major life events

Psycho-social factors can create vulnerability due to a number of differing conditions that have a high influence on mental illness: poor social skills, poor coping skills, communication problems, etc.

Family history of mental illness creates strong vulnerability for a person experiencing mental illness or symptoms themselves. Studies suggest this influence relates primarily to genetics as opposed to early family environments (Goldberg, 2001).

Biological factors that can increase vulnerability to mental illness include: family history of certain psychosis, brain abnormalities, neurodevelopmental problems, disease, poor prenatal nutrition and health, etc.

Slide 21

Criteria

1. **When behavior is abnormal by virtue of quantitative or qualitative differences.**
2. **When behavior cannot be explained on the basis of developmental delay alone.**
3. **When behavior causes significant impairment in functioning.**

This definition applies to individuals who have an intellectual disability.

Three criteria are required to identify mental illness in persons with IDD:

- Maladaptive behavior is observed and there is a difference in frequency or content of the behavior from baseline.

- The maladaptive behavior, which is a change from baseline, is not directly a result of the IDD.

- Maladaptive behavior, which is a change from baseline, results in impairment in day-to-day functioning over time (Einfeld & Aman, 1995).

Slide 22

Exercise

What did you learn from this section regarding people who have IDD/MI?

Suggest that people break into small groups to discuss highlights and prominent points.

Slide 23

Two to four times a typical population
(Corbett 1979)

32.9% of people with IDD have co-occurring MI
(NCI 2011-2012)

55% of people with IDD have MI
(NCI, 2016)

Researchers have found that one-third or more of people with IDD have significant behavioral, mental or personality disorder requiring mental health services.

Research studies have had a varied range of mental illness in persons with IDD. This is because of differing research methods (assessment methodology, inpatient or outpatient populations, differing definitions, etc.). However, the research and professional community have recognized and accepted a prevalence rate of at least one-third of individuals who have IDD would warrant having a co-occurring psychiatric disorder.

Slide 24

Total U.S. Population:

(U.S. Census Bureau, Census 2020)

330,017,895

Number of People in Total Population with IDD:

5,280,286

(1.6% – NADD)

Number of People with IDD Who Have MI:

1,737,214

(32.9% of ID – NCI, 2012)

Recent census indicates there are more than 330 million people in the United States.

Research indicates that approximately 1.6% of the general population have IDD, which accounts for more than 5 million people.

NADD has embraced the prevalence rate of one-third of people with IDD having a co-occurring MI disorder, resulting in an estimate of somewhat over a million and a half people with a dual diagnosis in the U.S.

Slide 25

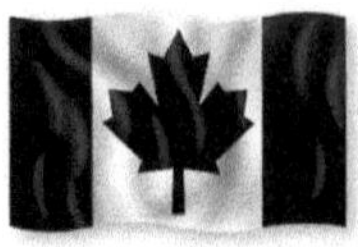

Total Canadian Population

37,766,314

(Government of Canada, Statistics Canada, 2018)

Number of People in the Total Population with IDD:

604,261

(1.6% NADD)

Number of People with IDD Who Have MI:

198,802

(32.9% ID- NCI, 2012)

Slide 26

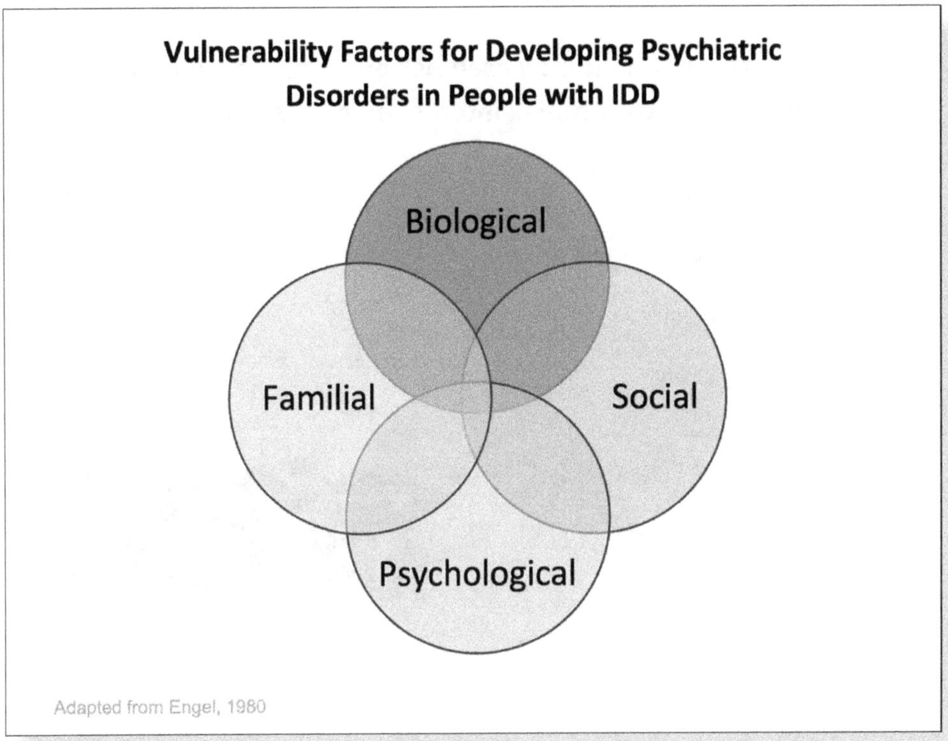

Very little is known about the causes of mental illness in people with IDD. However, it is proposed that there are both internal and external influences that contribute to the high rate of mental disorders in persons with IDD.

There are several risk factors that predispose people with IDD to develop psychiatric disorders. There are biological, psychological and social circumstances that contribute to vulnerability to mental health disorders in persons with IDD.

Slide 27

People with IDD are at increased risk of developing psychiatric disorders due to complex interaction of multiple factors:

- Biological
- Psychological
- Social
- Family

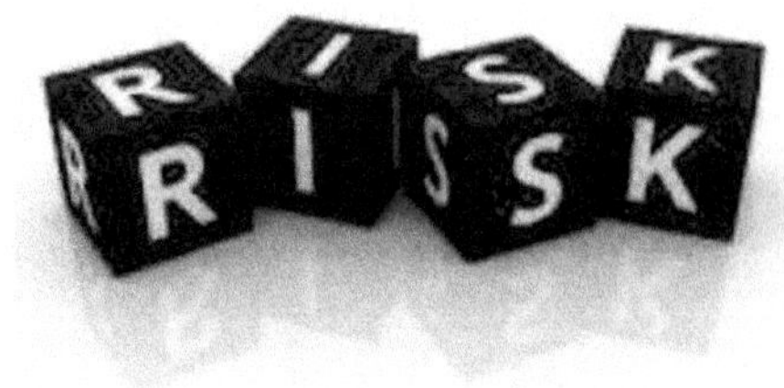

Royal College of Psychiatrists, 2001

There are a number of circumstances causing or contributing to mental health disorders in persons with IDD. People with IDD are at risk for developing psychiatric disorders at higher rates than the general population. This is due to interweaving influences based on a person's biology, psychology and environment.

Slide 28

Vulnerability factors for psychiatric disorders

Biological

- Brain damage/epilepsy
- Vision/hearing impairments
- Physical illnesses/disabilities
- Genetic/familial conditions
- Drugs/alcohol abuse
- Medication/physical treatments

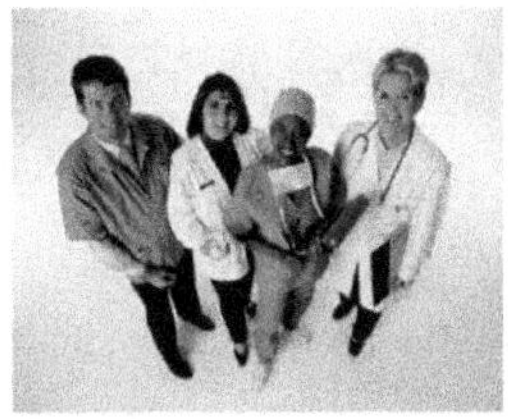

Royal College of Psychiatrists, 2001

People with IDD frequently have a host of health-related problems. As a group, persons with IDD have an increased prevalence of brain damage and seizure disorders.

At least 25% of all causes of IDD are known to be associated with biological abnormalities that affect the brain and often affect other body systems. Seizure disorders are increased proportionally as the level of IDD becomes more severe.

Some genetic syndromes associated with IDD are related to increased risk for certain psychiatric disorders (e.g., mood and anxiety disorders in persons with autism and Down syndrome). Some genetic syndromes as well as some psychiatric disorders can have a genetic predisposition (family history).

As a group, there is a greater prevalence of physical illnesses such as sensory deficits or disorders such as autism, congenital heart disease and gastrointestinal disorders. Additionally, they are at risk for medical and psychiatric misdiagnoses.

It is important to identify an individual's biological vulnerabilities as this offers opportunities to design and implement appropriate interventions.

Slide 29

Psychological

- Rejection/deprivation/abuse
- Life events/separations/losses
- Poor problem-solving/coping strategies
- Social/emotional/sexual vulnerabilities
- Poor self-acceptance/low self-esteem
- Devaluation/disempowerment

Royal College of Psychiatrists, 2001

A person with IDD is often excluded from normative activities experienced by the general population (e.g., sport activities, parties). He/she may have to endure stigmatizing perceptions and negative social reactions and comments made by others.

Overdependence, lack of confidence, poor self-identity or low self-esteem are characteristic in this population.

People with IDD have prolonged exposure to negative social conditions such as:

- **Labeling** – People with IDD are vulnerable to experiencing psychologically devastating labels such as "retard," which create a perception of inferiority, difference and exclusion.

- **Rejection and social disruption** – People with IDD are often socially rejected or neglected by their peers, and feelings of loneliness are common.

- **Segregation** – This can have severe psychological negative impacts. Segregation occurs across the life span from school through adulthood.

- **Restricted Opportunities** – The majority of people with IDD will not have the usual opportunities for a rewarding life. For example, the vast majority will not have romantic relationships, will not marry and will not experience parenthood.

- **Victimization** – People with IDD are at risk for physical, sexual and emotional abuse.

Slide 30

Social

- Negative attitudes/expectations
- Stigmatization/prejudice/social exclusion
- Poor supports/relationships/networks
- Inappropriate environments/services
- Financial/legal disadvantages

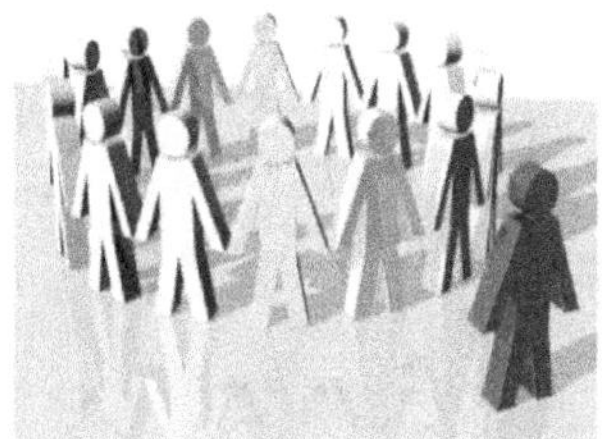

Royal College of Psychiatrists, 2001

People with IDD are often socially isolated or do not have social networks that are common in the general population. Their social networks are usually made up of family members and caregivers ("artificial friendships").

These individuals are less likely to have natural developing friendships and thus identify staff as friends. This can be problematic because a staff member who has become a "significant other" may leave and the individual may feel repeatedly rejected and/or experience a significant loss.

Due to lack of experience in social situations, people with IDD are vulnerable to being taken advantage of sexually, financially and in many other ways. This is partly because the person is taught to comply and can be easily intimidated and/or coerced. Additionally, in many cases they would appreciate the attention, even when it's inappropriate.

The person with IDD who has a poor self-image or low self-esteem may have a life that, by comparison to others, may feel unhappy, unsuccessful and defeated.

Slide 31

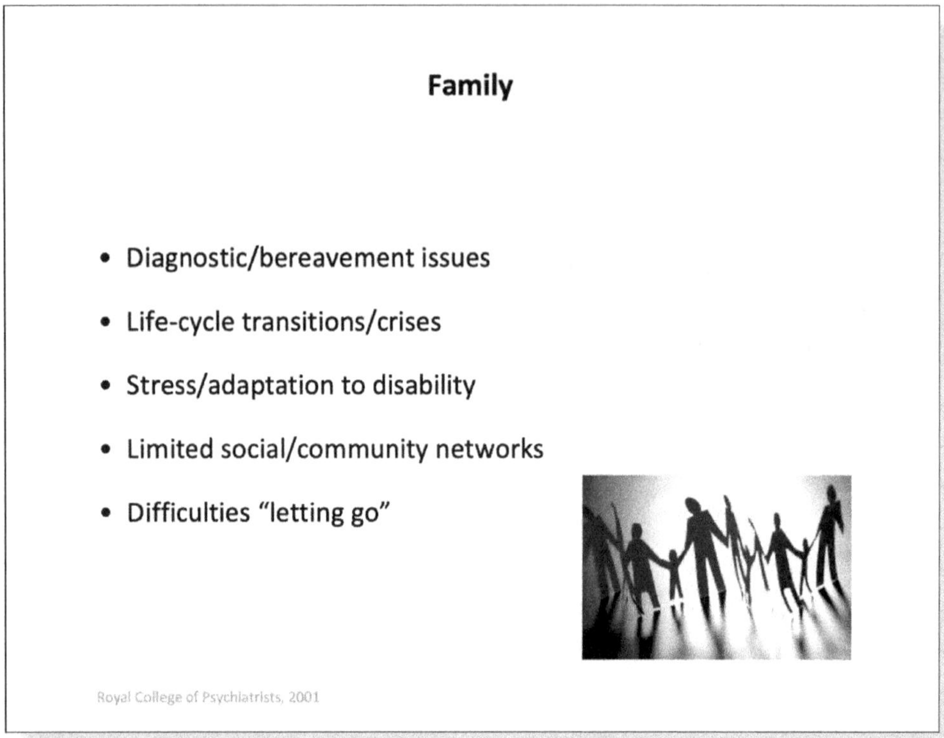

The reaction of families to having an individual with a disability can be a risk factor, combined with other variables, in the development of psychiatric disorders. When parents give birth to a child who has a disability, they generally go through a bereavement process.

Individuals with IDD and their families go through a series of life transitions, each of which can lead to a crisis situation. Some of these transitions are:

- Identification of giving birth to a person with IDD
- Beginning school
- Being surpassed by younger siblings
- Transitioning out of school
- Being in the adult world
- Onset of psychiatric disorder
- Death of parents

Parents sometimes have difficulty in letting go and can tend to overprotect.

Slide 32

Consider This Person

Tran is a 41-year-old woman who was diagnosed with mild IDD at age 12. She has recently moved from her family home to group living after the sudden death of her sister, with whom she spent nearly all her time.

Tran has been refusing to go to bed at night, spending hours awake sitting in the living room of her new home. Normally, Tran is not a fussy eater, but since moving, she has been leaving most of her meal on her plate and declining snacks when offered.

The Direct Support Professionals (DSPs) who support Tran are concerned about her. What do you think Tran could be experiencing?

Slide 33

High Vulnerability to Stress

The impact of a minimally or moderately stressful situation can be experienced as significant.

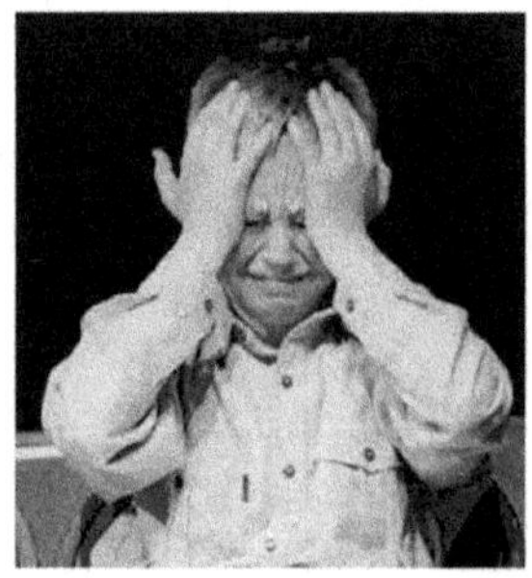

Hartley and MacLean, 2009

Recent research has indicated that people with IDD are more vulnerable to stress than people who do not have IDD. Situations that may not result in stress for a neurotypical person may cause a great deal of stress for a person with IDD.

For example, meeting new people and interacting is a normative behavior for the neurotypical person. However, for a person who has IDD, meeting new people and interacting with them may create a very stressful situation.

Vulnerability to stress can also be a product of limited life experience, limited opportunities and options, expectations that can exceed their abilities and past learning experiences. People who have IDD can develop mental health problems when confronted with only minimal to moderate stress.

Slide 34

Vulnerabilities in Skill Acquisition

- Challenges with coping skills
- Stress-management difficulties
- Fewer wellness opportunities
- Frequently lack the basic skills required for everyday living, e.g., budgeting money, using public transportation, doing laundry, preparing meals, etc.

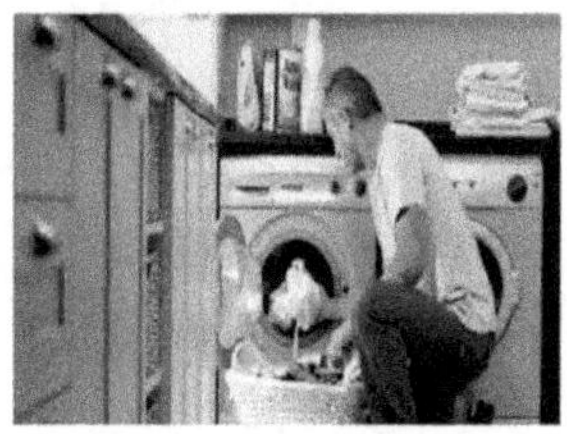

Individuals with IDD usually need instruction on how to perform basic responsibilities in daily life. This is particularly important for people living in the community. These tasks and functions need to be taught in a step-by-step manner with repetition as a method of learning. Instruction and teaching can be done either in the natural environment (home) or in a more formal environment (day program, school, work/employment).

Slide 35

Extreme Dependence

People who have IDD/MI can often experience themselves as quite helpless, thus requiring massive support from families or care providers to live successfully.

Hartley & Maclean, 2009

Due to dependency on caregivers, mental health may suffer if that support is removed or threatened. Helping the person develop their independence and resiliency as much as possible can assist with addressing this vulnerability.

Slide 36

Difficulty with Interpersonal Relationships

- With some exceptions, people with IDD/MI often have great difficulty in developing and maintaining close relationships with others.
- These interpersonal relationship problems can result in disruption in school, home, work and social environments.

Hartley & McLean, 2009

People with IDD/MI can have disruptions, across the lifespan, because of challenges associated with interpersonal relationships. These challenges can interfere in several domains involved in the individual's life.

For children, the challenge of interpersonal relationships can result in parent-child conflicts. For school-aged children, this challenge can occur with school-aged peers as well as with teachers. For adults, the problems associated with interpersonal relationships can interfere with social relationships and cause problems at work and in the residential environment.

People with a dual diagnosis have difficulty developing symmetrical relationships with others. These individuals often do not understand nor apply "give and take" relationships with others. In part this is due to a history of authority figures interacting with the individual. The nature of the relationship is usually unequal, and this inequality of relationships carries through the life span.

Individuals need to be taught how to engage in interpersonal relationships that are appropriate to the context in which the interpersonal relationship occurs. Formal social skills learning is needed to assist these individuals in developing and maintaining interpersonal relationships.

Additionally, the co-occurring mental illness can interfere with ongoing and appropriate interpersonal relationships. For example, an individual who has a psychotic disorder and is not stable is likely to have challenges in appropriate interpersonal relationships. The symptoms associated with an active psychotic disorder can significantly interfere with how the individual interacts with others.

Slide 37

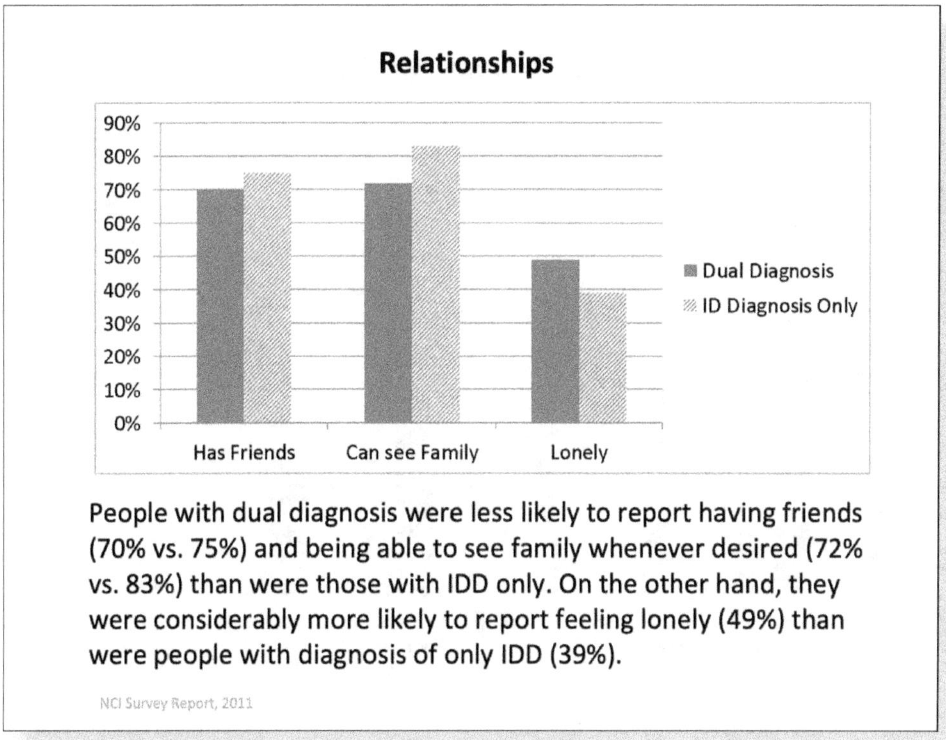

Developing meaningful relationships is difficult for people with a dual diagnosis. Also, the feeling of loneliness occurs in nearly 50% of people with IDD/MI.

It is important to assist people in nurturing and developing relationships. This can be accomplished in a variety of environments, including school and habilitative programs, as well as individual/group therapy.

Once individuals with a dual diagnosis begin to develop meaningful relationships, their feeling(s) of loneliness often subside.

Slide 38

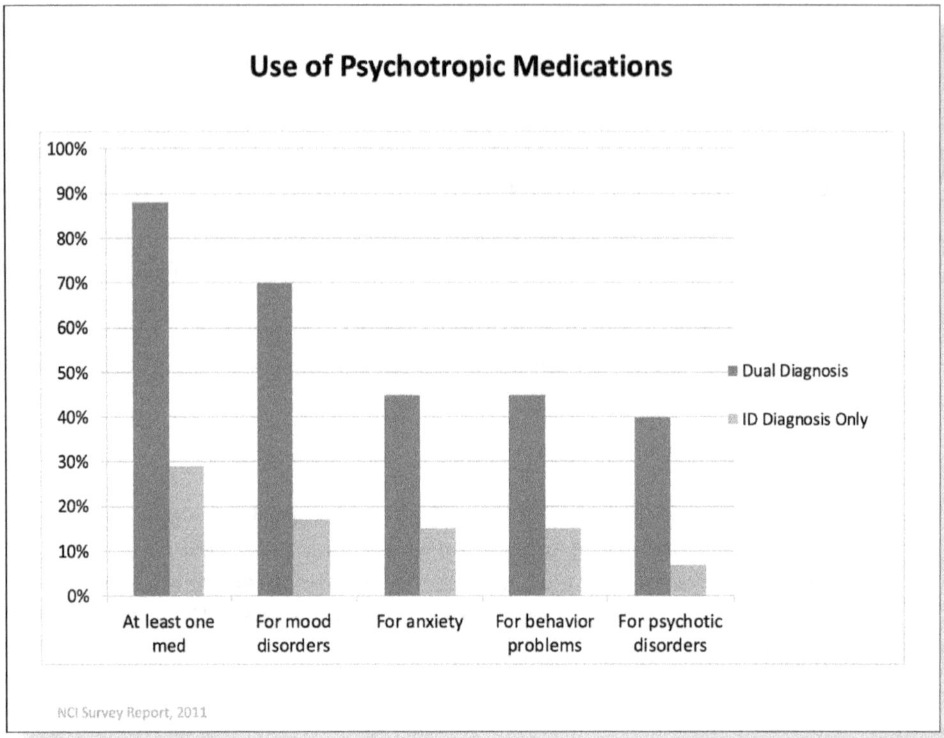

Not surprisingly, people with dual diagnosis were much more likely than people with only an IDD diagnosis to take at least one kind of psychotropic medication. The biggest difference was in the proportion of people taking medication for mood disorders — 70% of people with a dual diagnosis were taking them, compared to 17% with IDD diagnosis only.

What is more surprising is the finding that 29% of people without a diagnosis of mental illness take at least one type of psychotropic medication. This indicates that nearly one-third of people with IDD are being prescribed psychotropic medications for behavioral control. In the U.S., there has been a history of prescribing these kinds of medications for people with IDD to suppress behavioral problems.

Psychotropic medication treatment should be used only after a mental illness has been diagnosed. Prescribing medication treatment can be effective but should be used only when it is related to a specific psychiatric diagnosis.

Slide 39

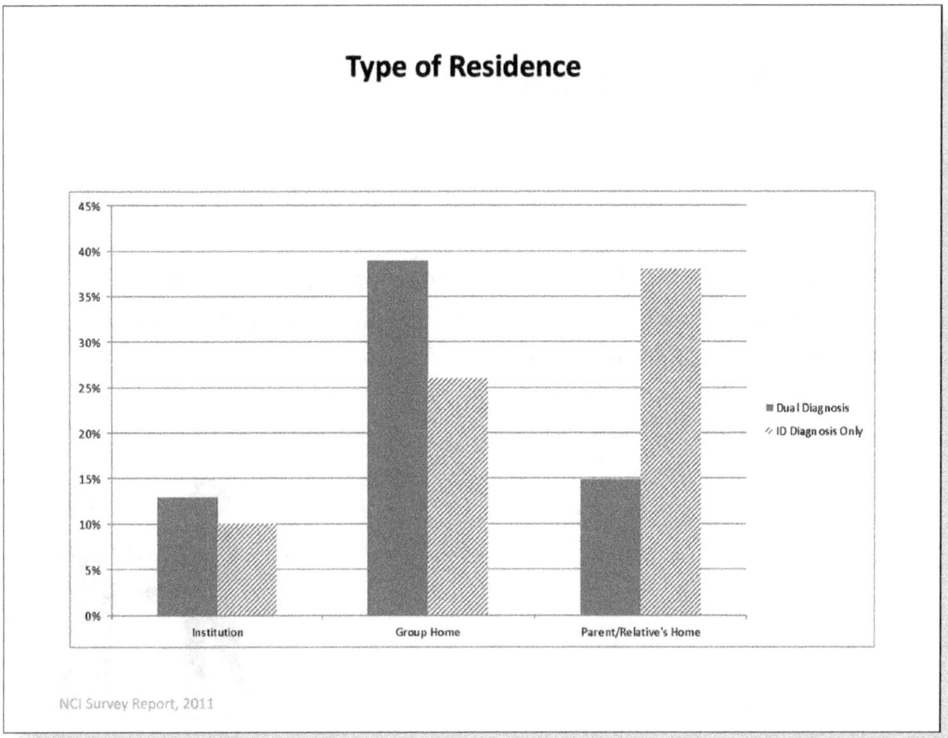

As a group, individuals with dual diagnosis were more likely to live in a group home, 39% compared to 26% for those with IDD only, and less likely to live in a parent/relative's home, 15% compared to 38%.

It is likely that behavioral/psychiatric problems are one contributor to why, as a group, individuals with a dual diagnosis are more likely to live in a group home than those who have IDD only. Similarly, this group of people are less likely to live with parents/relatives than people with IDD only. People with a dual diagnosis usually need a structured environment and a higher level of support with secondary issues, such as medication and symptom management. Group home living environments may offer more structure than living in parents'/relatives' home environments.

Slide 40

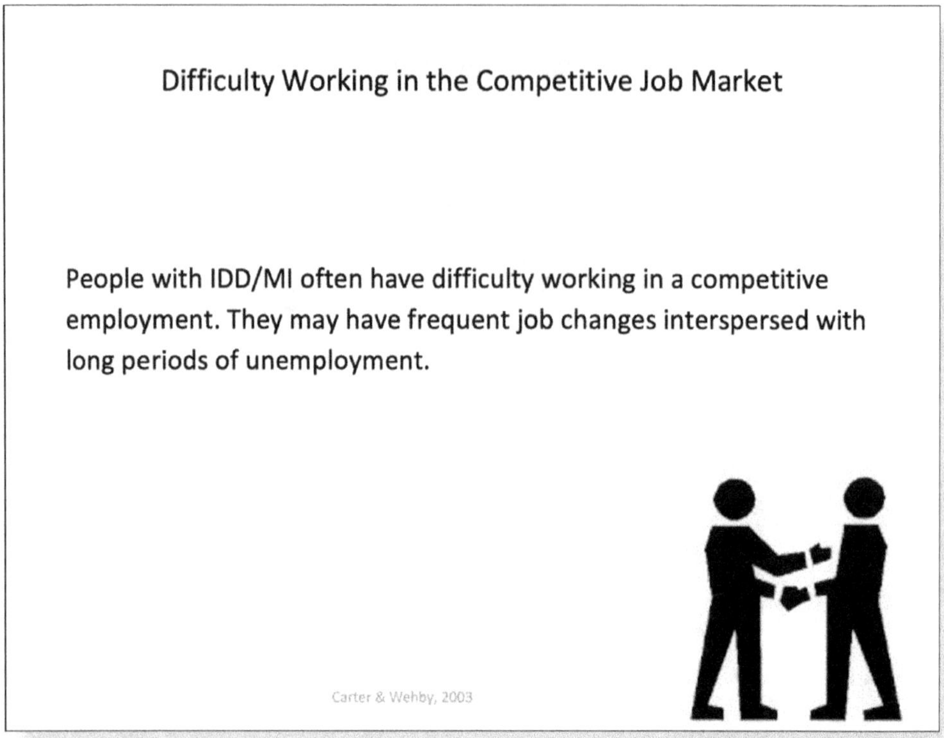

Persons with IDD/MI often have difficulty in both obtaining and sustaining employment in the competitive market. Behavioral problems often interfere with their ability to maintain job performance.

The behavioral problems may be triggered by perceived stress within the work environment or outside the work environment. Alternatively, the work distribution could be caused by an exacerbation or decompensation related to their mental illness.

Job coaching may help a person with IDD/MI in a work environment. The job coach would be able to assess if the person is experiencing stress and can also function as a liaison between the individual and the work environment.

Slide 41

Employment (community job)

	Hours worked in two weeks	Amount earned in two weeks (USD)	Hourly wage	Earning at or above minimum wage (%)	Length at current job
Dual Diagnosis	30.6	$170	$5.81	35%	56 months
IDD Only	31.5	$201	$6.40	43%	66 months

NCI Survey Report, 2010

Slightly fewer people with a dual diagnosis reported having a job in the community than people with an IDD diagnosis only (22% vs. 27%).

People with only IDD earned $201 on average in the most recent typical two-week time period preceding interview, whereas people with dual diagnosis earned $170 on average; the number of hours worked in the same time period was similar (31.5 and 30.6 respectively).

The data indicates that fewer people with a dual diagnosis are employed in the community compared to those with IDD only, and those with a dual diagnosis who are employed make less money than those who have IDD only.

Supported employment offers significant benefits for both the employer and the employee.

Slide 42

- People with IDD/MI may learn more slowly.
- They may have difficulty recalling information—especially newly acquired information.

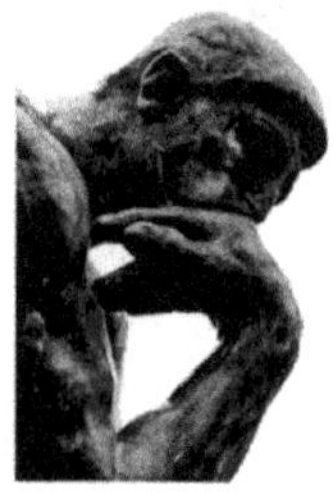

Memory issues and difficulty learning are quite common for people with IDD. Assisting them to learn to use memory tools and modifying learning/teaching requirements to their level of ability improves the person's ability to be successful with these tasks.

Slide 43

- **May have difficulty focusing, may have shortened attention span**
- **Difficulty in understanding some abstract concepts**
- **May have difficulty in considering alternative solutions. For example, may see things in black-and-white terms.**

Strategies to modify requirements about prolonged attention to task and decision-making skills can greatly assist a person who has IDD in these areas. Using concrete language and avoiding the use of slang and jargon can make a great difference in the person's ability to grasp concepts and communication.

Slide 44

- May have difficulty generalizing skills sets
- Developed skill sets may be very task-specific
- May have a passive learning style, which may make it difficult for the trainer to know what information is being retained
- Low expectations due to past difficulties. "Self-fulfilled prophecy" — the individual believes he/she cannot learn, thus preventing learning.

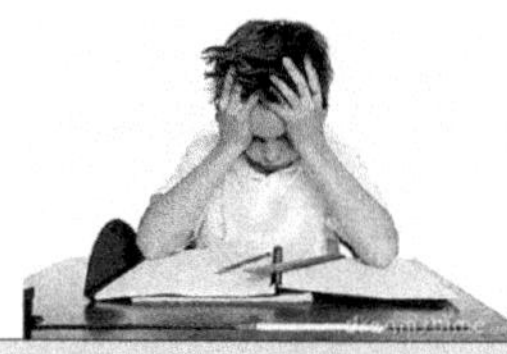

Slide 45

Exercise

Can you share examples of what might assist a person with IDD through some of the learning issues on the previous slide?

Ask the participants to give examples of what might assist a person with IDD through these learning issues.

Examples could include:

- Strategies to gain attention: using the person's name frequently
- Positive support strategies
- Errorless learning strategies (set the person up for success)

Slide 46

- May repeatedly do or think about the same thing
- Much harder to focus on things that are too difficult
- Problems with cognitive rigidity:
  - Difficulty changing from one task to another
  - Difficulty accepting alternative solutions or explanations
  - Difficulty shifting focus of attention

Transitions from a preferred activity to a less preferred activity can be very difficult for a person with IDD. Attention to how to set up transitions and shift focus can assist the person to move to a new task.

Slide 47

- Being different from peers
- More experience with losses rather than gains
- Social isolation although mainstreamed
- Rejected by peers
- Failure experiences dominate school histories
- Low social status

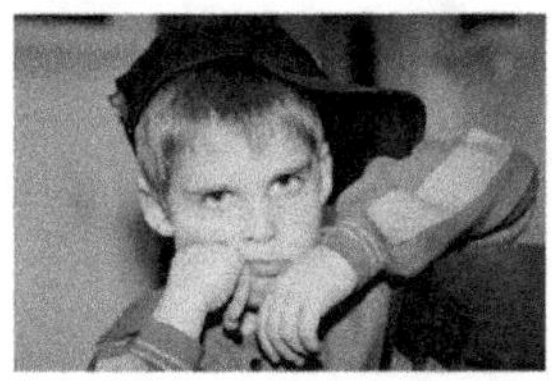

Heiman & Margalit, 1998

Ask the participants to give examples of how a person with IDD might experience each of these points.

Some responses might be:

- Being bullied and picked on or left out of activities
- Being picked last for teams
- Watching peers succeed academically much more quickly than they are

Slide 48

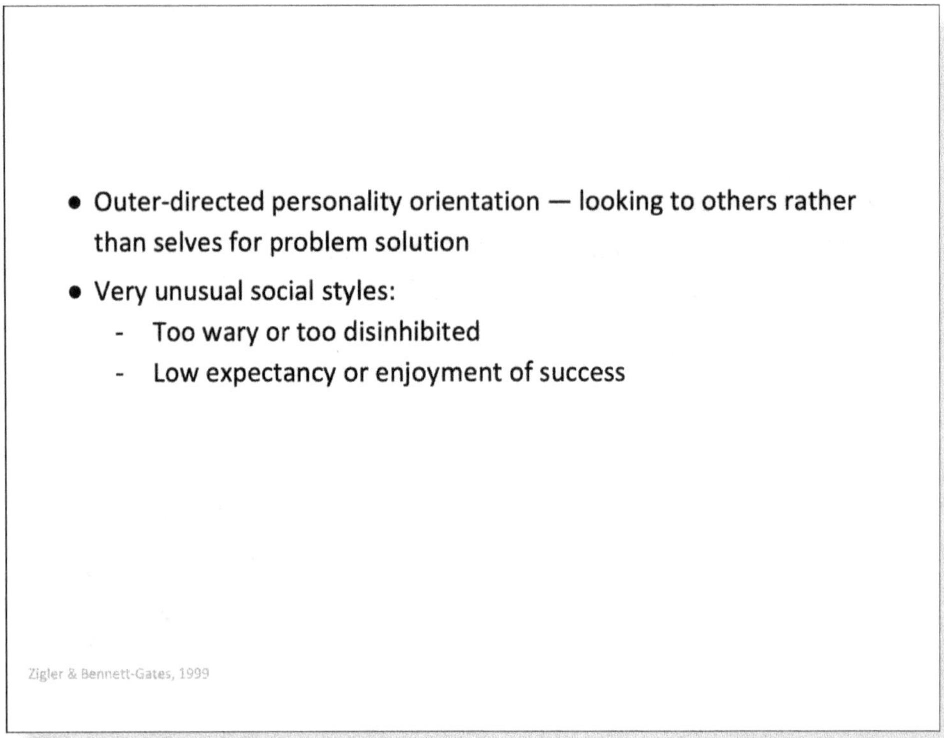

Issues related to higher dependency on caregivers, isolation from natural peer group and difficulty learning social skills create difficulty for a person with IDD when trying to fit in with a group or make friends. Skills that are learned typically through observing and imitating the actions of others may need to be taught more directly using positive reinforcement, modeling or verbal cuing in smaller steps.

Slide 49

- Low self-esteem
- Distrust of self
- Sadness, depression, dependency and withdrawal
- Helplessness
- Impulsivity

Zigler & Bennett-Gates, 1999

There is a large body of research showing that low self-esteem is a more significant issue for people who have an IDD than for their non-disabled peers.

Helping the person identify and focus on their strengths, as well as building skills in other areas, can assist in building self-esteem. This can have a large impact on preventing mental health issues related to low self-esteem.

Slide 50

Exercise

How can we support someone in improving their quality of life when one or more of these risk factors are present?

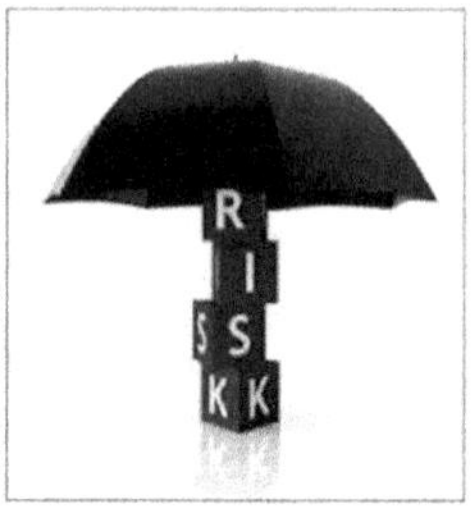

References: Module I

American Psychiatric Association. (2013). *Diagnostic and statistical manual of mental disorders* (5th ed.). https://doi.org/10.1176/appi.books.9780890425596.

Carter, W., and Wehby, J. (2003). Job performance of transition-age youth with emotional and behavioral disorders. *Exceptional Children,* 69, 449-465.

Corbett, J. A. (1979). Psychiatric morbidity and mental retardation. In F. E. James, & R. P. Smith (Eds.), *Psychiatric illness and mental handicap* (pp. 11-23). London: Gaskell Press.

Einfeld, S. L., & Aman, M. G. (1995). Issues in the taxonomy of psychopathology in children and adolescents with mental retardation. *Journal of Autism and Developmental Disorders*, 25, 143-167.

Einfeld, S. L., & Tonge, B. J. (1996). Population prevalence of psychopathology in children and adolescents with intellectual disability: II. Epidemiological findings. *Journal of Intellectual Disability Research*, 40, 99-109.

Engel, G. L. (1980). The clinical application of the biopsychosocial model. *American Journal of Psychiatry*, 137, 535–544.

Fisher, M. H., Moskowitz, A. L., & Hodapp, R. M. (2013). Differences in social vulnerability among individuals with autism spectrum disorder, Williams syndrome, and Down syndrome. *Research in Autism Spectrum Disorder,* 7 (8): 931-937.

Fletcher, R., Barnhill, J., & Copper, S. (Eds.). (2016). *Diagnostic manual – Intellectual disability (DM-ID-2): A textbook of diagnosis of mental disorders in persons with intellectual disability.* Kingston, NY: NADD Press.

Goldberg, D. (2014). Vulnerability factors for common mental illnesses. *British Journal of Psychiatry,* 178 (40), 69-71.

Harrison, P. L., & Oakland, T. (2000). *Adaptive behavior assessment system.* San

MODULE 1

Antonio, TX: The Psychological Corporation.

Hartley, S. L. & McLean, W. E. (2009). Depression in adults with mild intellectual disability: the role of stress, attributions, and coping. *American Journal of Intellectual and Developmental Disabilities,* 114 (3), 147-160.

Menolascino, F. J. (1977). *Challenges in mental retardation: Progressive ideology and services.* New York, NY: Behavioral Publications.

McBrien, J. A. (2003). Assessment and diagnosis of depression in people with intellectual disability. *Journal of Intellectual Disability Research,* 47 (1), 1-13. National Core Indicators Adult Consumer Survey 2015-16 Final Report. (2017). National Association of State Directors of Developmental Disabilities Services and the Human Services Research Institute. Retrieved from www.nationalcoreindicators.org.

Consumer Outcomes Final Report 2010-2011 NCI Adult Consumer Survey Data, August 2012. Alexandria, VA: National Core Indicators.

Royal College of Psychiatrists. (2001). *DC–LD: Diagnostic criteria for psychiatric disorders for use with adults with learning disabilities/mental retardation.* London: Gaskell Royal College of Psychiatrists.

Sparrow, S. S., Cicchetti, D. V., & Balla, D. A. (2005). Vineland Adaptive Behavior Scales, Second Edition (Vineland™-II). London, U.K.: AGS Publishing/Pearson Assessments.

Zigler, E., & Bennett-Gates, D. (1999). *Personality development in individuals with mental retardation.* Cambridge: Cambridge University Press.

Module II

The Genetics of IDD: Syndromes and Phenotypes

Slide 2

Learning Objectives

- Describe the many causes of IDD and identify five common syndromes.
- Describe what is meant by "behavioral phenotype."
- Understand the benefit of genetic testing and knowing the cause of the genetic disorder.

Slide 3

There are thousands of potential causes of intellectual/developmental disability. Among them:

- Chromosomal abnormalities
- Environmental genetic abnormalities
- Infections
- Metabolic issues/disorders
- Nutritional deficiencies/abnormalities
- Toxicity
- Trauma (prenatal and perinatal)
- Unknown

Whitaker, 2014

Infections (present at birth or occurring after birth), e.g., congenital cytomegalovirus, congenital rubella, congenital toxoplasmosis, encephalitis, HIV infection, listeriosis, meningitis, etc.

Chromosomal abnormalities

- Chromosome deletions (such as Cri-du-Chat syndrome)
- Chromosomal translocations (a gene is located in an unusual spot on a chromosome or located on a different chromosome than usual)
- Defects in the chromosome or chromosomal inheritance (such as Fragile X syndrome, Angelman syndrome, Prader-Willi syndrome)
- Errors of chromosome numbers (such as Down syndrome)

Environmental

- Deprivation syndrome can be caused by dysfunctional caregiver interaction, poverty, child abuse and parental ignorance about appropriate child care.
- Genetic abnormalities and inherited metabolic disorders such as adrenoleukodystrophy, galactosemia, Hunter syndrome, Hurler syndrome, Lesch-Nyhan syndrome, phenylketonuria, Rett syndrome, Sanfilippo syndrome, Tay-Sachs disease, Tuberous sclerosis, etc.
- Metabolic
- Congenital hypothyroid, hypoglycemia (poorly regulated diabetes), Reye syndrome, hyperbilirubinemia (very high bilirubin levels in babies)

Nutritional—Malnutrition

- Toxic prenatal exposure to alcohol, cocaine, amphetamines and other drugs or lead poisoning, methylmercury poisoning

Trauma (before and after birth)

- Intracranial hemorrhage before or after birth
- Lack of oxygen to the brain before, during or after birth
- Severe head injury

Unexplained (this is the largest category for occurrences of intellectual disability)

Slide 4

Advances in genetics over the past 30 years have lead to identification of previously unknown causes of intellectual/developmental disabilities. As a result, the number of identified genetic causes of IDD has grown exponentially into the thousands.

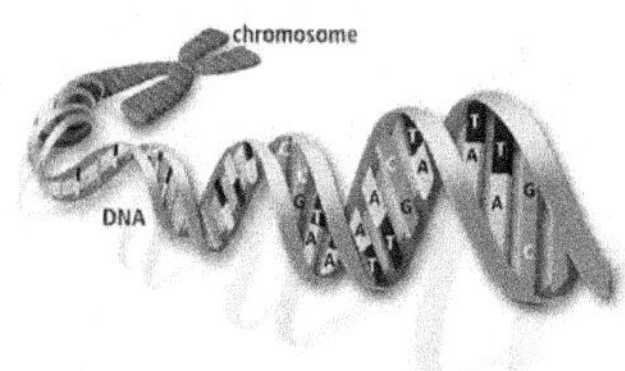

Deciphering Developmental Disorders, 2015

The genome is an organism's complete set of DNA. Genomes vary widely in size. The smallest known genome for a free-living organism (a bacterium) contains about 600,000 DNA base pairs, while human and mouse genomes have some 3 billion. Except for mature red blood cells, all human cells contain a complete genome.

DNA in the human genome is arranged into 24 distinct chromosomes — physically separate molecules that range in length from about 50 million to 250 million base pairs. A few types of major chromosomal abnormalities, including missing or extra copies or gross breaks and rejoinings (translocations), can be detected by microscopic examination. Most changes in DNA, however, are more subtle and require a closer analysis of the DNA molecule to find perhaps single-base differences.

Slide 5

Syndromes

A syndrome is a disease or disorder that has more than one identifying feature or symptom. Each particular genetic syndrome will have many typical, common features, depending on which aspects of development are affected by the abnormal genes or chromosomes.

The following are definitions (according to Webster's dictionary) for clarification:

Disease: A particular distinctive process in the body with a specific cause and characteristic symptoms.

Disorder: Irregularity, disturbance or interruption of normal functions.

Syndrome: A number of symptoms occurring together and characterizing a specific disease.

(www.med.umich.edu/yourchild/topics/genetic)

Slide 6

Advances in Genetic Testing

The study of genetics was advanced by the work of Gregor Mendel in the mid-nineteenth century.

Significant advancements in the understanding of genetics were made in the late twentieth century, including the ability to map the human genome and perform testing that can help identify what genetic changes are responsible for various aspects of disturbances in development.

Deciphering Developmental Disorders, 2015

Genetics is the study of heredity, which means the study of genes and factors related to all aspects of genes.

The discovery of the DNA structure in 1962 by Watson and Crick and the genetic code in 1966 made possible the development of new technologies and understanding about both heritable and non-heritable genetic disorders.

Rapid advancements in technology and in the understanding of the molecular background of genetics in the second half of the twentieth century have led to a greater understanding of genetics and the impact of genetic factors on life. Genetic testing is now accessible and feasible for most labs.

While deletions and duplications of chromosomes along a DNA strand are technically rare, they do collectively account for a significant minority of genetic causes of intellectual disability.

Slide 7

Definition of Phenotype:

The phenotype of a genetic syndrome is the set of physical characteristics produced by a genetic abnormality or genotype.

Definition of Behavioral Phenotype:

The specific and characteristic repertoire exhibited by people with a genetic disorder.

It is important to recognize the roles that behavioral phenotypes play. If we fail to pay attention to them, we can miss an important means for understanding the nature of challenges that some people present — not all people, but some.

Nyhan, W. L. Clinical features of the Lesch-Nyhan syndrome. *Archives of Internal Medicine*, 1972,130, 186–192. (a)

Slide 8

Behavioral Phenotypes

- Are not set in stone
- Look at syndromes rather than set diagnoses
- Behavioral manifestations arise from the interaction of genes and environment
- Present a wide range of symptoms
- Used as clues, not as expectations

Watson & Griffiths, 2016

Characterizing behavioral phenotype of a specific genetic disorder is a relatively recent approach.

Advances in behavioral phenotype research occur in two ways:

1. Studying individuals with known genetic disorders (such as Fragile X syndrome) and developing syndrome characterizations based on the observation.

2. Looking for a genetic marker in people with behavioral commonalities For example, the behavioral phenotype and developmental course of Rett syndrome has been well documented, but until recently the genetic marker had not been identified. As Rett syndrome previously had an identifiable phenotype without a genetic marker, it remained in the DSM-IV as an acceptable psychiatric diagnosis. Since the discovery of the genetic marker, it does not appear as a psychiatric diagnosis in the DSM-5. This has been the case with other genetically based

syndromes, such as Down syndrome or Fragile X syndrome, which are not included.

Etiologically based diagnosis is beneficial in driving clinical treatment and the related individual supports for a person. It is much easier to develop a unified support system when professionals, the family and the individual are operating from a common unifying concept, such as an etiological diagnosis.

Slide 9

The Importance of Genetic Testing

Genetic testing can lead to identification of a specific syndrome that may have associated

- **Medical vulnerabilities**
- **Behavioral phenotypes or specific behavioral patterns**

Watson & Griffiths, 2016

Identification of specific medical vulnerabilities can lead to a planned approach toward preventive health that considers both ongoing screening prevention, where possible, for health issues for which the person is predisposed.

For example, people who have 22q11.2 deletion syndrome (DiGeorge syndrome) are predisposed to congenital heart defects, airway obstructions, increased risk of pneumonia, hearing loss and other significant medical and dental issues. Identification of the genetic syndrome can lead to testing for these conditions and preventative health care.

Similarly, people with 22q11.2 deletion syndrome are also predisposed to anxiety disorders and have an increased likelihood of developing schizophrenia in adolescence. The knowledge of these predispositions allows the primary care provider the opportunity to be attentive for changes in behavior and seek earlier assessment, diagnosis and treatment.

Due to the range of intellectual disability exhibited across behavioral phenotypes, early assessment and intervention are important to assess cognitive functioning, so that educational intervention can be tailored to meet the person's needs and maximize the person's potential.

Challenging behavior can be a primary behavioral feature of a particular syndrome. On occasion, the underlying origin of these behaviors can sometimes be linked to a biological mechanism, such as a deficiency in the enzyme hypoxanthineguanine phosphoribosyltransferase (HPRT) in Lesch-Nyhan syndrome. However, in most conditions, the pathway from gene to behavior is less clear.

(http://www.intellectualdisability.info/mental-health/articles/behavioural-phenotypes-in-adulthood)

Slide 10

8 Benefits of Syndrome Identification

1. Increased understanding of mental health risks and development of resilience.
2. Cross-discipline collaboration to develop more effective treatment strategies.
3. Increased attention to understanding people from a bio-psycho-social perspective.
4. Allows people to make informed decisions about reproductive choices.
5. Increased support for families, care providers, and the person.
6. Along with challenges, early diagnosis allows early identification of strengths.
7. Early identification of learning challenges and educational adaptations.
8. Preventative health care.

Watson & Griffiths, 2016

Slide 11

Common Types of Intellectual Developmental Disability

- Down syndrome
- Fragile X syndrome
- Prader-Willi syndrome
- Williams syndrome
- Smith-Magenis syndrome
- 22q11.2 deletion syndrome
- Angelman syndrome
- Smith-Lemli-Opitz syndrome
- Autism Spectrum Disorders (ASD)
- Fetal Alcohol Spectrum Disorder (FASD)

DM-ID 2, 2016

The most common syndromes associated with intellectual disabilities are Autism Spectrum Disorder, Down syndrome, Fragile X syndrome and Fetal Alcohol Spectrum Disorder (FASD). While FASD is not a genetic syndrome, it does have an associated behavioral phenotype, medical vulnerabilities, cognitive implications and recommended support strategies. Additionally, recent studies indicate epigenetic changes also associated with FASD, which can be difficult to study as they are cell-specific and transient in nature. Nonetheless, they do have long-term consequences on gene expression and differentiation (Ungerer, Knezovich, & Ramsay, 2013).

Slide 12

Down Syndrome

Down syndrome is a genetic condition causing a set of delays in physical and intellectual development as a result of having an extra copy of chromosome 21.

All people with Down syndrome experience cognitive delays, but the effect is usually mild to moderate.

National Down Syndrome Society (NDSS, 2012)

Down syndrome is a non-hereditary genetic mutation caused by an error in cell division that occurs at conception. It causes lifelong developmental delays and health complications of varying severity. According to the NIH, Down syndrome occurs in about one of every 1,000 to 1,100 live births worldwide.

(CDC 2019, https://www.cdc.gov/ncbddd/birthdefects/downsyndrome/data.html)

Slide 13

People who have Down syndrome have increased risk for certain medical conditions such as:

- congenital heart defects
- respiratory and hearing problems
- Alzheimer's disease
- childhood leukemia
- thyroid conditions

A few of the common physical traits of Down syndrome are low muscle tone, small stature, an upward slant to the eyes and a single deep crease across the center of the palm.

CDC, 2019

Early interventions in specialized health care, speech therapy, physical therapy and occupational therapy will improve outcomes for people who have Down syndrome.

Slide 14

Down Syndrome Phenotype

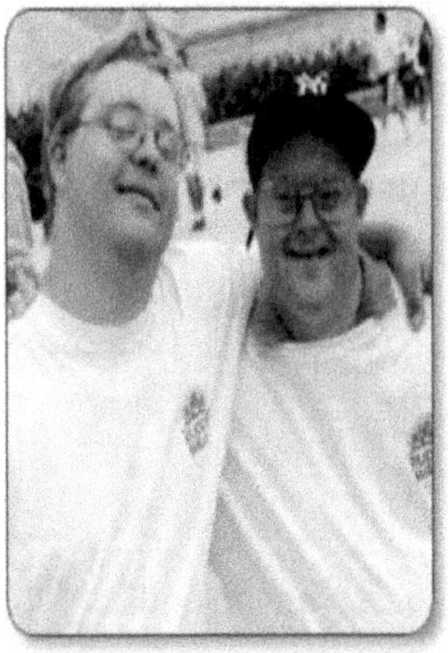

People who have Down syndrome typically have a smaller-than-average head, upward-slanting eyes, a broad neck and a tendency toward obesity.

DM-ID-2, 2016

TRISOMY 21–DOWN SYNDROME

Major malformations

- Cardiac
- GI

Minor malformations

- Facial, skin, etc.

Developmental pattern

- IDD
- Learning pattern

Slide 15

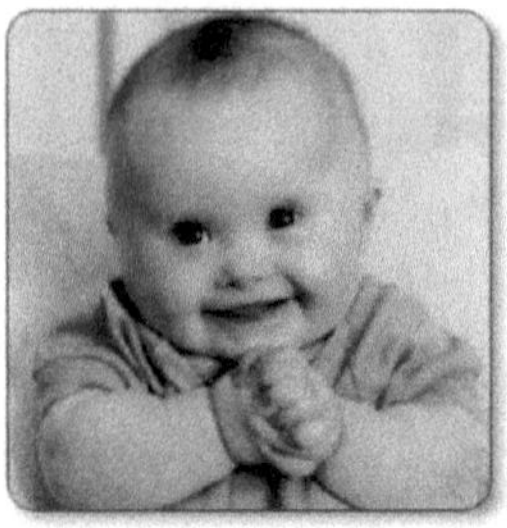

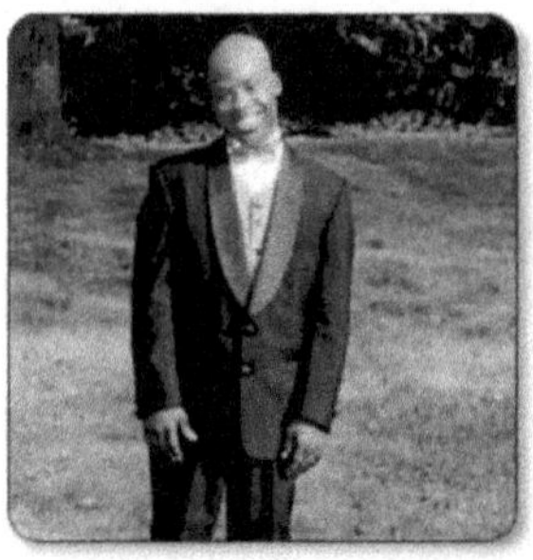

Behavioral Phenotypes
Down Syndrome

- Tendency to be noncompliant with requests
- Single-minded and tenacious
- Inattentive
- Overactive
- Argumentative
- Withdrawn
- Predisposition to depression and dementia among adults
- ADHD

ADHD

Autism

- In about 8% of people

Alzheimer's/Dementia

- 16-50% depending on criteria for diagnosis
- May require different programs than typical for IDD

Slide 16

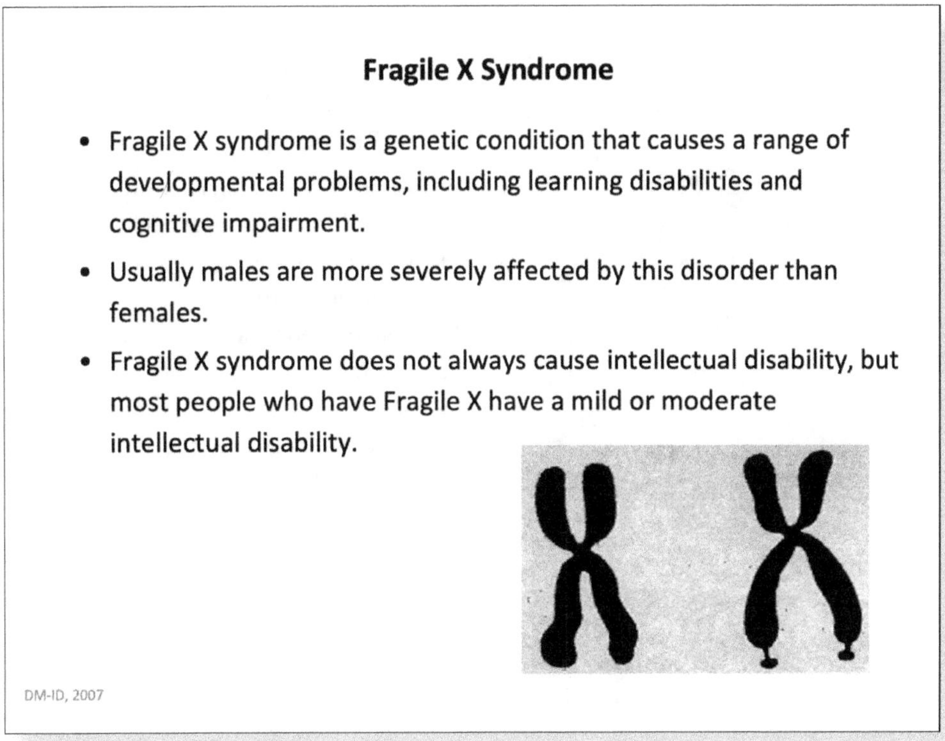

Fragile X usually causes a mild to moderate intellectual disability, predisposition to anxiety and hyperactive behavior. About one-third of people who have Fragile X also have features of an Autism Spectrum Disorder, such as impairments with communication and social interactions.

There is a great deal of ongoing research into the use of drug therapies to address the cellular and behavioral abnormalities of Fragile X.

Current therapies address the needs of a person who has Fragile X: speech and language, behavior, cognitive development and sensory integration. Medication is also often used to address some of the symptoms of Fragile X.

Slide 17

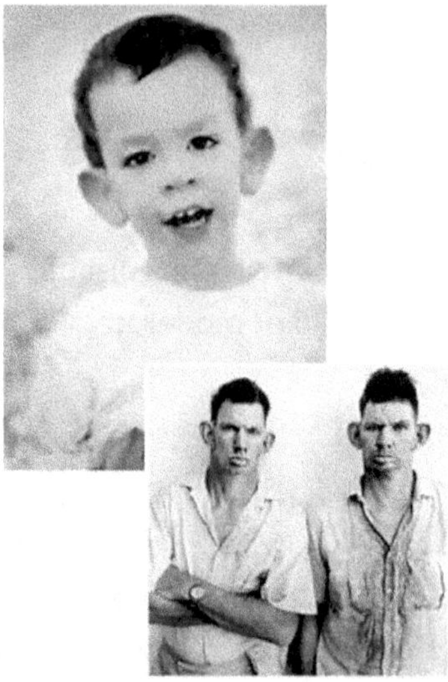

Fragile X Phenotype

People who have Fragile X often have common physical features such as:

- A long face
- Prominent ears
- High arched palate
- Flat feet
- Soft skin
- Other connective tissue abnormalities

DM-ID 2, 2016

Anxiety: hyperarousal

Early signs: self-injury (hand/wrist biting), mouthing objects, hand-flapping; escalate to task refusal, leaving the area, verbal aggression with imitated phrases

Triggers: forced eye contact, personal space issues, tactile defensiveness, emotional tone of peers/staff, changes in routine, auditory stimuli
Other contributors: auditory processing deficits, delayed emotional processing, hypersensitivity to negative correction, poor concept of time

A "cure" for Fragile X that targets pharmaceutical treatments is undergoing human clinical trials. It will target the underlying biochemical pathway affected by the Fragile X gene mutation. Families diagnosed with Fragile X syndrome will be able to benefit from this medical breakthrough.

Slide 18

Behavioral Phenotypes
Fragile X Syndrome

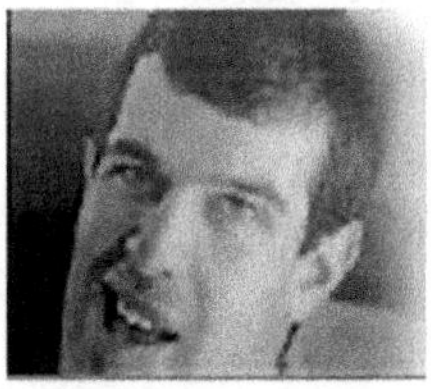

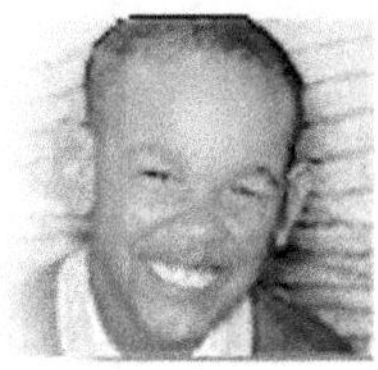

- Social anxiety
- Shyness
- Gaze aversion
- Perseveration
- Autism/PDD
- Inattention, hyperactivity, sadness or depression (primarily females)
- Attention Deficit Disorder

Dykens et al., 2000

X-linked (carriers: F-1:259; M-1:800)

1:2000 males; 1:4000 females

FMR1 gene on X chromosome (Xq27.3)

- Normal 0 to 25 repeats
- Premutation-25 to 200 repeats
- Mutation >200 repeats
- Diagnosis: DNA testing for mutation via PCR

MODULE 2

FRAGILE X SYNDROME

Facial features:

- Long face
- Large, protuberant ears

Hyperextensible joints especially fingers

Flat feet

Large size

Macroorchidism

Cognition:

- Males: most with IDD
- Females: one-third to one half with IDD, others with learning disability (LD)

ADHD (Males: 80-90%)

Anxiety disorders

Mood disorders, e.g. bipolar disorder/ depression

Autism (15-33%)/Autistic characteristics

- Hand-flapping/pica
- Poor social judgment/ interaction
- Sound/light/texture sensitivity
- Poor eye contact/perseverative speech

Slide 19

Prader-Willi Syndrome

Prader-Willi syndrome (PWS) is a genetic disorder that is complex in origin but results from an abnormality of the 15th chromosome.

PWS causes a wide range of development problems including learning disabilities and cognitive impairment.

The genetic mutation that causes PWS generally occurs randomly but can be heritable.

DM-ID 2, 2016

At this time, the mechanism by which the lack of functional genetic material on chromosome 15 leads to the symptoms associated with PWS is not understood. Scientists are actively studying the normal role of the genetic sequences in the PWS region and how their loss affects the hypothalamus and other systems in the body.

(http://www.fpwr.ca/about-prader-willi-syndrome)

Slide 20

Prader-Willi Syndrome Phenotype

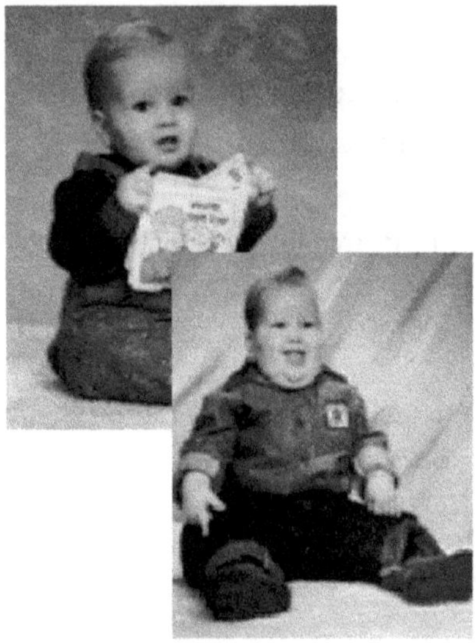

People who have PWS typically share common physical features including:

- short in stature
- hyperphagia
- obesity
- small hands and feet
- dysmorphic facial features
- hypogonadism
- low muscle tone

Hyperphagia refers to an abnormal, increased sensation of hunger that is not satisfied by eating and typically leads to significant overeating and weight gain.

PWS is often described in two contrasting stages. Infants typically experience poor feeding and a failure to thrive. As they develop, the second stage of hyperphagia develops, often resulting in childhood obesity.

Hypotonia (decreased muscle tone) can be detected in utero as decreased fetal movement. Failure to thrive in first year of life is often observed to include a weak cry, delayed motor milestones and delayed walking until two years.

While exercise will help people prevent excessive weight gain, there is evidence that people who have PWS have reduced resting metabolic rates, which means they have a lower rate of energy expenditure. Obesity can be prevented with a calorie-restricted nutrition plan and daily exercise. Locking up food is often needed to prevent overeating. There is some indication that hormone therapy may assist with the appropriate medical consultation.

Slide 21

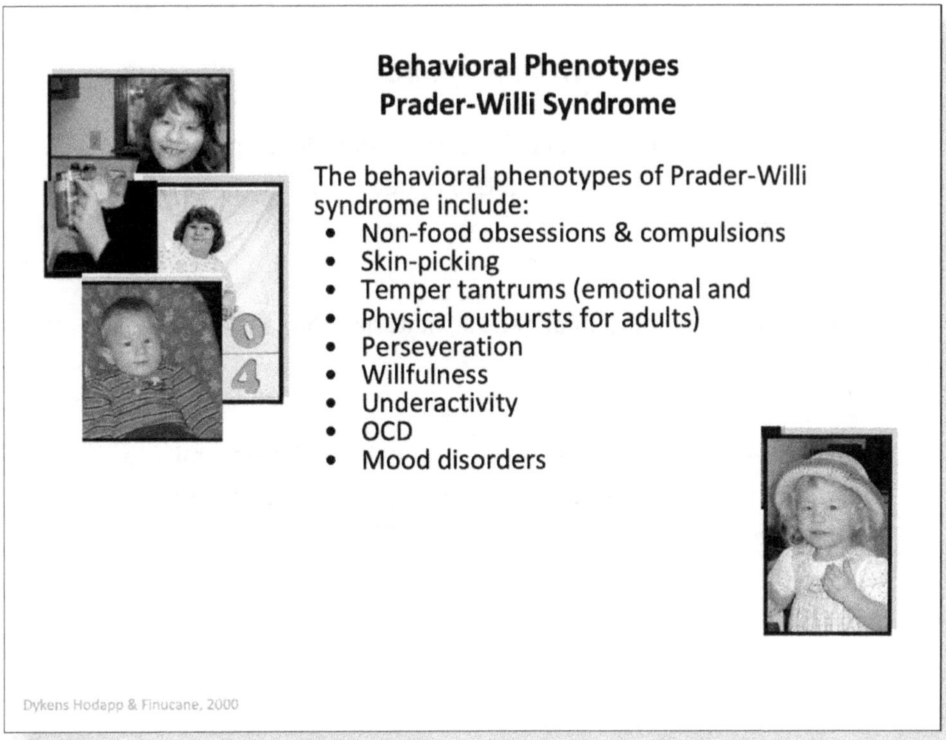

The prevalence rate for Prader-Willi syndrome is 1 in 15,000 general population. Of those, 1 in 100 also have an intellectual disability.

People with PWS tend to have a low tolerance for teasing and getting stuck on topics. People who overeat are inclined to hide their overeating. People with PWS are no exception.

Slide 22

Williams Syndrome

Williams syndrome is a genetically caused neurodevelopmental disorder that results in a wide variety of health, developmental and cognitive challenges.

It is caused by the deletion of genetic material from a specific region on chromosome 7.

Most people with Williams syndrome probably will have a mild to moderate intellectual disability or learning challenges. It is also characterized by a distinct personality profile.

DM-ID 2, 2016

Williams syndrome is generally caused by a random genetic mutation occurring during the formation of reproductive cells in one or both of the parents of the affected person.

(https://ghr.nlm.nih.gov/condition/williams-syndrome#genes)

Slide 23

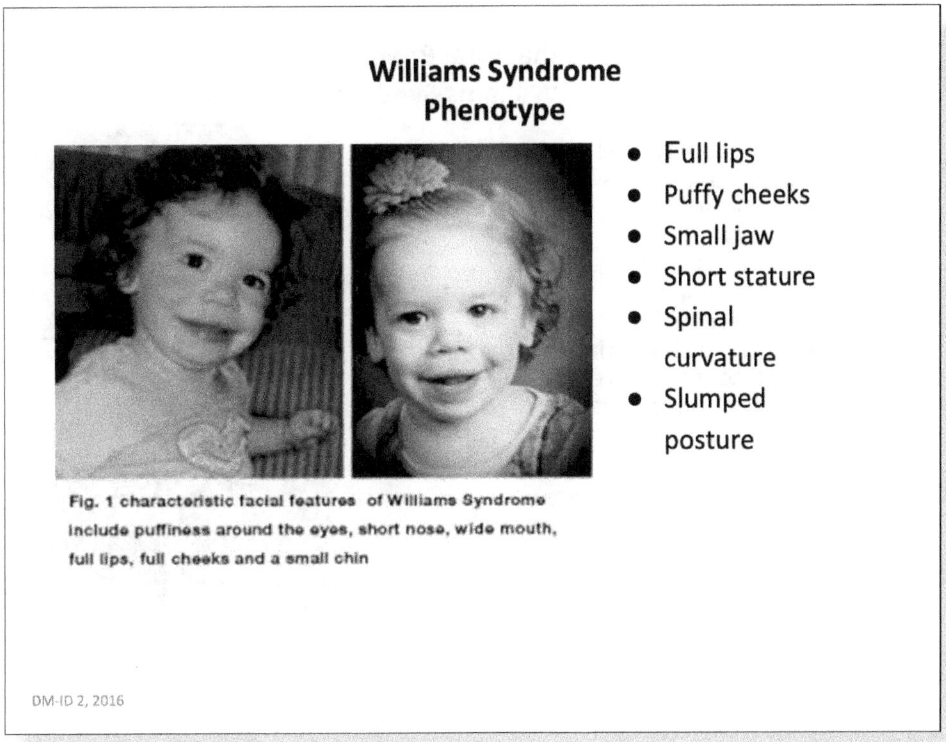

Young children with Williams syndrome have distinctive facial features including:

- a broad forehead
- a short nose with a broad tip
- full cheeks
- a wide mouth with full lips

Many people have dental problems. Cardiovascular problems are frequent.

(https://williams-syndrome.org/what-is-williams-syndrome)

Slide 24

Behavioral Phenotypes
Williams Syndrome

Williams syndrome has the associated behavior phenotype:

- Anxiety
- Fears
- Phobias
- Inattention
- Hyperactivity
- Social disinhibition/overly friendly
- Indiscriminate relating
- Attention Deficit Disorder

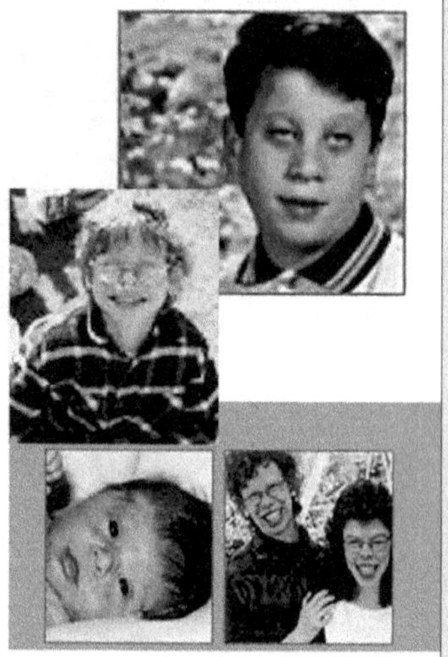

DM-ID 2, 2016

- Appealing face and engaging smile, auditory processing strength; strength in musical ability and facial recognition
- Short attention span/ADHD
- Cocktail party chatter: well-developed verbal skills, no fear of strangers
- Obsessive compulsive characteristics, e.g. topic of conversation
- Unusually sensitive to noise (hyperacusis), fear of heights
- Difficulty building friendships, poor visual motor integration, medically fragile
- Nail-biting, skin-picking behaviors
- Anxiety/anxiety disorders
- Autism/autistic features

Slide 25

Smith-Magenis Syndrome

Smith-Magenis syndrome is a genetic condition causing a set of delays in physical and intellectual development as a result of a chromosome deletion.

DM-ID 2, 2016

Smith-Magenis syndrome is a result of the deletion of chromosome 17p11.2. It causes a variety of physical and developmental delays and is associated with a specific behavioral genotype.

Slide 26

Smith-Magenis Syndrome

All people with Smith-Magenis syndrome will have an intellectual disability, most commonly in the mild to moderate range.

However, there is also a predisposition to strength in:

- Long-term memory for places, things and people
- Letter/word recognition
- Simultaneous processing skills

DM-ID 2, 2016

Slide 27

Smith-Magenis Syndrome Phenotype

A person who has Smith-Magenis syndrome is likely to have:

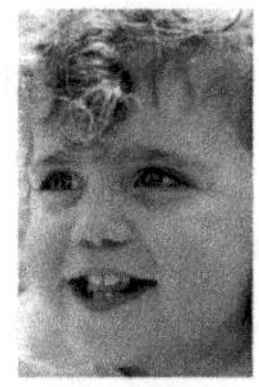

- A broad, square-shaped face with deep-set eyes
- Full cheeks
- A prominent lower jaw
- The appearance of flattened middle of the face and bridge of the nose
- Mouth will tend to turn downward
- Full, outward-curving upper lip
- Dental abnormalities are common

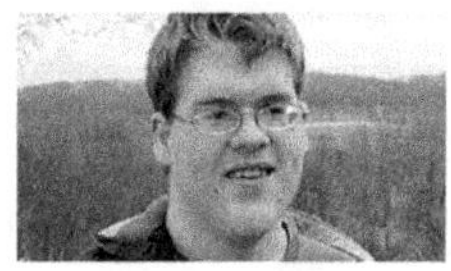

Poisson, et al, 2015

Physical indicators of Smith-Magenis syndrome include short stature, abnormal curvature of the spine (scoliosis), reduced sensitivity to pain and temperature and a hoarse voice. Some people have ear abnormalities that lead to hearing loss. Affected individuals may have eye abnormalities that cause nearsightedness (myopia) and other vision problems. Although less common, heart and kidney defects also have been reported in people with Smith-Magenis syndrome.

People who have Smith-Magenis syndrome have increased risk for certain medical conditions such as:

- Scoliosis
- Cardiac problems (25%)
- Dental and periodontal problems

- Peripheral neuropathy
- Heightened risk of hypothyroidism
- Urinary tract anomalies
- Frequent ear infections and vision problems

Facial differences can be subtle in early childhood, but they usually become more distinctive in later childhood and adulthood. Dental abnormalities are also common.

Disrupted sleep patterns are characteristic of Smith-Magenis syndrome, typically beginning early in life. Affected people may be very sleepy during the day, but they have trouble falling asleep and awaken several times each night.

(https://ghr.nlm.nih.gov/condition/smith-magenis-syndrome)

Slide 28

Behavioral Phenotypes
Smith-Magenis Syndrome

The chromosome deletion responsible for Smith-Magenis syndrome also results in a behavioral phenotype.

Common behavioral challenges can include:

- Self-injury
- Aggression
- Anxiety
- Impulsiveness
- Difficulty paying attention

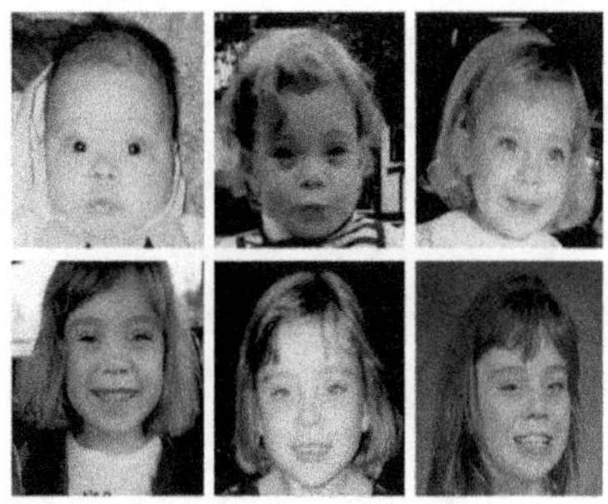

People with Smith-Magenis syndrome are inclined to have affectionate, engaging personalities but are also inclined to have behavioral problems. These include frequent temper tantrums and outbursts, aggression, anxiety, impulsiveness and difficulty paying attention. Self-injury, including biting, hitting, head-banging and skin-picking, is very common. Repetitive self-hugging is a behavioral trait that may be unique to Smith-Magenis syndrome. People with this condition also compulsively lick their fingers and flip pages of books and magazines (a behavior known as "lick and flip").

(https://ghr.nlm.nih.gov/condition/smith-magenis-syndrome)

Slide 29

22q11.2 Deletion Syndrome

22q11.2 Deletion syndrome is genetic disorder that can lead to a wide variety of physical and developmental delays. Features can vary widely, even in members of the same family.

22q11.2 Deletion syndrome can cause mild to moderate intellectual disability and causes a predisposition to mental health problems, particularly in adulthood.

Bassett, & Chow, 1999

Most people with 22q11.2 Deletion syndrome are missing a sequence of about 3 million DNA building blocks (base pairs) on one copy of chromosome 22 in each cell. Most cases of 22q11.2 Deletion syndrome are not inherited.

(https://ghr.nlm.nih.gov/condition/22q112-deletion-syndrome#genes)

Slide 30

22q11.2 Deletion Syndrome

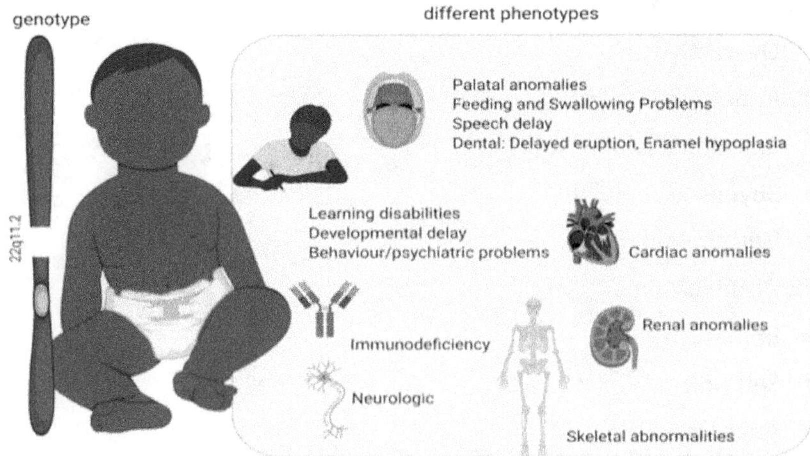

Slide 31

22Q Deletion Syndrome Phenotype

22q11.2 Deletion syndrome is associated with a number of physiological and physical differences including:

- Increased calcium levels
- Kidney abnormalities
- Immunodeficiency
- Problematic thyroid function
- Congenital heart defects
- Low platelet counts
- Velopharyngeal insufficiency (failure of palate to meet the throat during crying, swallowing and speech)
- Underdeveloped chin
- Low-set ears

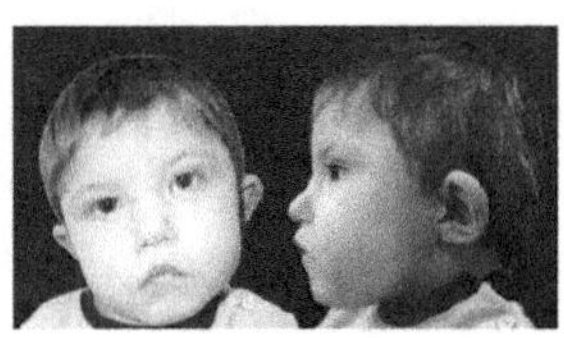

Slide 32

Behavioral Phenotypes
22q11.2 Deletion Syndrome

There are several common behavioral challenges observed in people who have 22q11.2 Deletion syndrome, including:

- Overactivity
- Impulsivity
- Emotional lability
- Shyness
- Withdrawal
- Disinhibition
- Immaturity
- Self-talk
- Anger issues
- Anxiety

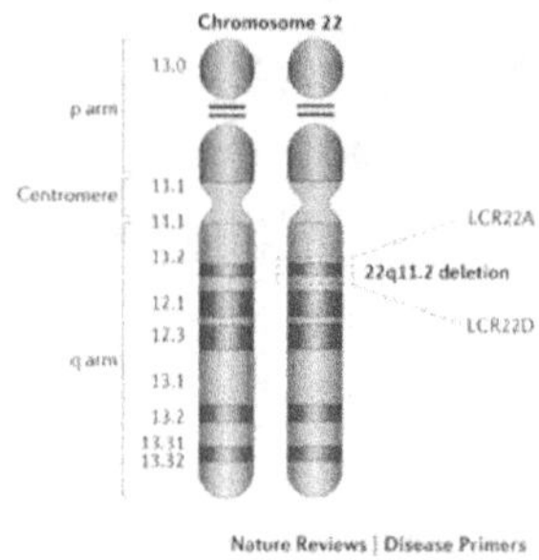

Mikhail et al, 2914

McDonald-McGinn et al, 2015

(Mikhail et al. (2014) https://www.ncbi.nlm.nih.gov/pmc/articles/PMC4586411/ Mikhail, F. M., R. D. Burnside, B. Rush, J. Ibrahim, R. Godshalk, S. L. Rutledge, et al. 2014. The recurrent distal 22q11.2 microdeletion are often de novo and do not represent a single clinical entity: a proposed categorization system. *Genet. Med.* 16:92–100.)

MODULE 2

Slide 33

Angelman Syndrome

Angelman syndrome (AS) is a genetic disorder that primarily affects the nervous system in a number of ways, including:

- Delayed development
- Severe speech impairment
- Ataxia (movement and balance problems)
- Microcephaly (in most cases)
- Epilepsy (in most cases)

It can be caused by a deletion, mutation or replication error in a portion of chromosome 15 or a mutation in the gene UBE3A.

AS causes a full range of intellectual/developmental disabilities.

Prevalence of Angelman syndrome is estimated to be between 1/10,000 and 1/20,000 live births worldwide.

There is generally a normal prenatal and birth history, with normal head circumference at birth and no major birth defects. The first signs of Angelman syndrome begin to appear between 6 and 12 months of age with delayed developmental milestones.

Slide 34

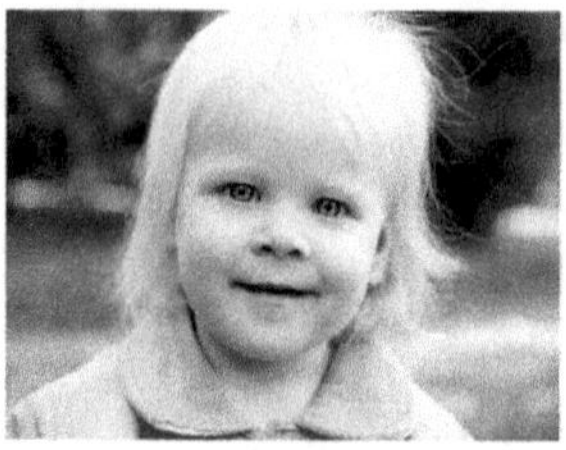

Angelman Syndrome Phenotype

- Hair, skin and eyes that are light in color (hypopigmentation)
- Scoliosis is common
- As children, appear thin with low or near-normal subcutaneous fat

MODULE 2

Complications associated with Angelman syndrome include:

- **Feeding difficulties.** Difficulty coordinating sucking and swallowing may cause feeding problems in infants. Your pediatrician may recommend a high-calorie formula to help your baby gain weight.

- **Hyperactivity.** Children with Angelman syndrome often move quickly from one activity to another, have a short attention span and keep their hands or a toy in their mouths. Hyperactivity often decreases with age and medication usually isn't necessary.

- **Sleep disorders.** People with Angelman syndrome often have abnormal sleep-wake patterns and need less sleep than most people. Sleep difficulties may improve with age. Medication and behavior therapy may help control sleep disorders.

- **Curving of the spine (scoliosis).** Some people with Angelman syndrome develop an abnormal, side-to-side spinal curvature over time.
- **Obesity.** Older children with Angelman syndrome tend to have large appetites, which may lead to obesity.

(https://www.mayoclinic.org/diseases-conditions/angelman-syndrome/symptoms-causes/syc-20355621)

Slide 35

Behavioral Phenotype Angelman Syndrome

Characterized by:

- A happy demeanor with prominent "smiling"
- Poorly specific laughing
- General exuberance associated with hypermotive behavior
- Reduced behavioral adaptive skills

Cassidy & Allanson, 2010

One of the first behavioral phenotypes to be observed in people with Angelman syndrome is early and persistent social smiling, which develops between ages one and three months.

In very rare instances, the predominantly happy demeanor is short-lived and replaced by irritability, crying, shrieking or screaming. In these cases, behavior that can be interpreted as aggressive is also observed: pinching, hitting, biting, grabbing.

For most people who have Angelman syndrome, facial grimacing, which is interpreted as a pleasant demeanor, is not necessarily an expression of mood. People who have Angelman syndrome experience a full range of emotions. Their expression is likely a motor reaction to physical or mental stimuli. It can be accompanied by laughter or laughter-like grimacing.

Slide 36

Smith-Lemli-Opitz Syndrome

Smith-Lemli-Opitz syndrome is a genetic disorder that causes intellectual/developmental disability and a range of physical problems.

It is characterized by distinctive physical, intellectual and behavioral characteristics.

Smith-Lemli-Opitz syndrome is caused by a mutation on the gene that is responsible for the activity of a cholesterol reductase and prevents cells from producing enough cholesterol.

Smith-Lemli-Opitz syndrome's prevalence rate is estimated around one in 29,000 live births based on studies in Canada, with higher incident rate in Canadians of European descent (Waye et al., 2002).

The severity of the condition varies greatly in affected people.

It is known by several other names as well:

- DHCR7 abnormality
- RSH syndrome
- SLOS
- SLO syndrome

Slide 37

Smith-Lemli-Opitz
Phenotype

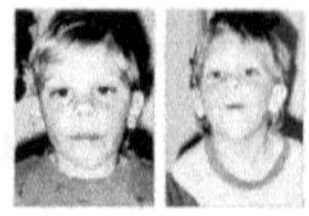

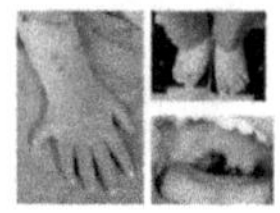

- Growth delay
- Microcephaly
- Extra fingers and toes
- Fused second and third toes
- Cleft palate
- Underdeveloped external genitals in males
- Distinctive facial features

Distinct facial features of Smith-Lemli-Opitz include:

- droopy eyelids
- nostrils that are turned forward
- long upper lip with an inverted V shape
- small jaw
- large external ears

Occasional findings include seizures, heart defects, low muscle tone (hypotonia) in young children, a narrowing in the distal opening of the stomach (pyloric stenosis) and bowel obstruction. Many individuals with SLOS have an unusual sensitivity to light (photosensitivity) (Bianconi, Cross, Wassif & Porter, 2015).

Slide 38

Smith-Lemli-Opitz
Behavioral Phenotype

- Repeated self-injury
- Prolonged temper tantrums
- Violent outbursts
- Hyperactivity

(Bianconi, Cross, Wassif, & Porter, 2015)

A common posturing behavior for people with Smith-Lemli-Opitz is a stretching motion of the upper body accompanied by hand-flicking. People may experience sensory hyper-reactivity, temperament dysregulation, sleep disturbance, and social and communication deficits (Tierney, Nwokoro, Porter, Freund, Ghuman & Kelley, 2001).

A person with SLOS may have low/normal intelligence and react negatively or with hypersensitivity to different sensory stimuli. This is particularly true for certain auditory and visual stimuli.

Other behaviors associated with SLOS can be linked directly to physical abnormalities. For example, infants often show challenges with feeding. Some may need increased caloric intake due to accelerated metabolism. Recurrent infections, including ear infections and pneumonia, are also common.

Slide 39

Autism Spectrum Disorder

Autism Spectrum Disorder (ASD) is a complex condition that impacts normal brain development and affects a person's social relationships, communication, interests and behavior across multiple contexts. ASD is a single condition with different levels of symptom severity.

DSM 5, 2013

According to the DSM-5, ASD diagnosis now encompasses the previous DSM-IV autistic disorder, Asperger syndrome, childhood disintegrative disorder and pervasive developmental disorder — not otherwise specified (PDD-NOS).

Under the DSM-5 diagnostic criteria, people with ASD must show symptoms from early childhood. This change in criteria encourages earlier diagnosis. People who have an ASD require different support levels depending on the severity of symptoms. Severity is based on social communication impairments and restricted, repetitive patterns of behavior.

There is ongoing research into causes of ASD, with a growing body of evidence for genetic causes in some cases.

Slide 40

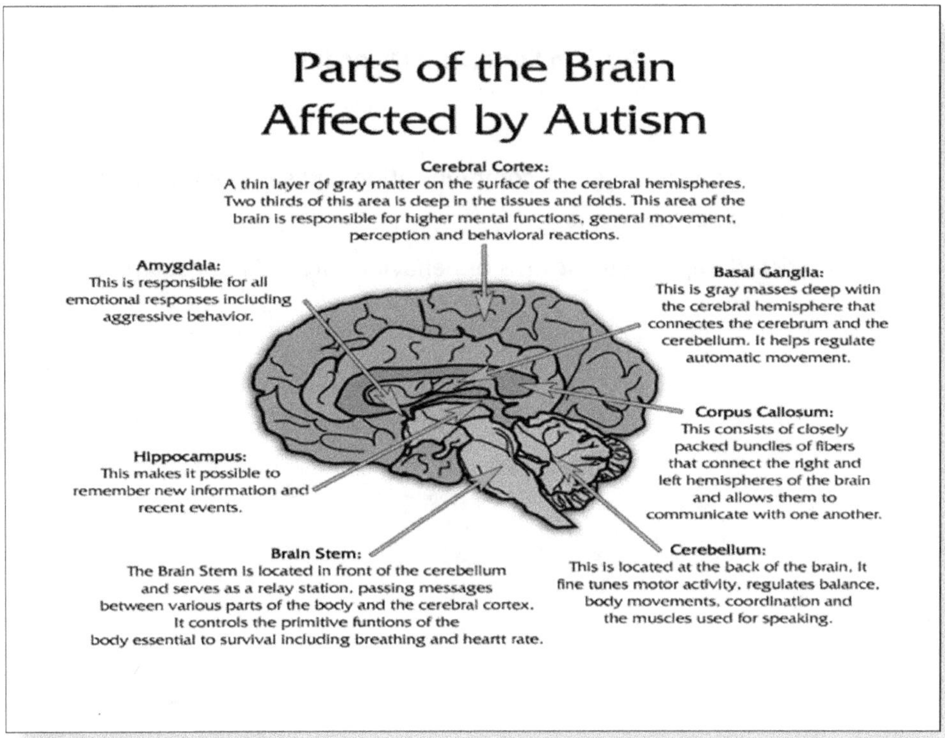

Magnetic resonance spectroscopy (MRS) can be used to detect regional concentrations of neuron-related molecules, a combination of altered molecular markers and an increase in white and gray matter (DiCicco-Bloom et al., 2006).

The core symptom domains likely involve widely dispersed neural systems and can imply generalized cellular abnormality. However, the differences in symptom severity and abilities can also suggest that not all brain systems are equally affected (DiCicco-Bloom et al., 2006).

Slide 41

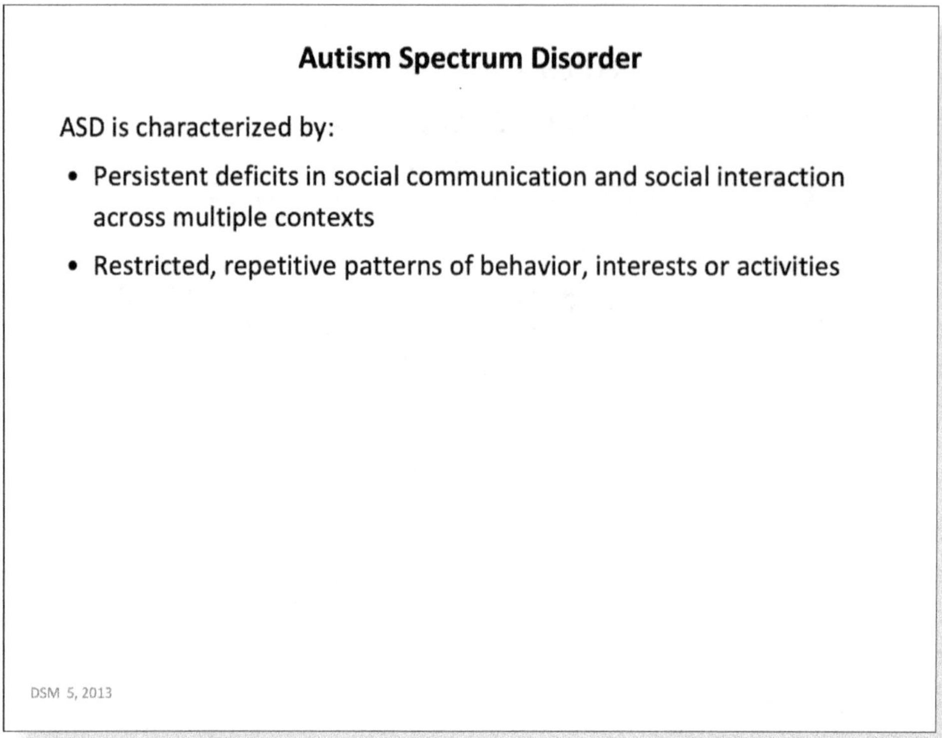

Diagnosis of ASD is based on the presence of both deficits in social communication and social interaction, as well as restricted, repetitive behaviors, interests and activities. Symptoms must be present in the early developmental period; cause clinically significant impairment in social, occupational or other important areas of current functioning; and are not better explained by intellectual disability or global developmental delay.

The diagnosis of ASD can now be made in children as young as 2, as well as adults, using a combination of standardized instruments: a parent interview (e.g., the Autism Diagnostic Interview–Revised) and an observational scale (e.g., the Autism Diagnostic Observation Schedule).

Diagnostic evaluation typically will involve a multidisciplinary team: doctors (pediatrician), psychologist, speech and language pathologist and occupational therapist. Genetic testing may likewise be recommended, as well as screening for related medical issues such as sleep difficulties.

Slide 42

Autism Spectrum Disorder

ASD is typically noticed in the first or second year of life with:

- Delay or abnormality in language and play.
- Repetitive behaviors, such as spinning things or lining up small objects.
- Unusual interests, such as preoccupations with stop signs or ceiling fans.

DiCicco-Bloom et al., 2006

Although some areas of development in a person who has autism are delayed, people who have an Autism Spectrum Disorder (ASD) often exhibit skills in other areas. These intellectual strengths may overshadow the developmental problems experienced.

Common Strengths

- nonverbal reasoning skills
- reading skills
- perceptual motor skills
- drawing skills
- computer interest and skills
- exceptional memory
- visual spatial abilities
- music skills

Slide 43

Autism Spectrum Disorder
Phenotype

People who have autism spectrum disorders often have difficulties with:

- Abnormal responses to sensory stimulation
- Behavior problems
- Variability of intellectual functioning
- Uneven development profile
- Difficulties in sleeping, toileting and eating
- Immune irregularities
- Nutritional deficiencies
- Gastrointestinal problems

McCray, Trevvett, & Frost, 2014)

Treatment of ASD usually focuses around early intervention with proper medical care, education/behavior therapy, language and speech therapy, occupational therapy and physical therapy. The most significant impairments associated with ASD are deficits in social relationships/interactions, deficits in communication and variability of intellectual functioning.

People with ASD also tend to have difficulty with:

- social relationships
- transitions
- communication/language
- perseveration on interests and activities
- dependence on routine

Slide 44

Autism Spectrum Disorder
Behavioral Phenotype

Deficits in social interaction can be observed in these areas:

- Failure to initiate or sustain conversations (e.g., turn-taking)
- Serious deficits in the ability to make friendships
- Failure to respond to their names when called
- Appearing not to listen when spoken to
- Difficulty identifying boundaries of others

McEvoy, Rogers, and Pennington, 2006

Autism is characterized by an impaired ability to engage in social relationships.

Slide 45

Autism Spectrum Disorder
Behavioral Phenotype

Restricted repetitive behaviors, interests and activities may be observed as:

- Perseveration of interests and activities—people who have ASD typically have a narrow range of interests
- Repetitive, stereotyped body movements such as hand-flicking, spinning or rocking
- Perseverations might extend to food
- Dependence on routine

McEvoy, Rogers & Pennington, 2006

Difficulties in sleeping, toileting and eating are common in people who have an ASD.

Abnormal responses to sensory stimulation are also common. Many people who have ASDs have unexpected reactions to stimuli. People may have hypersensitivity (cannot tolerate touch, can hear the sound of a light buzzing, can be fascinated with an object spinning, etc.) or hyposensitivity (can appear deaf or have extremely high pain tolerance to different sensory stimuli).

Slide 46

Fetal Alcohol Spectrum Disorder (FASD)

FASD is a term used to describe a range of disabilities caused by prenatal exposure to alcohol.

While each person impacted by FASD is unique, brain damage typically results in various symptoms commonly observed in people who have an FASD.

Astley, 2004

FASD is a diagnosis is based on a history of prenatal alcohol consumption by the mother, combined with a group of characteristics in the infant, including poor growth and neurological abnormalities. Accurate diagnosis of FASD requires the input of a multidisciplinary team.

Characteristic facial features may or may not be present and are not dependent on the severity of the disorder. They are representative of prenatal alcohol consumption during the time when the facial features were developing.

Primary challenges for people with FASD are connected to executive functions:

- planning actions toward a goal
- using information flexibly
- realizing consequences or outcomes of behavior
- making inferences based on limited information

Slide 47

FASD Phenotype

FASD is associated with several potential physical features and challenges that can include:

- Low birth weight and trouble gaining weight
- Smaller-than-average head circumference
- Heart defects
- Anomalies to ears, eyes, liver and joints

Facial features associated with FASD will occur only if there was exposure to alcohol during a specific period of pregnancy. The features are:

- Small eye openings
- Smooth, wide philtrum
- Thin upper lip

Astley et al, 2002

Slide 48

FASD Behavioral Phenotype

People with FASD often share common behavioral traits, including:

- Memory problems
- Difficulty storing and retrieving information
- Inconsistent performance ("on" and "off") days
- Impulsivity, distractibility, disorganization
- Ability to repeat instructions, but inability to put them into action
- Difficulty with abstractions, such as math, money management, time concepts
- Cognitive processing deficits (may think more slowly)
- Slow auditory pace (may only understand every third word of a normally paced conversation)
- Developmental lags (may act younger than chronological age)
- Inability to predict outcomes or understand consequence

Streissguth & Kanter, 1997

FASD is often called an invisible disorder. In the absence of facial features, it is observable only through behavior. These behaviors are the result of permanent damage to the brain and are typically not within the person's control. However, they are often interpreted as chosen behavior and intentional on the person's part (Streissguth & Kanter, 1997).

Slide 49

FASD

Preventable *Secondary* Characteristics

In the absence of accurate diagnosis, patterns of defensive behaviors commonly develop over time. These are called secondary characteristics of FASD:

- Fatigue, tantrums
- Irritability, frustration, anger, aggression
- Fear, anxiety, avoidance, withdrawal
- Shutdown, lying, running away
- Trouble at home, school and community
- Legal trouble
- Drug/alcohol abuse
- Mental health problems (depression, self-injury, suicidal tendencies)

Streissguth et al., 2004

Secondary characteristics can be prevented with proper diagnosis and support strategies.

Intervention strategies typically include concrete instructions, consistent messages, repetition, routine, simple tasks, explanations, supervision and decreased stimulation (Streissguth et al., 2004).

References: Module II

Astley, S. J. (2004). *Diagnostic guide for Fetal Alcohol Spectrum Disorders: The 4-Digit Diagnostic Code.* Third Edition. Seattle, WA: University of Washington.

Astley, S. J., Stachowiak, J., Clarren, S. K., & Clausen, C. (2002). Application of the fetal alcohol syndrome facial photographic screening tool in a foster care population. *Journal of Pediatrics.* 141(5):712-717.

Bassett, A. S., & Chow, E. W. (1999). 22q11 deletion syndrome: a genetic subtype of schizophrenia. *Biological psychiatry*, 46(7), 882-891.

Bianconi, S. E., Cross, J. L., Wassif, C. A., & Porter, F. D. (2015). Pathogenesis, Epidemiology, Diagnosis and Clinical Aspects of Smith-Lemli-Opitz Syndrome. *Expert opinion on orphan drugs*, 3(3), 267-280.

Buckley, R.H., Dinno, N., & Weber, P. (1998). Angelman syndrome: are the estimates too low? *American Journal of Medical Genetics*, 80(4), 385-389.

Capute, A.J., & Accardo, P. J. (Eds.) (1998). *Developmental Disabilities in Infancy and Childhood*, 2nd Ed., vols. I, II. Paul H. Brookes Publishing, Baltimore, MD.

Cassidy, S. B., & Allanson, J. E. (Eds.) (2010). *Management of Genetic Syndromes.* Hoboken, NJ. John Wiley & Sons, Inc.

Dagli, A.I., Mathews, J., & Williams, C.A. (2021). Angelman Syndrome. In: Adam, M.P., Ardinger, H.H., Pagon, R.A., et al., (Eds). *GeneReviews®.* Seattle: University of Washington, Seattle; 1993-2021. Available from: https://www.ncbi.nlm.nih.gov/books/NBK1144.

Deciphering Developmental Disorders Study (2015). Large-scale discovery of novel genetic causes of developmental disorders. *Nature, 519*(7542), 223-228.

DiCicco-Bloom, E., et al. (2006). The developmental neurobiology of autism spectrum disorder. *The Journal of Neuroscience: the Official Journal of the Society for Neuroscience,* 26(26), 6897-6906.

Driscoll, D. J., et al. (1998). Prader-Willi Syndrome. Updated 2017 Dec 14. In: Adam, M. P., et al., (Eds.). *GeneReviews*. Seattle: University of Washington, Seattle; 1993-2020.

Dykens, E. M., & Volkmar, F. R. (1997). Medical Conditions Associated with Autism. In: Cohen. D.J., Volkmar, F. R. (Eds.) (1997). *Handbook of Autism and Pervasive Developmental Disorders* 2. New York: John Wiley & Sons Inc: pp. 388-410.

Finegan, J. (1998). Study of behavioral phenotypes: Goals and methodological considerations. *American Journal of Medical Genetics*. 81(2): 148-155.

Fletcher, R., Barnhill, J., & Cooper, S. A. (Eds.) (2016). *DM-ID-2: Diagnostic Manual of Intellectual Disability: A textbook of diagnosis of mental disorders in persons with intellectual disability*. Kingston, NY: NADD Press.

Flint, Jonathan. (2002). Behavioral Phenotypes: Conceptual and Methodological Issues. *American Journal of Medical Genetics*. 81. 10.1002.

Genetic Alliance; The New York-Mid-Atlantic Consortium for Genetic and Newborn Screening Services. *Understanding Genetics: A New York, Mid-Atlantic Guide for Patients and Health Professionals*. Washington, DC: Genetic Alliance; 2009 Jul 8. Chapter 1, Genetics 101.

Griffiths, D., & King, R. (Eds.) (2004). *Demystifying Syndromes*. Kingston, NY: NADD Press.

Hagberg, B., & Witt-Engerström, I. (1985). Rett syndrome: a suggested staging system for describing impairment profile with increasing age towards adolescence. *American Journal Medical Genetics Supplement*. 1:47-59.

Kent, L., Evans, J., Paul, M., & Sharp, M. (1999). Comorbidity of autistic spectrum disorders in children with Down syndrome. *Developmental Medicine and Child Neurology*. March; 41(3):153-158.

Karbarz, M. (2020). Consequences of 22q11.2 Microdeletion on the Genome, Individual and Population Levels. *Genes, 11*(9). 977. MDPI AG. Retrieved from http://dx.doi.org/10.3390/genes11090977.

Landry, O., & Chouinard, P. A. (2016). Why We Should Study the Broader Autism Phenotype in Typically Developing Populations, *Journal of Cognition and Development*, 17:4, 584-595.

McCray, A. T., Trevvett, P., & Frost, H. R. (2014). Modeling the autism spectrum disorder phenotype. *Neuroinformatics*, 12(2): 291-305.

McDonald-McGinn, D., Sullivan, K., Marino, B., et al. (2015). 22q11.2 deletion syndrome. *Nature Reviews Disease Primers*. 1, 15071.

McEvoy, R. E., Rogers, S. J., & Pennington, B. F. (1993). Executive function and social communication deficits in young autistic children. *Journal of Child Psychology and Psychiatry and Allied Disciplines*. 34(4):563-578.

Mikhail, F. M., R. D. Burnside, B. Rush, J. Ibrahim, R. Godshalk, S. L. Rutledge, et al. (2014). The recurrent distal 22q11.2 microdeletion are often de novo and do not represent a single clinical entity: a proposed categorization system. *Genetic Medicine*. 16:92–100.

Nyhan, W. L. Clinical features of the Lesch-Nyhan syndrome. *Archives of Internal Medicine*, 1972, 130: 186-192. (a)

Opitz, J. M. Smith-Lemli-Opitz Syndrome. In: *The NORD Guide to Rare Disorders*, Philadelphia: Lippincott, Williams and Wilkins, 2003:253.

Pelc, K., Cheron, G., & Dan, B. (2008). Behavior and neuropsychiatric manifestations in Angelman syndrome. *Neuropsychiatric disease and treatment*, 4(3): 577–584.

Poisson, A., Nicolas, A., Cochat, P., et al. (2015). Behavioral disturbance and treatment strategies in Smith-Magenis syndrome. *Orphanet Journal of Rare Diseases*, 10: 111.

Steffenburg, S., et al. (1996). Autism in Angelman syndrome: a population based study. *Pediatric Neurology*. 14(2): 131-136.

Streissguth, A. P. & Kanter, J. (Eds.) (1997). *The Challenge of Fetal Alcohol Syndrome: Overcoming Secondary Disabilities* (300 pp.). Seattle: University of Washington Press.

Tierney, E., Nwokoro, N. A, Porter, F. D., Freund, L. S., Ghuman, J. K., & Kelley, R.I. (2001). Behavior phenotype in the RSH/Smith-Lemli-Opitz syndrome. *American Journal of Medical Genetics*. 98(2):191-200.

Ungerer, M., Knezovich J., Ramsay M. (2013). In utero alcohol exposure, epigenetic changes, and their consequences. Alcohol Research and Health. 35(1):37-46.

Vorstman, J. A., & Ophoff, R. A. (2013). Genetic causes of developmental disorders. Current Opinion in Neurology. Apr; 26(2):128-136.

Watson, S. L., & Griffiths, D. M. (Eds.). (2016). *Demystifying Syndromes II: Clinical and Educational Implications of Common Syndromes Associated with Persons with Intellectual Disabilities*. Kingston, NY: NADD Press.

Waye, J. S., Eng, B., & Nowaczyk, M. (2007). Prenatal diagnosis of Smith-Lemli-Opitz syndrome (SLOS) by DHCR7 mutation analysis. *Prenatal Diagnosis: 27*(7), 638-640.

Whitaker, S. (2013) Causes of Intellectual Disability. In *Intellectual Disability*. London: Palgrave Macmillan.

Wright, C. F., et al. (2015). Genetic diagnosis of developmental disorders in the DDD study: a scalable analysis of genome-wide research data. *Lancet* 385, 1305–1314.

Retrieved from: National Center on Birth Defects and Developmental Disabilities, Centers for Disease Control and Prevention on October 18, 2020 https://www.cdc.gov/ncbddd/birthdefects/downsyndrome/data.html.

Module III

Comprehensive Assessment Practices

Slide 2

This module includes content related to conceptual models related to behavior problems: integrative approach, functional assessment of behavior and assessment and diagnostic practices.

Slide 3

Learning Objectives

- Articulate the elements of behavioral, medical, communication and physical models of problem behavior.
- List the components and importance of the Integrative Model.
- Articulate the importance of medical assessments in the assessment process.

Slide 4

Conceptual Models Related to Behavioral Problems:

An Integrated Assessment Approach

In assessing an individual who has IDD, it is important to identify the reasons why the individual is exhibiting behavioral problems. The question is often raised as to whether the maladaptive behavior is related to the person having an intellectual disability or related to the person having a mental illness. This is a false dichotomy as it is usually not just one causal relationship. Also, there may be other comorbidities that contribute to the behavioral problem.

All potential problem areas and causes of the problem must be addressed by conducting an integrated assessment procedure.

Slide 5

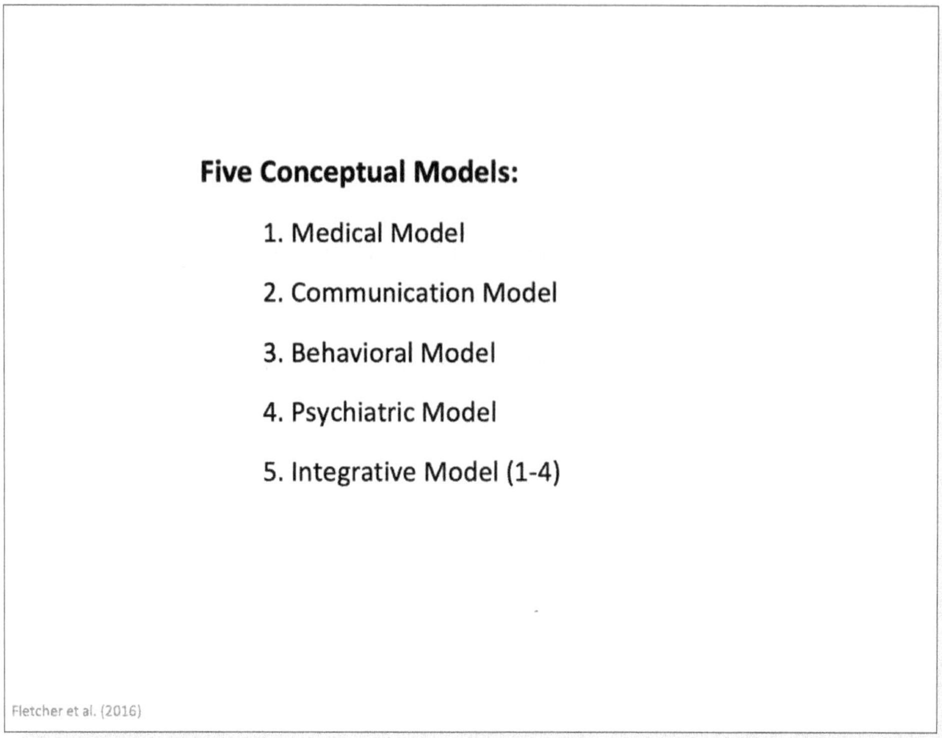

When we think of problem behaviors in people with IDD, we often look for the etiology or reason why an individual's behavior is maladaptive. There are generally four schools of thought that are associated with maladaptive behaviors. These are medical models, communication models, behavioral models and psychiatric models.

NADD has generally encouraged use of a fifth model, that being the integrative model. The integrative model assesses the dynamic influence of the previously mentioned four models to arrive at a multimodal or integrative model. Often, there are multiple determinants that influence the expression of maladaptive behaviors. The integrative model assesses these various "pieces" and puts the clinical puzzle together as a whole.

A bio-psycho-social framework considers the multiple determinants and how each may contribute to the function of behavior. An integrative model provides a person-centered method of assessment.

Slide 6

1. Medical Model

- Problem behaviors are exhibited because of coexisting medical problems
- Assessment of potential medical problems involves conducting a full medical workup
- Treatment focuses on addressing the underlying medical problem

Engel, 1977

Health disorders in people with IDD frequently differ from those encountered in the general population in terms of prevalence, age of onset, rate of progression, degree of severity and presenting manifestations. These disorders are also more likely to be multiple and complex in people with IDD (Haverman et al., 2009).

Medical conditions can mask as behavioral problems or psychiatric conditions. A person may "act out" as a way to express discomfort from a medical condition.

A full medical workup should be part of a mental health assessment process. Medical conditions should be assessed before looking at other causes of problem behaviors.

Slide 7

2. Communication Model

- Views behavioral problems as reflecting “challenging behaviors” in persons who have deficits in language skills.
- Treatment—teach communication skills.
- Assessment focuses on evaluation of skills, deficits and communicative intent.

McClintock, Hall & Oliver, 2003

Individuals with IDD often come from backgrounds that are impoverished of life-enriching experiences, especially in the area of communication.

Maladaptive behavior can be an attempt to communicate. Limited verbal repertoires reduce a person’s ability to express feelings and communicate what they want verbally, leading to behavioral attempts to communicate. For example, a person who has IDD may experience the stress of an office visit. Without the verbal repertoire to express their discomfort verbally and indicate they wish to leave, the person must rely on attempts to communicate physically through what could be perceived as aggressive behavior.

Slide 8

3. Behavioral Model

- Problem behaviors are viewed according to learning principles
- Assessment identifies the antecedent and consequences of the problematic behavior
- Treatment focuses on changing or eliminating behavior though behavioral approaches
- Does not usually identify people's needs/emotions

Baer, Wolf & Risley, 1968

In the traditional behavioral model, the problem behavior is studied and then the environment is manipulated in such a way as to increase, decrease or maintain the behavior. The problem or, as it is otherwise called, the target behavior is described, and then the antecedents and/or the consequences of the behavior are examined. This is known as the ABC approach.

The behavioral model is used extensively in the developmental disability field. Traditionally, the focus is on changing an unwanted behavior to a behavior that is more appropriate. The behavioral approach does not usually address people's feelings or emotions that are associated with the behavior. Rather, the focus of treatment is simply to change the behavior.

Slide 9

4. Psychiatric Model

- **Views problem behavior as a possible manifestation of a mental disorder**
- **Presentation of problem behaviors may be associated with a psychiatric disorder**
- **Assessment based on a bio-psycho-social model**
- **Treatment focuses on underlying psychiatric disorders**

Engel, 1977

The psychiatric model essentially mirrors the medical model. The clinician identifies psychopathology in the individual, i.e., identification of a specific psychiatric disorder. The manifestation of the psychiatric disorder — for example, sleep disturbance or loss of interest in preferred activities — is viewed as a manifestation of the identified psychiatric disorder. The treatment focuses on the underlying psychiatric disorder.

In the psychiatric model, the first line of treatment typically would include a specific medication or psychiatric intervention associated with a particular psychiatric diagnosis.

Slide 10

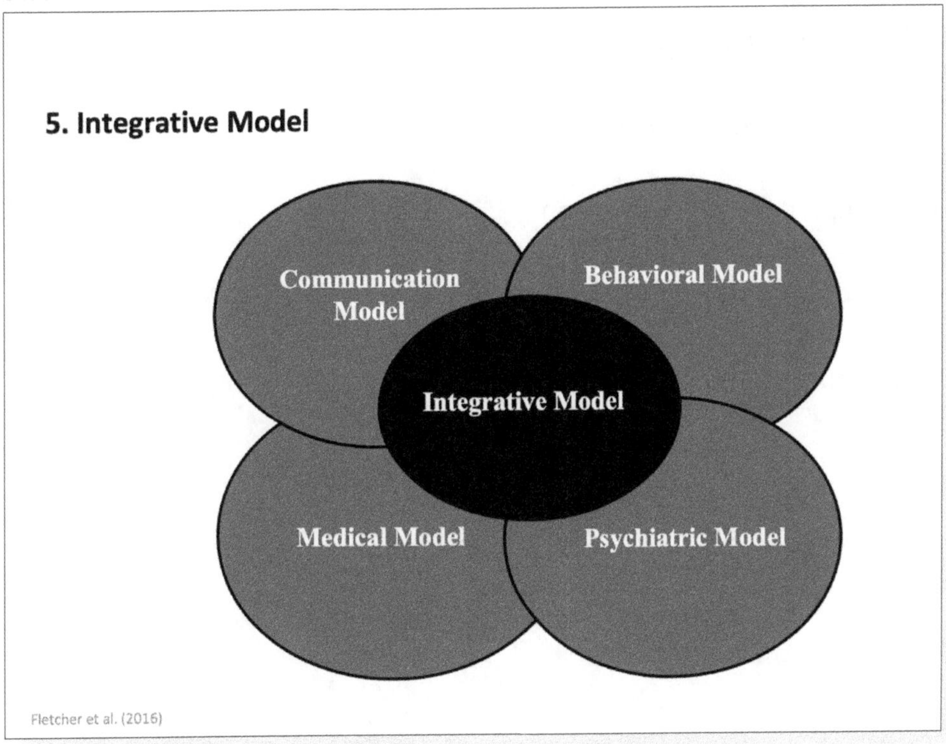

The integrative model assesses the individual's communication skills, assesses whether the individual is displaying maladaptive behaviors associated with learned behaviors, assesses the individual's medical conditions and assesses whether the individual has a psychiatric disorder.

The integrative model assesses the dynamic overlapping influences and, after a comprehensive bio-psycho-social assessment, arrives at an integrative approach with regard to assessment and diagnosis.

Multiple determinants of problem behaviors are common in persons with IDD. Therefore, a multidimensional approach is critically important in conducting a comprehensive assessment in persons with IDD.

Positive Behavior Supports (PBS) is one model that integrates the four aspects proposed in the integrated model: medical/biological considerations, psychiatric considerations, communication considerations and behavior considerations.

A PBS approach includes:

- Functional assessment
- Comprehensive Intervention
- Focus on quality of life and wellness (Carr & Sidener, 2002)

PBS is discussed in detail in Module VII.

Slide 11

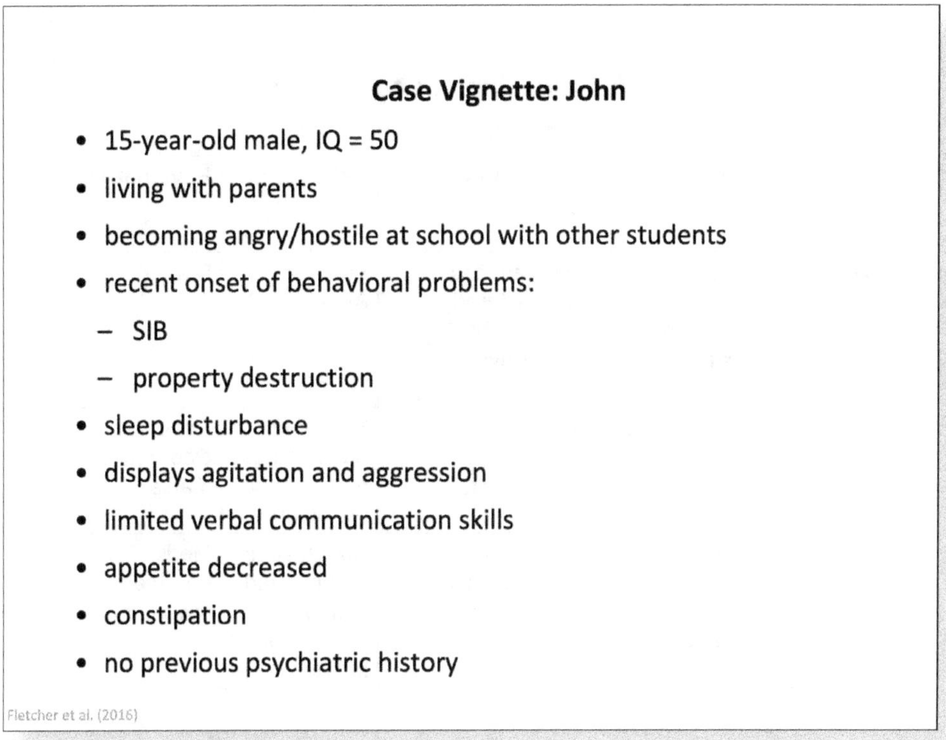
Case Vignette: John
• 15-year-old male, IQ = 50
• living with parents
• becoming angry/hostile at school with other students
• recent onset of behavioral problems:
– SIB
– property destruction
• sleep disturbance
• displays agitation and aggression
• limited verbal communication skills
• appetite decreased
• constipation
• no previous psychiatric history
Fletcher et al. (2016)

Slide 12

The Relationship of Challenging Behavior and IDD

Type of Model	Medical	Communication	Behavioral	Psychiatric
Assessment	Medical evaluation by primary care physician	Standardized administered measure of expressive language	Functional Analysis	DM-ID
Problem Identification	Constipation	Speech and language impairment	Function/ need being met through behavior	Affective disorder, mania
Treatment	Medication for bowel movement (laxative)	Functional communication skill training	Addressing unmet need, supporting appropriate behavior	Medication treatment, psychotherapy

Fletcher et al. (2016)

In John's case, we conducted a bio-psycho-social assessment employing the integrative model. Therefore, we assessed the medical, communication, behavioral and psychiatric domains. Each domain involved an assessment of the problem followed by a treatment protocol that corresponded to the medical, behavioral, communication and psychiatric aspects of the problem.

It is very important to conduct this assessment within an interdisciplinary framework. As such, a holistic perspective is maintained throughout the assessment and treatment process.

Outcome: John has made significant improvement. His sleep and appetite are at normal levels. There has been a significant decrease in intensity and frequency of challenging behaviors.

Slide 13

The Function of Behavior

Behaviors may persist because the individual...

- enjoys the sensory experience — it feels better, satisfies a need or impulse (internal triggers, internal rewards)
- escapes or avoids demands or things he or she doesn't like to do
- gains attention from others
- obtains tangible items or opportunities — access to something he or she prefers

Beavers, Iwata & Lerman, 2013

Professionals describe the possible functions in different ways and this outline avoids using a single word but does organize around the four major categories highlighted in much of the literature:

- Tangibles
- Attention
- Escape
- Sensory, or as many refer to it, automatic reinforcement. In describing this category, we try to emphasize that the behavior is generally triggered by internal stimuli and the reinforcing consequences also tend to be internal.

Slide 14

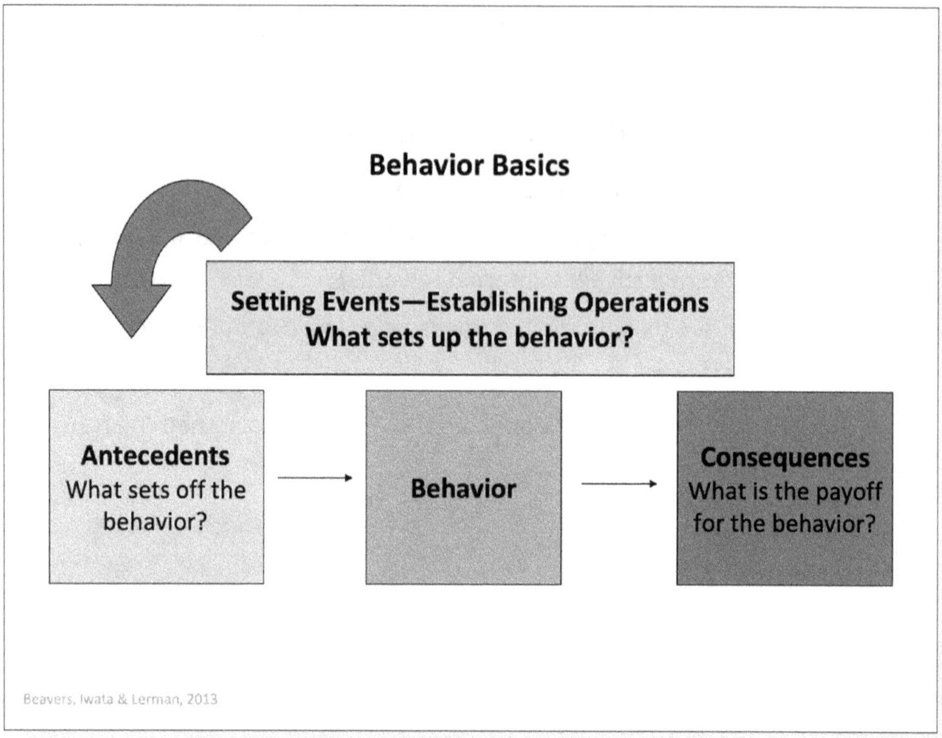

This is a visual representation of the ABC model of behavior and categories we described above.

Slide 15

Considerations of Functional Assessment

- A pattern of behavior that repeats
- Understand why the behavior occurs
  - What are the antecedents/precursors; what "sets off" the behavior?
  - Are there any setting events, things that set the person up to do the behavior?
  - What are the consequences/outcomes; what does the person get as a result?
- Is the behavior:
  - an attempt to communicate?
  - a way to avoid or obtain something?
  - the result of a medical condition or other factor?

Iwata et al., 1994

The slide introduces FBA, which is a way to understand the function of the behavior. The goal is to figure out what purpose a behavior serves for the individual; in other words, what makes it rewarding for them.

The big difference between understanding the function of a behavior and traditional interpretations of behavior is the perspective from which the behavior is viewed. Direct support professionals and clinicians need to understand the behavior through the eyes of the person who engages in it, rather than talking about the problems it causes for other people. Most of the time, people talk about the behavior as inappropriate or inconvenient. For the person, it meets a need they do not have met in other ways.

This perspective is helpful through the remainder of the section.

The main points to learn are:

1. Direct support professionals and clinicians need to focus on an observable behavior; something they can see the person doing.

2. There are basic elements that need to be understood and investigated in order to understand behavior. These include antecedents and consequences, which are discussed further in this section.

3. Behavior can meet the needs of a person and can make sense from the person's perspective. Direct support professionals and clinicians need to be able to identify what need the person is attempting to meet and if the behavior is the most appropriate, effective way the person can meet the need.

Slide 16

The Steps to a Functional Assessment

- Describe what the target behavior is, the operational definition.
- Interview the person or care providers.
- Observe the person to see what else might be happening.
- Use the interview and observation to make some guesses about the antecedents and consequences.
- Identify antecedents, setting events and consequences (outcomes).
- Look for patterns to identify function.

Iwata et al., 1994

Now we make the transition. Before we start using antecedent-based interventions, it is important to know what the function is and which antecedents to address.

Slide 17

Look for Patterns

- The same type of triggers tend to set the behavior off.
- People respond in similar ways to maintain the behavior; the person gets the same kind of outcome.
- Setting events (establishing operations) make behavior more likely to occur when trigger is present.
- The behavior doesn't have to happen every time the trigger is present but work enough to make the behavior "worth it" for the individual.

Iwata et al., 1994

Setting events and triggers can act as cues for the person to engage in a specific behavior.

The identification of patterns of triggers and responses assists in the functional assessment of behavior by helping to identify the conditions under which a specific behavior is likely to occur. If similar conditions lead to similar responses with high frequency, the conditions to analyze the function are present.

Slide 18

Involving Direct Support Professionals (DSPs) and Caregivers in Plan Development

- DSPs often work closest to and spend most time with people
- Encourage contributions, observations, hypotheses, ideas, intervention strategies
- DSPs can identify trends and missing puzzle pieces that managers and behaviorists often cannot
- Foster control and confidence
- Promote participation and involvement in planning
- Consider opinions and answer questions
- Provide ongoing support and guidance

Direct support professionals and caregivers are the people who generally spend the most time with the person. They can have valuable and insightful contributions to make about observations of the person, ideas around why the behavior occurs and possible intervention strategies based on their knowledge and experience with the person.

The benefits of including direct support professionals and caregivers:

- Opportunity for staff to take ownership in planning for the individuals they support
- More likely to follow plans and strategies if involved in development
- Increases staff self-efficacy in following plans or implementing strategies
- Greater consistency

- Staff learn to be more observant and more comfortable contributing information
- More accurate and useful information will emerge
- Individuals will associate staff with progress and challenging behavior will decrease

Slide 19

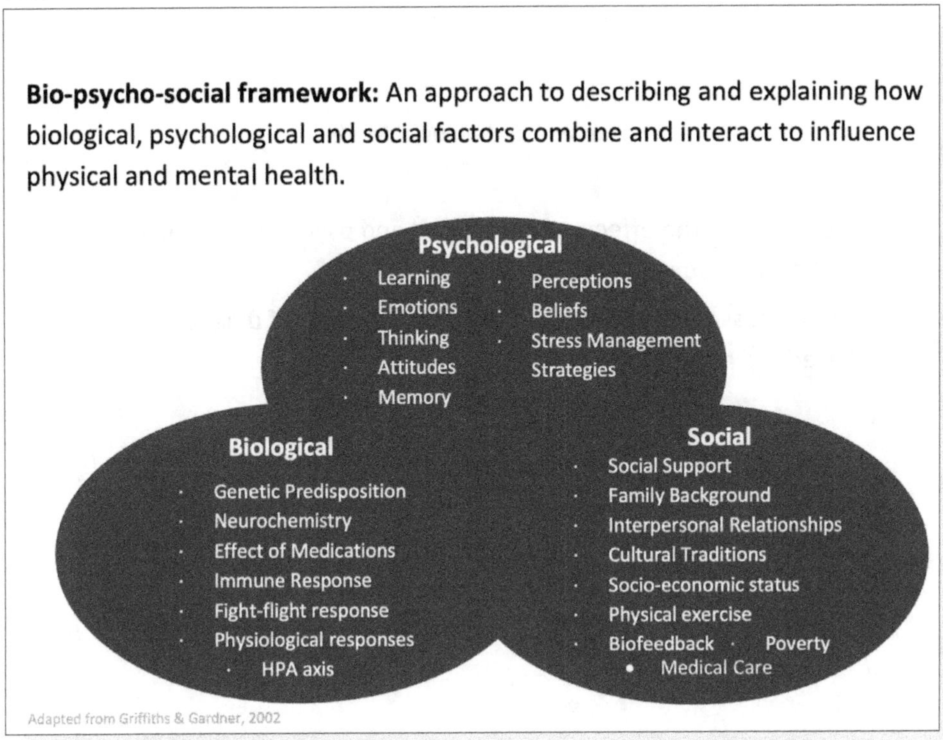

The bio-psycho-social framework provides an integrated model of assessment. If we limit ourselves to a single way to try to understand the challenges posed in supporting a person with IDD/MI, we will miss the mark in most cases and fail to understand the true complex nature of needs. One of the philosophical difficulties we encounter in supporting this population is that many professionals only consider their specific discipline and professional training and, as such, don't consider other ways to view the challenges of the person.

Exacerbating this is the fact that many assessment tools are based on the practices of a specific discipline. For example, a behavior analytic assessment tool may primarily ask questions leading to a functional assessment of behavior, considering setting events, discriminative stimuli and maintaining consequences, but not delving into physiological events or asking why certain events have such a degree of salience. Similarly, a mental health assessment may fail to take into account a person's culture. The bio-psycho-social assessment is an effort to address these problems by creating an assessment model that includes and embraces multiple disciplinary perspectives.

Slide 20

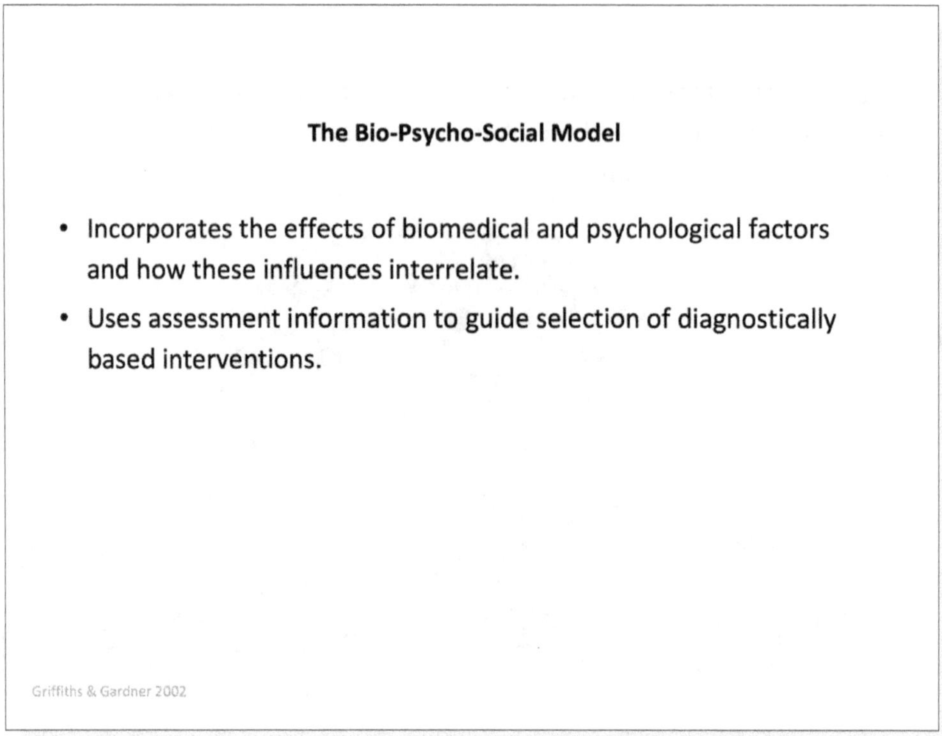

Bio-psycho-social assessment specifically considers the factors listed on the prior slide. In complex situations in supporting a person with IDD/MI, all of these factors overlap and interrelate. For example, if a person takes a decongestant that causes insomnia (bio), gets very frustrated by being awake at night and copes by watching horror movies at high volume (psycho) and awakens family members leading to family stress (social), all three factors need to be considered in taking a comprehensive look at understanding these difficulties. The bio-psycho-social assessment model will guide subsequent design of intervention. In the example, all three areas would need to be considered, with both short- and long-term goals being of clinical necessity.

Slide 21

The Bio-Psycho-Social Model

- Identifies skills and related supports required by the individual to cope effectively with multiple bio-psycho-social influences.
- Is proactive in focus.
- Provides for translation of multiple modalities of influence in a common model.

Griffiths & Gardner 2002

The bio-psycho-social model identifies skill deficits as possible causes of behavior, anticipates needs and makes accommodations for biomedical and psychological factors identified in assessment.

The bio-psycho-social model also considers the supports in place and the supports needed. Skill deficits, such as communication and stress management, are significant contributors to mental health challenges and related problems. Related supports are equally relevant.

A person's environment generally determines how severe a problem is perceived or becomes. Supports can buffer against a problem behavior or can assure an effective, rapid response to a mental health problem. Consider the example from the prior slide. Skills for self-management during nocturnal wakefulness are needed, as well as a quick end to the decongestant use. The bio-psycho-social model seeks to promote a proactive mode of addressing challenges by heading them off rather than reacting to them.

Slide 22

The Bio-Psycho-Social Model

- Provides an integrated multimodal treatment plan.
- Recognizes that mental health consists of both the presence of personal contentment and the relative absence of psychological distress.

Griffiths & Gardner 2002

The inclusion of different perspectives into a single model directly leads to an integrated multimodal treatment plan. Having a unified understanding of a person's support needs in a single assessment increases the likelihood of having a single plan of intervention and treatment, which will promote coordination of intervention and simplicity of support provision.

Finally, the bio-psycho-social model recognizes that mental health isn't just the absence of a disorder. It include the presence of positive emotion. In this framework, personal contentment is a valid consideration, as are other forms of mental wellness and positive experiences and character traits.

Slide 23

A comprehensive assessment includes:

1. **Reviewing reports**
2. **Interviewing family**
3. **Interviewing care provider/DSP**
4. **Completing direct observation**
5. **Conducting a clinical interview**

Morrison & Gillig, 2012

A comprehensive assessment process involves gathering existing data and background information. Additionally, interviewing the individual as well as relevant others are also essential components of the assessment process. Making observations in the natural environments is also important.

Conducting a comprehensive assessment takes much more time than an assessment of a person from the general population. The interview with the client is important, but insufficient in conducting a comprehensive assessment.

The clinician first needs to get releases to obtain information from a variety of sources such as:

- School
- Foster home/group home
- Residential institutions
- Outpatient mental health services
- Primary care physician
- Other

Slide 24

A comprehensive assessment includes:

- Obtain records in advance
  - School, medical, development and family
- Become familiar with collateral informants who attend the interview
  - Parents, care provider, service coordinators
- Understand that the assessment interview can be stressful for all involved
  - Interviewer will need to be alert for increased distress on part of the client

Morrison & Gillig, 2012

When completing a mental health assessment, there are a number of tips the interviewer would find helpful in completing the assessment process.

By obtaining records in advance of the assessment, the interviewer is able to review information and history pertinent to the current situation. It may also provide a more thorough history than the person is able to relate themselves.

Good sources of information are staff, caregivers, family members, etc. They probably spend the most time with the person and have a helpful knowledge of their history and current condition.

Slide 25

- Assessment interview probably will take more time than with a neurotypical person
- Examiner needs to use language that correlates with the expressive and receptive language skills of the client
  - Simple language
  - Reflection
  - Stay away from abstract concepts and analogies

Morrison & Gillig, 2012

When completing the mental health assessment, the clinician will want to be sure to:

- Use simple language, avoiding jargon and slang.
- Use reflection to ensure the accurate message is conveyed.
- Avoid abstract concepts and comparisons. Language should be concrete and direct.

Slide 26

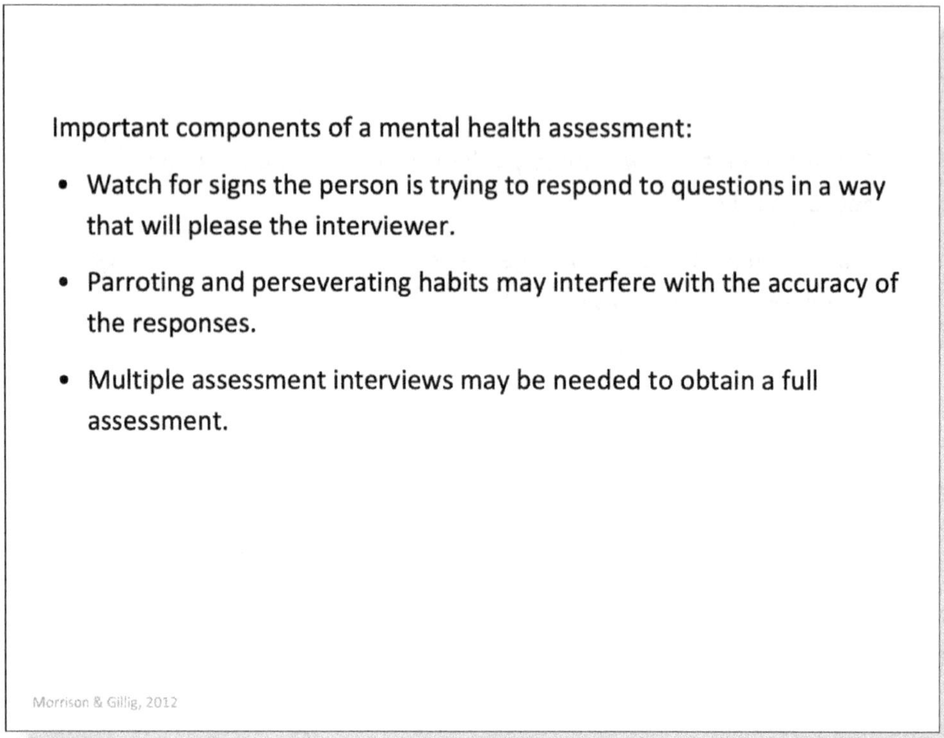

People with IDD often want to please the interviewer and will answer questions in ways that are perceived to please.

People with IDD may repeat words and language they have heard but don't fully understand in an attempt to mask their disability.

Attention to detail may be difficult for the person in a prolonged interview. The clinician may want to break the interview into shorter sessions that are more manageable for the client with IDD.

Slide 27

Historical Data Gathering

- Source of information and reason for referral
- History of presenting problem and past psychiatric history
- Family health history
- Social and developmental history

Fletcher et al. (2016)

The purpose of an assessment is to identify the developmental, biological, psychological and environmental factors that might be associated with precipitating and/or maintaining the maladaptive behavior.

It is important to obtain information from multiple sources. These assessments frequently require a multidisciplinary approach as there may be multiple factors at play and no one approach can truly develop the necessary holistic level of understanding.

As the person with IDD may have limitations with regard to communication skills, it is important to rely on reports from others. These reports should convey current as well as historical information. Arriving at an understanding of why a particular maladaptive behavior has developed or establishing whether there has been an apparent change in mood, mental state or general well-being, may therefore be a considerable challenge to the person(s) conducting the assessment.

Inadequate assessment may lead to ill-informed interventions. Many factors must be considered in the assessment process: culture, gender identity, ethnicity, traumatic experience, living arrangements, education/employment status, goals, person-centered plans, modes of communication, etc.

Slide 28

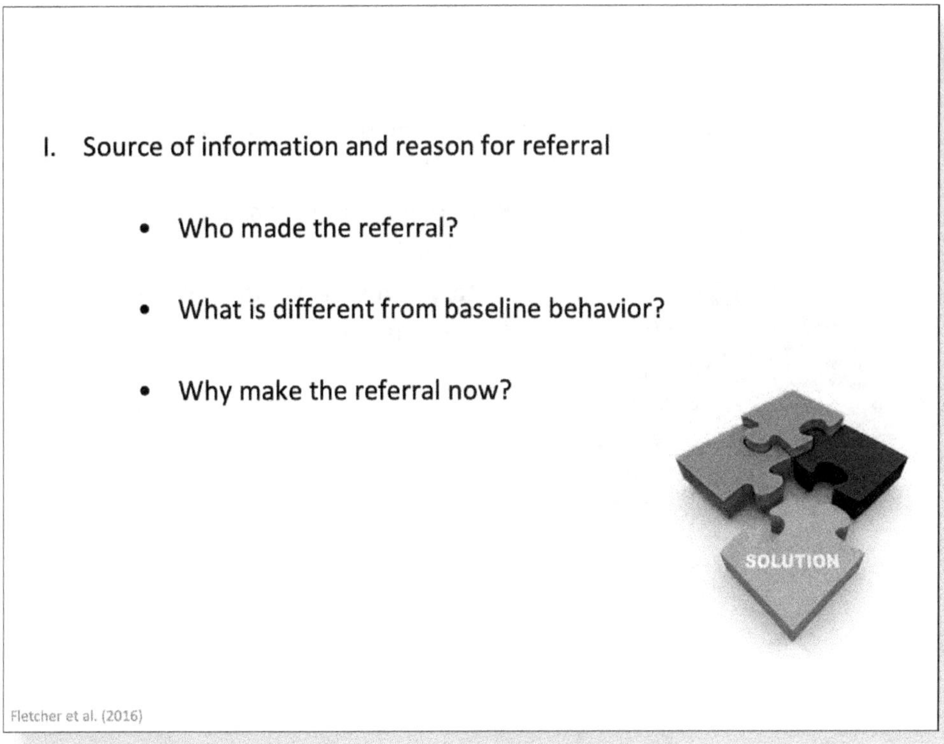

It is important to know who made the referral and the reason for the referral for the assessment. Unlike with the neurotypical person, referrals for mental health assessments are generally not made by the client but by care providers involved in the individual's life.

There are occasions when it has been determined that the actual problem does not primarily involve the person being referred, but instead the person or environment who referred the client for a mental health assessment. The following questions should be asked:

- Who made the referral (e.g., agency, parent)?
- Why is the referral being made now?
- What is the presenting problem?
- What are the expectations of the referring source?
- What is the person's perception of the problem?

Slide 29

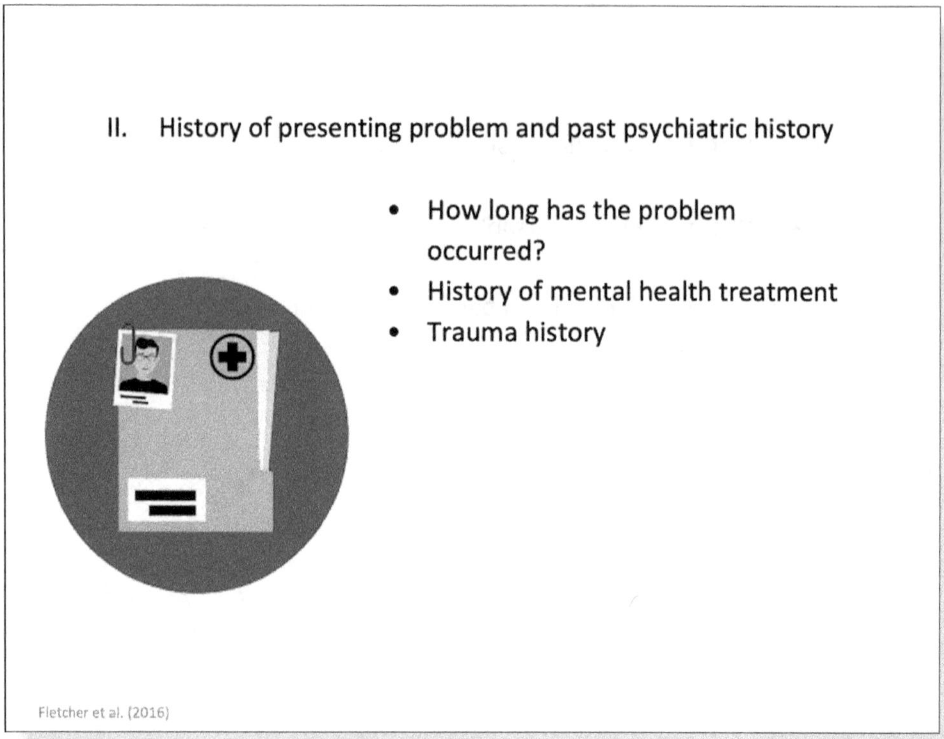

The assessment process needs to include obtaining information regarding the history of the presenting problem. It is, therefore, important to obtain background history such as:

- Chronological history of problem
- Precipitating factors
- Significant symptomology

If the person has had a past psychiatric history, the assessment should include the following:

- Outpatient mental health services including diagnosis, therapies, medications and response to treatment
- Inpatient mental health services including diagnosis, therapies, medications and response to treatment

Slide 30

III. Personal and family health history

- **Medical, psychiatric and substance abuse history**
- **Psychotropic medications**
- **Medical conditions**
- **Genetic disorders**
- **Hypo/hyperthyroid condition**
- **Constipation**
- **Epilepsy**
- **Diabetes**
- **Gastrointestinal problem**

Fletcher et al. (2016)

The assessment process needs to obtain information regarding personal and family health history. Medical conditions as well as mental health disorders can have a genetic predisposition. For example, affective disorders tend to have a genetic predisposition and therefore can be passed from one generation to another.

Physical illnesses are important differential diagnoses for most psychiatric presentations in people with IDD. People with IDD have a higher prevalence of physical illness compared to other population groups.

Full blood count, measures of thyroid, kidney and liver function and blood glucose are important routine blood tests and should be ascertained as part of a comprehensive mental health assessment.

In fact, a physical health assessment should be conducted first in order to determine whether a behavioral problem is caused by a physical health problem.

Slide 31

IV. Social/developmental history

- Developmental milestones
- Relevant school history
- Work/vocational history
- Current work/vocational status
- Legal issues
- Relevant family dynamics
- Drug/alcohol history
- Abuse history (emotional/physical/sexual)
- Trauma history

Fletcher et al. (2016)

An important part of the assessment process is gathering information regarding social and developmental history. Some of this information, such as developmental milestones, can be obtained from parents. Other information can be obtained from other resources. The clinician may have to obtain records from various sources, such as school and residential and/or day programs.

Research has indicated that the majority of people with IDD have experienced some type of abuse, including sexual abuse. Therefore, obtaining information about abuse history is very important. This can be a delicate matter if family members or other significant others are suspected of the abuse. Depending on the level of functioning of the individual, the use of anatomical dolls, pictures and other nonverbal forms of communication can be useful.

Slide 32

Myth: Individuals with IDD Cannot Have a Verifiable Mental Health Disorder

PREMISE
Maladaptive behaviors are a function of IDD.

REALITY
The full range of psychiatric disorders can be represented in persons with IDD.

DIAGNOSTIC IMPLICATIONS
Psychiatric diagnosis can be made using the DM-ID, DSM-5 records, service providers, family input and client interview.

Adapted from Sovner & Hurley ,1989

This myth is based on the historical notion that behavioral problems in people with IDD are directly associated with having the condition of IDD.

The reality is that the full range of psychiatric conditions that are expressed in the general population are also represented in persons with IDD. In fact, there is a higher prevalence rate of psychiatric disorders in persons with IDD as compared to the general population.

An appropriate diagnostic procedure is both complex and time-consuming. It involves obtaining and gathering multiple sources of information. The use of either the DSM or DM-ID is needed.

Slide 33

8 Diagnostic Principles for Recognizing Psychiatric Disorders in People with IDD

1. **People with Intellectual/Developmental Disabilities suffer from the full range of psychiatric disorders.**
2. **Psychiatric disorders usually present as maladaptive behavior.**
3. **The origin of psychopathology has multiple etiologies.**

Adapted from Sovner & Hurley, 1989

1. Psychiatric disorders in people with IDD are considered to be at a higher prevalence rate than in the general population. This includes disorders in children, adolescents and adults, as well as older adults.

2. Behavioral problems or maladaptive behaviors are often associated with the manifestation of a psychiatric disorder. This is different than what occurs in the general population, as people with IDD usually manifest a psychiatric disorder through observations of their behavior, and these behaviors are often maladaptive.

3. There can be internal as well as external contributing factors to the origin of a psychiatric disorder in a person with IDD. There are interwoven influences from a bio-psycho-social-family perspective.

Slide 34

8 Diagnostic Principles for Recognizing Psychiatric Disorders in People with IDD

4. An acute psychiatric disorder may present as an exaggeration of longstanding maladaptive behavior.
5. Maladaptive behavior rarely occurs alone.
6. The severity of the problem is not diagnostically relevant.

Adapted from Sovner 1989

4. Maladaptive behaviors that previously existed may increase in frequency and intensity during the onset of a mental illness. For example, an individual might have a low rate of mild self-injurious behavior, but during the time of stress, the frequency and intensity of this behavior can escalate. This may be when a psychiatric diagnosis is made.

5. Generally, the occurrence of repeated maladaptive behaviors in a person with IDD is a clear clue to the presence of a psychiatric disorder. People with IDD usually don't have serious and persistent maladaptive behaviors as part of having IDD. Rather, these maladaptive behaviors are more likely to be a manifestation of a psychiatric disorder. Therefore, maladaptive behaviors rarely occur alone.

6. The severity of a maladaptive behavior, such as an act of aggression, does not lead to a mental health diagnosis. In fact, aggression is a nonspecific behavior that may or may not be related to a diagnosis (Sovner & Hurley, 1989).

Slide 35

8 Diagnostic Principles for Recognizing Psychiatric Disorders in People with IDD

7. The clinical interview alone is rarely diagnostic.
8. It is very difficult to diagnose psychotic disorders in people with very limited verbal skills.

Adapted from Sovner 1989

7. Interviewing the client is a condition of, but insufficient for, a comprehensive diagnostic assessment. People with IDD tend to acquiesce, as they want to please the interviewer. Also, people at the lower end of the intellectual range may not have expressive and receptive language skills or may have limited vocabulary. Multiple sources of data collection are therefore necessary to obtain relevant information that will assist in the assessment and diagnostic process.

8. Psychotic disorders such as schizophrenia usually require the client to provide a self report of signs and symptoms. For example, the person would express experiencing hallucinations and delusions. These are internal states that are difficult, if not impossible, to observe. Therefore, verbal skills are helpful, if not essential, for the diagnosis of psychotic disorders.

Slide 36

Barriers to Diagnosis and Treatment:
15 Complicating Diagnostic Factors

1. Diagnostic overshadowing
2. Problems with polypharmacy
3. Communication deficits
4. Atypical presentation of psychiatric disorders
5. Limited life experiences
6. Medical conditions
7. Acquiescence
8. Learned behavior
9. Aggression and SIB (self-injurious behavior)
10. Sensory impairment
11. Behavioral overshadowing
12. Medication masking
13. Episodic presentation
14. Division of services
15. Lack of expertise

McGilvery & Sweetland, 2011

Diagnosis of mental illness in people with IDD can be complicated by a number of factors, as indicated above.

1. **Diagnostic Overshadowing** – Reiss, Leviton & Szyszko (1982) developed the term "diagnostic overshadowing" to indicate the tendency to attribute many of the possible symptoms of a psychiatric disorder to the intellectual/developmental disability. For example, when a person with an IDD communicates being upset by "acting out," it can be defined as a behavioral challenge.

2. **Problems with Polypharmacy** – Individuals with IDD are sometimes on multiple medications, and some are on multiple medications of the same class. That is to say they may be on multiple medications treating the same symptom. This can present medical as well as behavioral problems. Some of the side effects of the medication can produce symptoms that are similar to a psychiatric disorder. For example, fatigue, confusion, agitation, lethargy, short attention span or changes in sleep or

appetite are common medication side effects. They are also symptoms of mental health disorders.

3. **Communication Deficits** – Individuals with IDD often have difficulty in expressive language skills. Additionally, they frequently come from backgrounds that are impoverished of life-enriching experiences, especially in the area of communication. If the individual's verbal ability or insight is limited, that person is not likely to provide an accurate presentation of symptoms.

4. **Atypical Presentation of Psychiatric Disorders** – Persons with IDD may manifest a psychiatric symptom in a different way than a person from the general population. Often, the expression of a psychiatric disorder is through behavioral disturbances rather than through a self report of symptoms. It is not uncommon for a person with IDD to "act out" in a maladaptive manner. Severe behavioral disturbances in the form of verbal or physical aggression are not uncommon and may be related to a psychiatric disorder. Therefore, observing behavior is very important.

5. **Limited Life Experiences** – Due to a narrow range of life experiences, it may be difficult to detect some of the symptoms of a psychiatric disorder. For example, a typically developing individual with bipolar disorder who is in a manic phase may spend excessively and run up charges on credit cards or increase social activity, sometimes to an unsafe level. An individual with an intellectual disability may not have the financial resources for overspending, promiscuous relationships, travel, etc. Therefore, the diagnosis may be missed because the symptoms look different.

6. **Medical Conditions** – Medical conditions often co-occur with psychiatric disorders in persons with IDD. Medical conditions can mask psychiatric disorders; it is therefore very important to assess medical conditions as one of the first areas in conducting a mental health assessment. Limited communication skills make it difficult for the person to express pain and discomfort. Typical signs and symptoms of a mental health disorder can reflect signs and symptoms of a medical condition.

7. **Acquiescence** – Interviewing someone who has an intellectual disability and obtaining accurate information about the individual's symptoms can be confounded by an increased tendency for the person to agree quickly. The person may tell the clinician or care provider what they think the interviewer wants to hear or agree to things in order to avoid the risk of disapproval. The person may be more likely to report "yes" or "no" to all questions despite the true response.

8. **Learned Behavior** – An individual with IDD may exhibit behaviors that have been learned and modeled from others. For example, a person may begin a spitting behavior after observing and thus learning this behavior from another individual in the group home. A person may learn task avoidance behaviors from others in their environment. For example, at an adult group home for people with mild levels of IDD, a person might refuse to do dishes when it's their turn, and this behavior may be modeled on others in the group home. This can be considered a secondary function of behavior.

9. **Aggression and SIB** – Self-injurious behavior and aggression are often displayed by people with IDD. However, they are not diagnostically related to any one psychiatric diagnosis. SIB and aggressive behaviors can result from either internal or external triggers and setting events. For example, a person can display aggression or SIB associated with a specific psychiatric disorder such as mania or could display these behaviors associated with stress from the external environment.

10. **Sensory Impairment** – It is important to consider whether the individual has any sensory impairments (sight, hearing, touch, etc.). For example, it is not unusual for an individual who is totally blind to have disruptions in sleep. Therefore, diagnosing depression based on changes in sleep as one criterion or diagnosing a sleep disorder in light of these disruptions may be inaccurate. Similarly, it is not unusual for a person with a hearing impairment to become agitated with changes in a schedule because, not having heard the conversation about making new plans, the person finds the changes unexpected.

11. **Behavioral Overshadowing** – Behavioral overshadowing refers to a tendency to identify psychopathology as learned behavior while failing to recognize it as an indicator of mental illness. For example, a person's behavioral challenges may be thought to be related to "task avoidance" rather than loss of motivation due to schizophrenia.

12. **Medication Masking** – The sedative effects of certain medications (e.g., typical antipsychotic medications) can suppress or mask the presence of significant mental health symptoms. For example, a person may be experiencing agitation related to depression but, due to limited communication skills, be unable to describe symptoms of their depression. If the person is prescribed a typical antipsychotic medication, the agitation may stop. However, the medication has not effectively treated the person's illness and they may continue to suffer with symptoms of depression.

13. **Episodic Presentation** – Significant mental health symptoms may come and go in an unpredictable manner. If a person is not displaying symptoms when they are assessed by a mental health professional, the presence of a mental health disorder may go undetected. As an example, an individual with bipolar disorder may be in a manic episode when an appointment is scheduled with their psychiatrist. By the time of the appointment, however, they may have cycled out of the manic episode, and thus the symptoms of mania may no longer be present when examined by the psychiatrist.

14. **Division of Services** – Even today, there exists a tendency for the administration and funding of mental health and intellectual/developmental disability services to be separate. Each system may expect the other to serve the individual who has a dual diagnosis. In addition, there may be a perception by staff in both types of systems that they are poorly equipped to provide appropriate services. Due to these factors, many individuals may be unable to access appropriate and comprehensive services.

15. **Lack of Expertise** – Typically, professionals receiving formal training in

the realm of mental health (e.g., psychiatry, social work) receive minimal training regarding the issue of intellectual/developmental disability. Conversely, professionals trained to work with people with intellectual/developmental disability (e.g., psychologists, special education teachers) may receive extremely limited training in the realm of mental health disorders in persons with IDD. As a result, collaboration among professionals is required to ensure all significant issues in a person's life are understood and appropriately addressed.

Slide 37

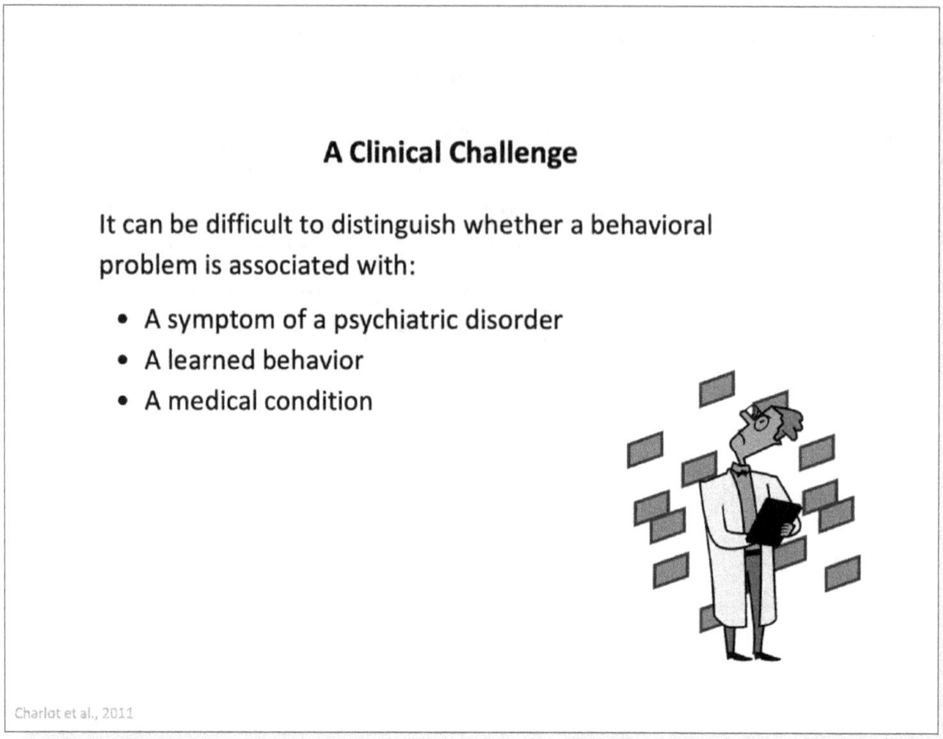

Challenging behaviors may at times be related to the person's mental illness, while at other times they may be an expression of learned behavior. Often psychiatric symptoms and learned behaviors coexist. Also, a medical condition can be a strong influence on challenging behavior. Mental illness and physical illness can both contribute to the function of behavior.

Slide 38

12 Indications That a Behavioral Pattern May Be the Result of a Psychiatric Condition

1. The behavior occurs in all environments; it is not just exhibited in specific settings.
2. Behavioral strategies have been largely ineffective.
3. The individual doesn't appear to have control over their behavior. They don't appear to be able to start or stop the behavior at will.

Adapted from McGilvery & Sweetland, 2011

The following four slides present a list of different "tips" or "clues" that a behavior pattern may have a psychiatric origin. First, does the behavior occur in all settings? If the behavior does not seem to have any connection to the environment or features of the environment (school, home and community; occurs with all different care providers and family), then the cause of the behavior might be internal. Second, have competent behavior intervention strategies been used with no effect? This is the most difficult one to judge, as simply having tried behavioral interventions may be meaningless if they were not well-constructed. Third, does the person seem to make efforts to control the behavior with no success? Many patterns of behavior that do occur as a means for manipulating the environment or others do seem purposeful.

Slide 39

4. There are changes in sleep patterns; increased, decreased or disturbed sleep.
5. The individual is experiencing excessive mood or unusual mood patterns.
6. There are changes in the individual's appearance and a decline in their independent living skills.

Adapted from McGilvery & Sweetland,

MODULE 3

Significant change in sleep patterns may represent a sign of a psychiatric condition, though there are a legion of other causes, such as a side effect of a decongestant. When there is a change in behavior along with a change in sleep, that information may be of diagnostic use. Different types of psychiatric conditions may cause different disturbances in sleep. Changes in mood are a symptom of some kinds of psychiatric illness, and mood tracking may be suggested by clinical professionals. Changes in appearance and self-care are of similar import. If someone is normally quite fastidious but suddenly stops bathing or combing their hair, that may be an important bit of information.

Slide 40

7. The person may start to engage in purposeful self-harm (cutting, hitting, scratching, pulling out hair).

8. The person may start to show signs of hallucination, such as staring to the side or corners and not appear to track conversations.

9. There may be changes in eating patterns such as eating less or more.

Adapted from McGilvery & Sweetland,

Items No. 7 and No. 8 are important and direct symptoms of some kinds of mental illness, and information about these should be immediately shared with clinical professionals. Chronic, low-level pulling out hair ("trichotillomania") may be more akin to a bad habit such as nail-biting in some people and is not a particularly significant warning sign in and of itself. Changes in eating, like changes in sleep (No. 4) should be monitored.

Slide 41

10. **The individual has a history of a psychiatric disorder that was in remission.**

11. **There is an acute onset of the behavior. If there is a particularly rapid onset with a significant change in mental status or cognitive functioning, rule out a possible delirium with an underlying medical cause.**

12. **There is an unusual change in behavior patterns, such as a significant change from baseline behavior.**

Adapted from McGilvery & Sweetland, 2012

Item No. 10 is very important, as psychiatric illnesses do go into and out of remission in some cases. Keeping a thorough record of prior psychiatric illness is necessary for this reason. If a person lives in a setting where staff turnover is frequent, prior knowledge of illness history can easily be forgotten. Good recordkeeping and review is important, as is knowledge of behavior patterns. Acute onset of changes in behavior is always of concern and should always be considered.

Slide 42

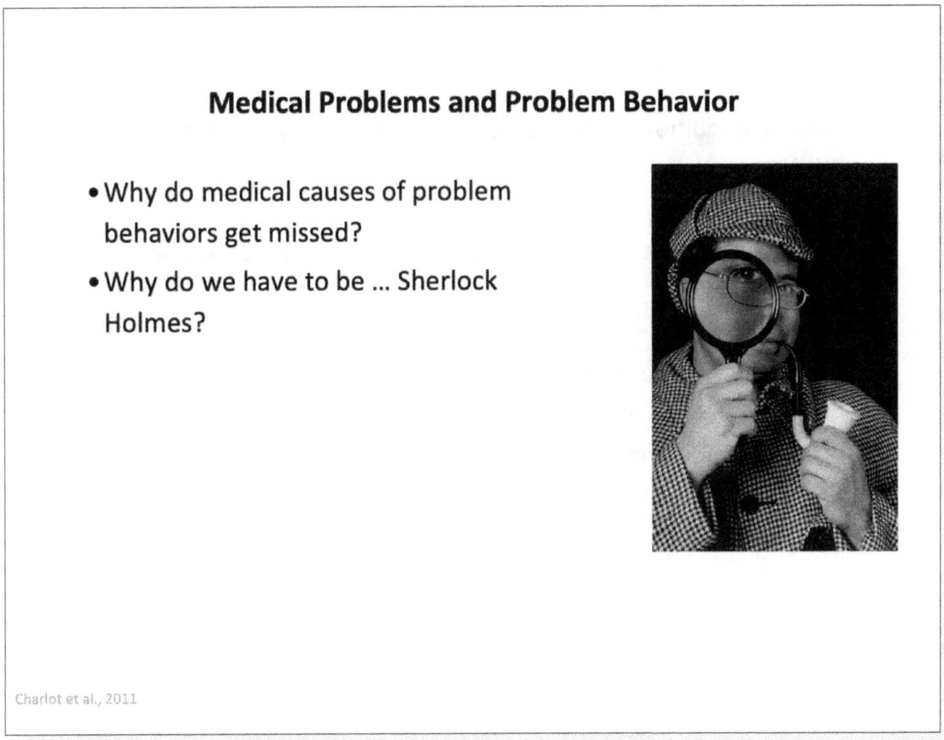

Ask the participants to offer suggestions as to why medical problems are often missed in assessing behavior and mental health.

Slide 43

- **Medical conditions can be present when behavioral problems are exhibited.**
- **Medication effects/reactions can be present when behavioral problems are exhibited.**
- **Medical conditions are often underdiagnosed.**
- **Medical conditions can mask as behavioral problems.**

Charlot et al., 2011

Medical conditions, including those associated with medications, can be present when an individual with IDD exhibits a behavioral problem.

Limited verbal skills in persons with IDD complicate the diagnosing of comorbid medical problems. Frequently, the involved individual is not able to communicate his/her discomfort, distress or pain.

Behaviors may be associated with a known health problem or a previously unrecognized health problem. General medical conditions of importance are pain or other discomfort, sleep disorders, atypical seizure disorders and tic disorders, as well as problems associated with alcohol use, abuse or abrupt withdrawal and use of illegal drugs. Individuals with other health problems may have behavior problems associated with their general medical condition, such as behavior problems often seen with low blood sugar in people with diabetes; various behavioral symptoms associated with thyroid disease; or problems related to dental pain or discomfort expressed as behavioral symptoms.

Slide 44

- Drug side effects
  - Akathisia, delirium, dyskinesia
- Endocrinological problems
  - Thyroid problems, diabetes
- Neurological problems
  - Epilepsy, other movement problems
- Other
  - Dental pain, sleep apnea, headaches, hearing and vision problems, back pain

Charlot et al., 2011

People with IDD can experience a variety of medical conditions, and these medical conditions can influence the manifestation of behavioral problems.

There are a number of medical conditions that can present as psychiatric symptoms or behavioral problems. It is therefore very important to assess medical conditions as part of the overall bio-psycho-social assessment. The following are some medical causes that can present as psychiatric symptoms:

- Endocrine disorders
- Nutritional deficiencies
- Neurological disorders
- Cardiovascular disorders
- Cancers
- Gastrointestinal disorders
- Sensory disorders

Slide 45

Group Exercise

- How do you look at potential medication side effects as part of an assessment?
- Who provides information?
- Who has expertise?

Ask attendees to answer these questions as a group or in small groups. You are giving the attendees a chance to practice looking at how they would get an exhaustive list of medications, determine what side effects are possible from that list and determine if any of those side effects may be present.

Slide 46

- Medical problems often underrecognized
- Dental problems often underrecognized
- Medical/dental problems can cause SIB
- Need to identify if there is an underlying physical problem

Charlot, et al, 2011

Ruling out physical causes of challenging/problem behavior is a critical component of any bio-psycho-social assessment, especially given the challenges a person with IDD has in self-reporting pain or discomfort caused by an underlying medical or dental problem.

Slide 47

Case Example of Discomfort and SIB

- 28-year-old female with IDD referred to behavior specialist for self-injurious behavior.
- Mother noted that she scratches at her arm until it bleeds and won't leave that spot alone.
- Medical exam showed dry skin during a cold winter and recommended lotion.
- Mother subsequently reported that scratching ceased.

Slide 48

Condensed Medical Data in Chart

It is essential that all earlier medical data be available.

It is important that the past and present medical history be condensed in a format that can be easily read and placed in the person's chart.

Poindexter, 2005

Gathering medical information and placing it in the chart often occurs as a list of medical diagnoses in the past, as well as all treatments for these conditions, usually in some sort of timeline form. While this list may take a great deal of time to develop and condense, it is usually time well spent.

A copy of the information should always be retained in files for whatever the current living situation may be but should move with the individual. Copies can be provided to consultants as appropriate. Information should, of course, be updated frequently.

Slide 49

Medical problems may cause significant alterations in mood and behavior that mimic acute psychiatric illness.

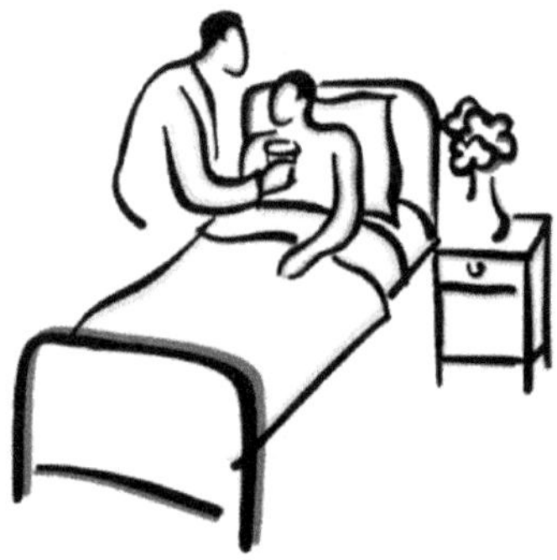

Charlot et al., 2011

Medical conditions can, and often do, mask as mental health problems in people with IDD. This is a result of three variables:

1. Medical problems are often not adequately diagnosed in persons with IDD.

2. Limited communication skills make it difficult for the persons to express pain and discomfort.

3. Typical signs and symptoms of a mental health disorder can reflect signs and symptoms of a medical condition.

Slide 50

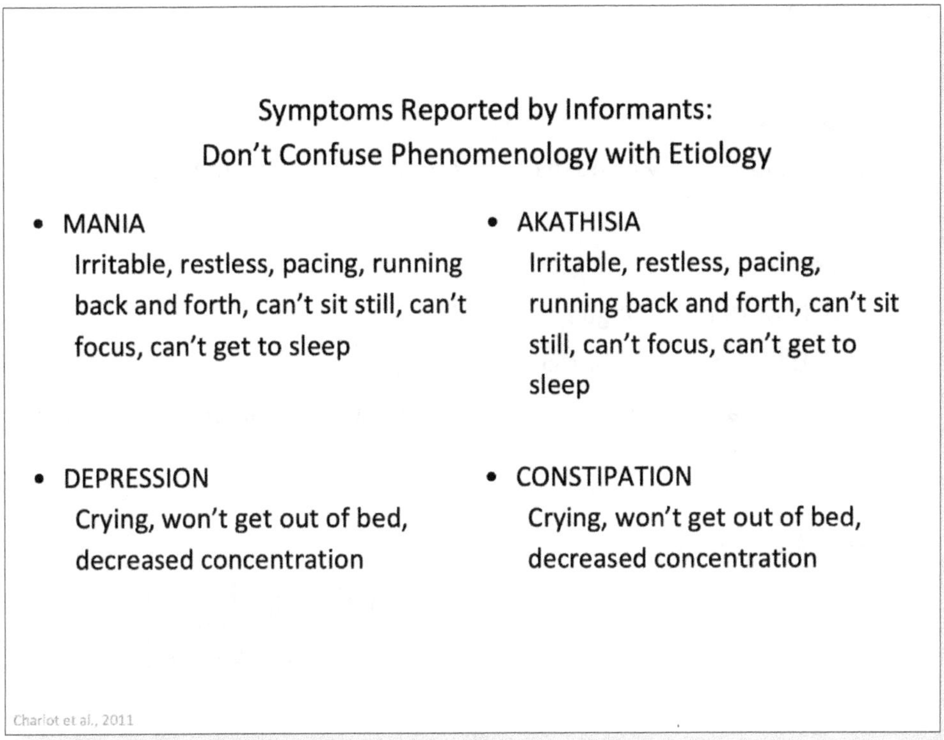

The fact that medical conditions and mental illness can look similar reinforces the need for an integrated model to ensure a comprehensive assessment and symptom tracking over time/settings to differentiate conditions.

For example, as indicated in this slide, symptoms of mania are the same as symptoms of akathisia.

Symptoms of depression can be the same as symptoms of constipation.

Slide 51

1. Sleep Pattern:

   Quality and quantity of sleep can affect physical and mental health

   For example:

   a. Poor sleep ⇨ fatigue ⇨ irritability

   b. Depression ⇨ poor sleep ⇨ irritability

   c. Medical problem (discomfort caused by constipation) ⇨ poor sleep ⇨ irritability

Assessment Strategy:

Maintain sleep data.

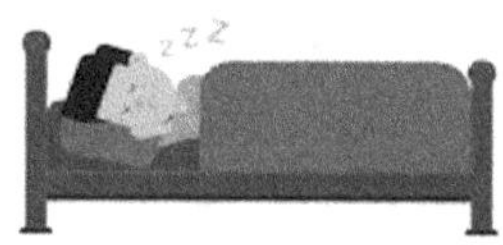

Charlot et al., 2011

The issue of poor sleep has the final pathway of resulting in irritability. It is important to assess the determinants that are causing the poor sleep and irritability. Is it a medical problem or is it a psychiatric problem? The answer to this question is based on collecting other information in addition to maintaining sleep data.

Slide 52

2. Appetite pattern:

   Changes in appetite can be clues in the assessment of mental health or physical problem.

   Significant weight change may indicate a medical or mental health problem.

   Assessment strategy:

   Monitor and document a person's weight on a weekly basis.

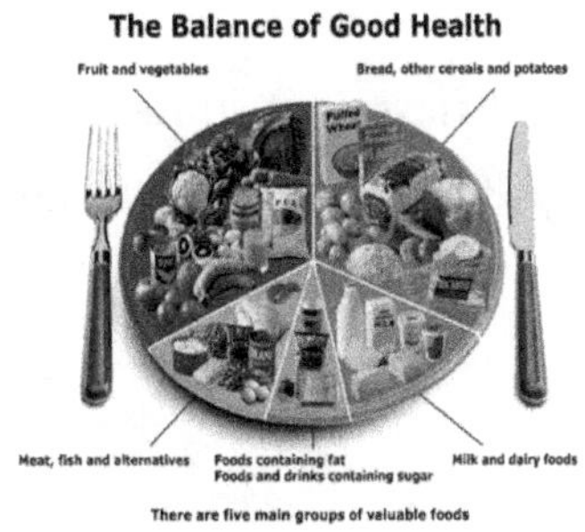

Charlot et al., 2011

A change in appetite can be a clue to either a medical or psychiatric problem. The key to assessment of change in appetite is to monitor and document eating patterns and use this data along with other sources of information. This will help to determine the primary cause of a change in food consumption.

Slide 53

3. Activity level:

   Activity level refers to the things a person usually does during the day. For example:

   - going to work
   - completing chores
   - leisure time pursuits

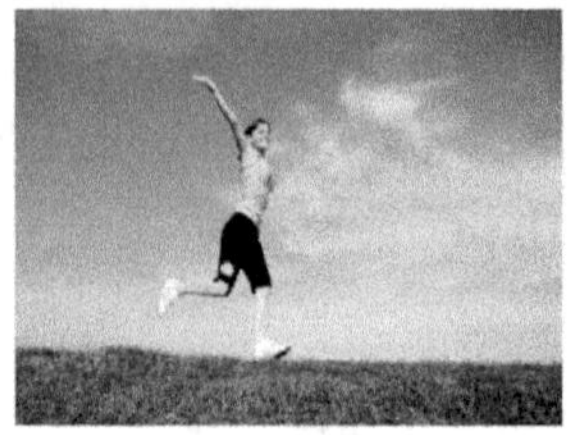

Assessment strategy:

If a person's activity level changes drastically, it may be an unrecognized medical or mental health problem.

Charlot et al., 2011

A change in activity level from baseline behavior may be indicative of either a medical or psychiatric problem. It is, therefore, important to monitor and document changes in activity level as well as to monitor other signs and symptoms.

Slide 54

3. Activity level (continued):

Examples:

Arthritis ⇨ decreased activity ⇨ refuses to go to work ⇨ could be viewed as non-compliant

Depression ⇨ decreased activity ⇨ refuses to go to work ⇨ could be viewed as noncompliant

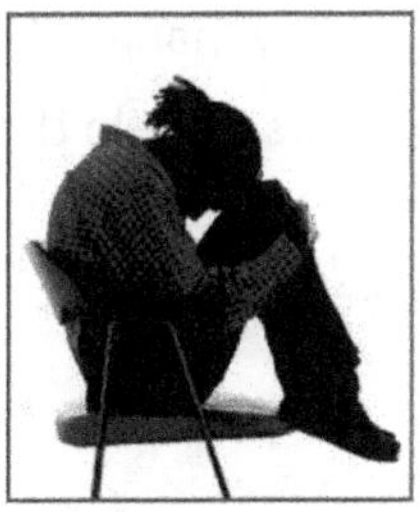

Charlot et al., 2011

A person who has IDD and has a decreased activity level from baseline may be exhibiting a medical problem or a psychiatric symptom. A change in one's level of activity needs to be assessed from a holistic perspective.

The final pathway in this example, noncompliant behavior, could be caused by either a medical problem or psychiatric condition.

Slide 55

BEAMS

- Are there any changes in the current conditions?
- Are there any changes in:
  - B = behavior
  - E = energy level*
  - A = appetite
  - M = mood
  - S = sleep patterns
- How long have the symptoms/changes been occurring?
- Is there anything that appears to help the person feel better when these signs are present?
- In what context have these changes occurred?

The BEAMS assessment can act as a pre-screening for mental illness. Direct support professionals can collect data on observations of changes in current conditions to mental health/health professionals to help direct assessment for medical/mental health issues.

* While previous slides refer to change of activity level as an indicator, energy level is used in this tool but can be used in the same manner as activity level, although it does include factors such as lethargy and hyperactivity.

References: Module III

Appleton, H., Roberts, J., & Simpson, K. (2020). How is Anxiety Identified and Diagnosed in Individuals with Autism Spectrum Disorder and Intellectual Disability? A Scoping Review. *Journal of Mental Health Research in Intellectual Disability*, 13, 152-175.

Baer, D. M. Wolf, M. M. Risley, T.R. (1968). Some current dimensions of applied behavior analysis. *Journal of Applied Behavior Analysis, 1*(1), 91–97.

Barnhill, J. (2015). Thinking about epidemiology of self-injury. *The NADD Bulletin*, 18,123, 3-7.

Barnhill, J. (2019). The problem of irritability in IDD. *The NADD Bulletin*, 22, 63-67.

Beasley, J. B., Kroll, J., & Sovner, R. (1992). Community-based crisis mental health services for persons with developmental disabilities: The START model. *The Habilitative Mental Healthcare Newsletter,* 11 (9), 55-57.

Beavers, G. A., Iwata, B. A., & Lerman, D.C. (2013). Thirty years of research on the functional analysis of problem behavior. *Journal of Applied Behavior Analysis*, 46(1), 1-21.

Carr, J. E., & Sidener, T. M. (2002). On the relation between applied behavior analysis and positive behavioral support. *The Behavior Analyst*, 25, 245-253.

Charlot, L., Abend, S., Ravin, P., Mastis, K., Hunt, A., & Deutsch, C. (2011). Non-psychiatric health problems among psychiatric inpatients with intellectual disabilities. *Journal of Intellectual Disability Research,* 5, 199-209.

Cook A., & Angkhavong, S. (2018). Non-pharmacological management of challenging behaviors in adults with intellectual disabilities. *The NADD Bulletin*, 21, 3-7.

Engel, G. (1977). The need for a new medical model: a challenge for

MODULE 3

biomedicine. *Science.* 196(4286), 129-196.

Fletcher, R., Barnhill, J., & Cooper, S-A. (2016). *Diagnostic Manual – Intellectual Disability (DM-ID-2): A Textbook of Diagnosis of Mental Disorders in Persons with Intellectual Disability* (2nd ed.). Kingston, NY: NADD Press.

Griffiths, D. & Gardner, W. (2002). The integrated biopsychosocial approach to challenging behaviours. In Griffiths, D., Stavrakaki, C., & Summers, J. (Eds.). *Dual diagnosis: An introduction to the mental health needs of persons with developmental disabilities.* Sudbury, ON: Habilitative Mental Health Resource Network.

Hawkins, B. (1999). Rights, place of residence and retirement: Lessons from case studies on aging. In S. Herr & G. Weber (Eds.), *Aging, rights and quality of life.* Baltimore, MD: Brookes.

Haveman, M. J., Heller, T., Lee, L. A, Maaskant, M. A., Shooshtari, S., & Strydom, A. (2009). Report on the State of Science on Health Risks and Aging in People with Intellectual Disabilities. IASSID Special Interest Research Group on Ageing and Intellectual Disabilities/Faculty Rehabilitation Sciences, University of Dortmund.

Iwata, B. A., Dorsey, M. F., Slifer, K. J., Bauman, K. E., & Richman, G. S. (1994). Toward a functional analysis of self-injury. *Journal of Applied Behavioral Analysis*, 27(2), 197-209.

Kildahl, A., Helverschou, S., Bakken, T., & Oddli, H. (2020). Driven and Tense, Stressed Out and Anxious": Clinicians' Perceptions of Post-Traumatic Stress Disorder Symptom Expressions in Adults with Autism and Intellectual Disability. *Journal of Mental Health Research in Intellectual Disability*, 13, 201-230.

McClintock, K., Hall, S., & Oliver, C. (2003). Risk markers associated with challenging behaviours in people with developmental disabilities: a meta-analytic study. *Journal of Intellectual Disability Research*, 47, 40-416.

McGilvery, S., & Sweetland, D. (2011). *Intellectual disability and mental health: A training manual in dual diagnosis.* Kingston, NY: NADD Press.

Mevissen, L., Didden, R., de Jongh, A., & Korzilius, H. (2020). Assessing Posttraumatic Stress Disorder in Adults with Mild Intellectual Disabilities or Borderline Intellectual Functioning. *Journal of Mental Health Research in Intellectual Disability*, 13, 110-126.

Morrison, A. K., & Gillig, P. M. (2012). Psychiatric assessment. In J. P. Gentile. & P. M. Gillig (Eds.), *Psychiatry of intellectual disability: A practical manual* (pp. 14-25). Oxford, UK: John Wiley & Sons, Ltd.

Poindexter, A. R. (2005). *Assessing medical issues associated with behavioural/ psychiatric problems in persons with intellectual disability.* Kingston, NY: NADD Press.

Reiss, S., Leviton, G. W., Szyszko, J. (1982). Emotional disturbance and mental retardation: diagnostic overshadowing. *American Journal of Mental Deficiency*, 86(6), 567-574.

Sovner, R., & Hurley, A. D. (1989). Ten diagnostic principles for recognizing psychiatric disorder in mentally retarded persons. *Psychiatric Aspects of Mental Retardation Reviews*, 8, 9-14.

Valdovinos, M., Seibert, H., Piersma, D., Wilkinson, A., Griffith, G., Hillring, S., & Boyle, B. (2019). Characterizing Mood States in Individuals Diagnosed with Bipolar Disorder and Intellectual Disability. *Journal of Mental Health Research in Intellectual Disability*, 12, 26-44.

Module IV

Mental Status Exam

Slide 2

This module includes information about best practices in mental health evaluation for persons with IDD with a focus on mental status examination (MSE).

Slide 3

Learning Objectives

- Summarize the importance of assessing the cognitive developmental level of the person with IDD as it pertains to Mental Status Examination.
- Describe the 11 domains and how they are pertinent to the assessment process.
- Describe how the developmental level of the person is related to the assessment process.

Slide 4

Definitions

Affect: The observable expression of emotion

Psychomotor activity: Movement or muscle activity related to mental processes

Thought process: Brain processing information to form concepts, make decisions, reason and problem-solve

Cognitive functions: The mental processes involved in gaining knowledge and comprehension—thinking, knowing, remembering, judging and problem-solving. These are higher-level functions of the brain and encompass language, imagination, perception and planning.

Judgment: Process by which people make decisions and form conclusions based on available information and material combined with thought and experience

Insight: Self-understanding—the awareness of own attitudes, feelings and behavior

Slide 5

Effects of IDD in Clinical Presentation

The interaction between IDD and MI is a result of four factors that reflect the profound bio-psycho-social effects of developmental disabilities:

1. Intellectual distortion
2. Psycho-social masking
3. Cognitive disintegration
4. Baseline exaggeration

Sovner,1986

All four of these factors are critical to examine in the clinical presentation of a person with IDD who also has MI. Part of the traditional difficulty in proper diagnosis in this population comes from these four concerns. Each will be discussed in turn.

Slide 6

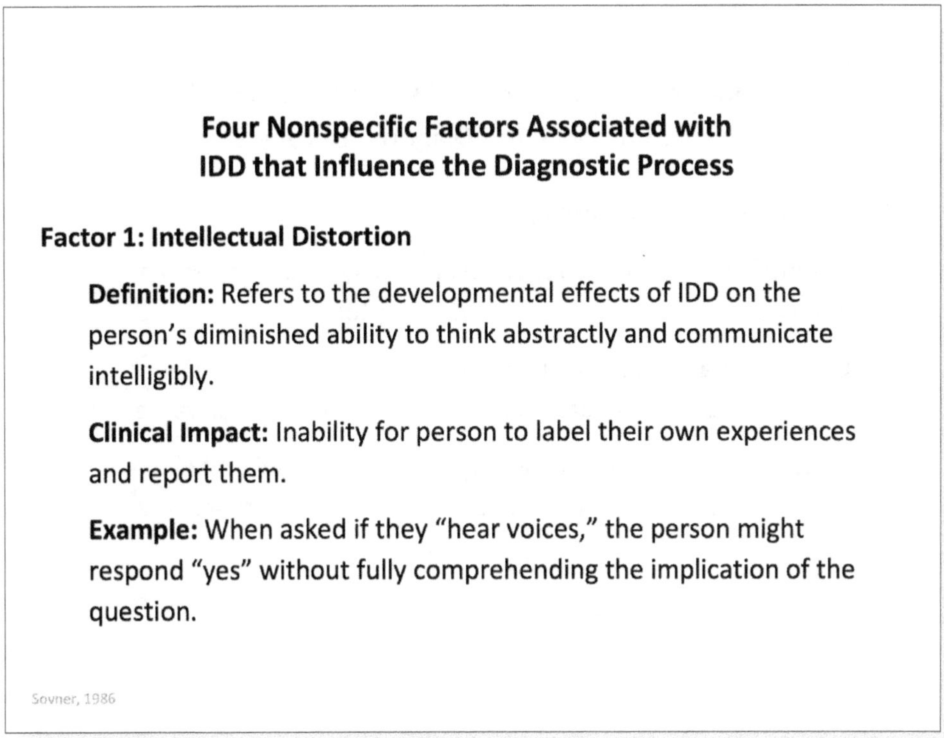

In the general population, diagnosis of an MI often is made based on an interview of the person with a standard set of questions. A person with IDD may not have the intellectual function to understand the question, communicate about experiences, remember experiences or have the self-awareness to reflect on changes in perception or what is "normal." One of the common interview questions is about hearing voices. What might happen if a person answers "yes" because they hear the interviewer asking the question?

Slide 7

Four Nonspecific Factors Associated with IDD that Influence the Diagnostic Process

Factor 2: Psycho-social Masking

Definition: Impoverished social skills and life experiences can influence the content of psychiatric symptoms.

Clinical Impact: The person with IDD might present significant symptomatology that occurs within the developmental framework.

Example: A person with a moderate level of IDD might believe they can drive a car, and this can be a manifestation of grandiosity.

Sovner, 1986

This refers to differences in the psycho-social lives of persons with IDD masking the presence of an MI. The lives of people with IDD are often very different from those of the general population. Knowledge of the lives of people with IDD is crucial in understanding enough to make a competent diagnosis.

Slide 8

Four Nonspecific Factors Associated with IDD that Influence the Diagnostic Process

Factor 3: Cognitive Disintegration

Definition: Stress-induced disruption of information processing—Tendency of person with IDD to become disorganized under stress.

Clinical Impact: Bizarre presentation and psychotic-like state may be misdiagnosed as schizophrenia.

Example: Vulnerability to high levels of stress and overload of cognitive functioning may lead to atypical clinical presentation.

Sovner, 1986

While it is true that many people under stress experience some degree of cognitive disintegration, due to the overall difficulties in cognition and typically less developed stress management skills, this is a more significant problem for people with IDD. Cognitive disintegration has resulted in many misdiagnoses. Pressurized speech can occur under conditions of stress, but it is also a symptom of schizophrenia, and in our clinical experience, people with IDD have ended up on neuroleptics as a result.

Slide 9

Four Nonspecific Factors Associated with IDD that Influence the Diagnostic Process

Factor 4: Baseline Exaggeration

Definition: Preexisting maladaptive behaviors that were not attributed to mental illness may increase in frequency and intensity with the onset of a psychiatric disorder.

Clinical Impact: Creates difficulty in establishing illness features, target symptoms and outcome measures.

Example: SIB (Self-Injurious Behavior) or aggression that occurred infrequently may suddenly increase in severity at onset of a psychiatric disorder.

Sovner, 1986

Baseline exaggeration can be a significant problem with making a good diagnosis, as the frequency of problem behavior may go up, and then care providers only see the escalating problem behavior and only want to respond to that, rather than paying attention to other symptoms which also may be occurring.

Slide 10

- The Mental Status Exam can only be administered by a regulated health or mental health professional such as a physician, nurse, psychologist or psychiatrist.

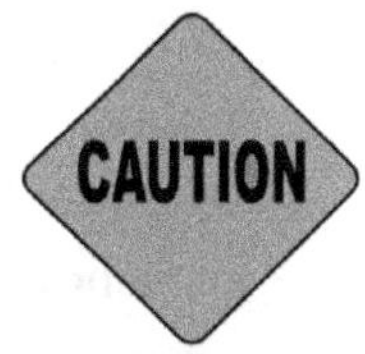

- A direct support professional can contribute to the process by being familiar with the components of the exam and the information they may need to assist the person to receive an accurate assessment.

The mental status examination is intended to be one part of a comprehensive assessment of a person's overall condition. It is infrequent that this process would be completed by a physician or nurse, but they are qualified to administer it. More frequently, this will be completed by a mental health professional: a psychologist or psychiatrist.

It is outside the scope of practice for a direct support professional to conduct this examination. However, it is important to be familiar with the components of the exam to be able to provide thoughtful and informed contributions to the assessment process. A direct support professional needs to be prepared to provide a comprehensive history of the person, their medical conditions, normative behavior/baseline behavior and any previous assessment results including results of functional assessment/analysis of behavior. The clinician will need to understand the nature of a presenting problem, who defined it and how, the history of the problem, how long it has been observed, in what environments it is observed, if it is long-standing and why assessment is being sought (Fletcher, Loschen, Stavrakaki & First, 2007).

Slide 11

A Mental Status Exam is a brief assessment intended to provide a snapshot of the mental status of the person at the time of the assessment.

Levitas, Hurley & Pary, 2001

Slide 12

- Systematic observation and recording about a person's thinking, emotions and behavior
- MSE for people with IDD needs to be modified
- Useful way to organize and standardize the data of patient observation
- MSE is a snapshot of the mental status at the time of the assessment. The MSE can be used as a tool to note change in the status from one point in time to another.
- MSE is a diagnostic measurement. Data from care providers and patient history can be helpful.

Levitas, Hurley & Pary, 2001

Along with other components such as the history of the presenting complaint, family history and current and past medical history, the mental status examination can provide more detailed information to formulate a psychiatric diagnosis and to direct any further assessments which need to take place: adaptive functioning assessment, cognitive assessments, psychometric testing, etc.

Slide 13

I. General appearance and behavior
II. Mood and affect
III. Psychomotor activity and speech
IV. Thought process and content
V. Cognitive function
VI. Judgment and insight

Levitas, Hurley & Pary, 2001

The purpose of a Mental Status Exam (MSE) is to get a comprehensive cross-section of the person's mental state.

An MSE is essentially the equivalent of a physical health exam but focuses on the behaviors and the mental state of the patient as opposed to the physical health. It provides a quick snapshot of the mental state at the time of the assessment and can be used as a tool to note change in status from one point in time to another.

The MSE records both the clinician's observation of the person's mental and emotional functioning at the time of assessment and responses to specific questions. The direct support professional's input may be required for the observational process as well as the interview process when the person being assessed has an intellectual/developmental disability. Contributions would be needed to assist the clinician to understand what baseline behavior looks like for the person, i.e., what the person's behaviors are like in general, as they may appear quite different from those of a person who does not have an intellectual/developmental disability. Assistance may also be needed during the question/answer portion of the assessment for any number of reasons that are explicated further in this section.

Slide 14

Case Study

As we work through each section of the mental status exam, we will consider the case of Ms. Thao. This is the examiner's first appointment with Ms. Thao. The results of the assessment will serve as the baseline for noting change in Ms. Thao's mental health.

Levitas, Hurley & Pary, 2001

Slide 15

I. General appearance and behavior

- Assess person's attentiveness and effective participation in interview
- Note person's attitude toward examiner
- Assess posture and general motor activity
- Note facial expression
- Note personal hygiene and grooming
- Assess weight status

Levitas, Hurley & Pary, 2001

Note: All of the above are based on the cognitive developmental level of the individual with IDD.

- Level of consciousness: if person is awake, alert or sedated
- Participation in interview: The person with IDD may have significant limitations with regard to his/her participation in the interview. This is associated with limitations in expressive and receptive language skills.
- Attitude toward examiner: e.g., cooperative, guarded, suspicious
- Posture and general motor activity: e.g., rigid, tense, restless, pacing
- Facial expression: e.g., tearful, laughing, smiling, angry
- Personal hygiene and grooming: e.g., unkempt appearance, meticulous grooming
- Weight status: e.g., obesity, extreme thinness

Slide 16

I. General appearance and behavior (cont.)

- The clinician may need to rely on collateral information about the person's baseline appearance and behavior.
- Baseline for a person with IDD may be very different from the neurotypical person. For example, in a person with ASD, body posturing, self-hugging and finger-flicking may be the typical baseline behavior for a person on the spectrum.

Levitas, Hurley & Pary, 2001

Note: All of the above are based on the cognitive developmental level of the individual with IDD.

For a person with an IDD, direct support professionals may be needed to provide baseline information on all the above observations so the assessor has information on what the person's general appearance and behavior are like. Baseline appearance and behavior can differ significantly from that of the general population. For example, for a person with ASD, the examiner may note the person's lack of eye contact. However, lack of eye contact is relatively "typical" for a person with ASD, so this behavior is baseline for them. Similarly, body posturing, self-hugging, finger-flicking and other behavior may be "typical" for the person but be interpreted differently if the assessor does not have information about what is general behavior for the person.

Slide 17

I. General appearance and behavior — Ms. Thao

- Wearing loose-fitting T-shirt and dress customary for her ethnicity
- The examiner has no further ability to determine gender
- Eye contact averted for first 10 minutes of the exam
- Following first 10 minutes, Ms. Thao was attentive and engaged, speaking freely and unguarded.
- Ms. Thao was neatly groomed with unremarkable hygiene.

Levitas, Hurley & Pary, 2001

Different patterns of eye contact are more common for people of Ms. Thao's ethnicity.

Slide 18

- Ms. Thao appears to be underweight.
- She displayed a high level of motor activity. Her facial expression appeared worried.
- She fidgeted and squirmed frequently.
- Ms. Thao did smile and laugh periodically.
- Ms. Thao's care providers reported her appearance and behavior as typical.
- Ms. Thao's posture and appearance of muscle tone were unremarkable.
- Ms. Thao wrung her hands and adjusted her clothing repeatedly

Levitas, Hurley & Pary, 2001

Slide 19

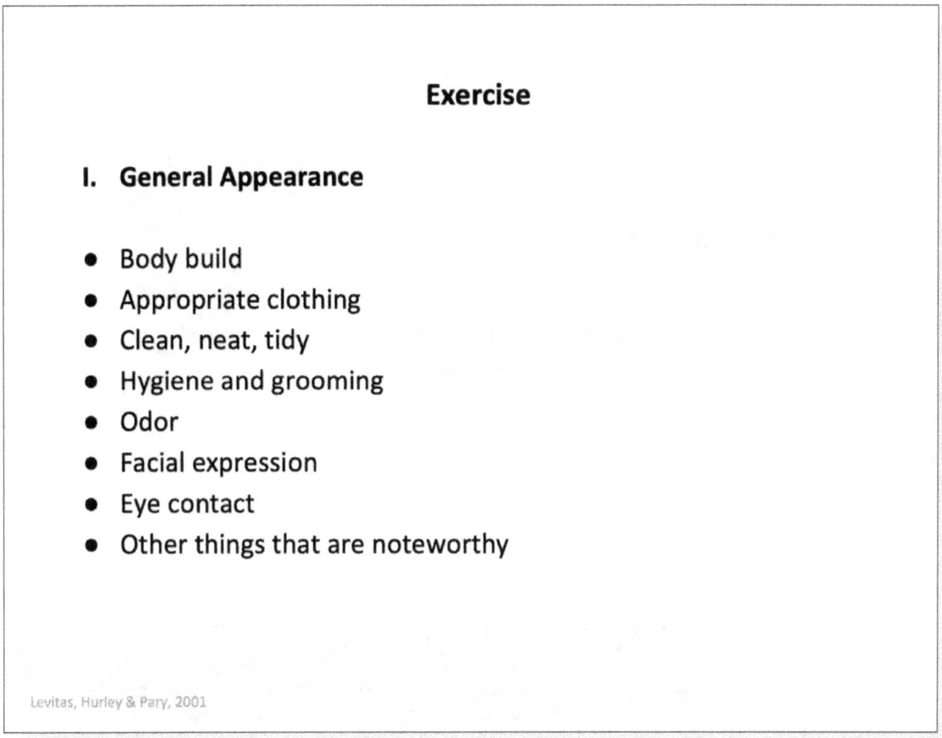

Have the participants list examples of possible observations on appearance and behavior. Ask the participants to think of various people with IDD they have known and generate things that might have been observed about them for each question.

Slide 20

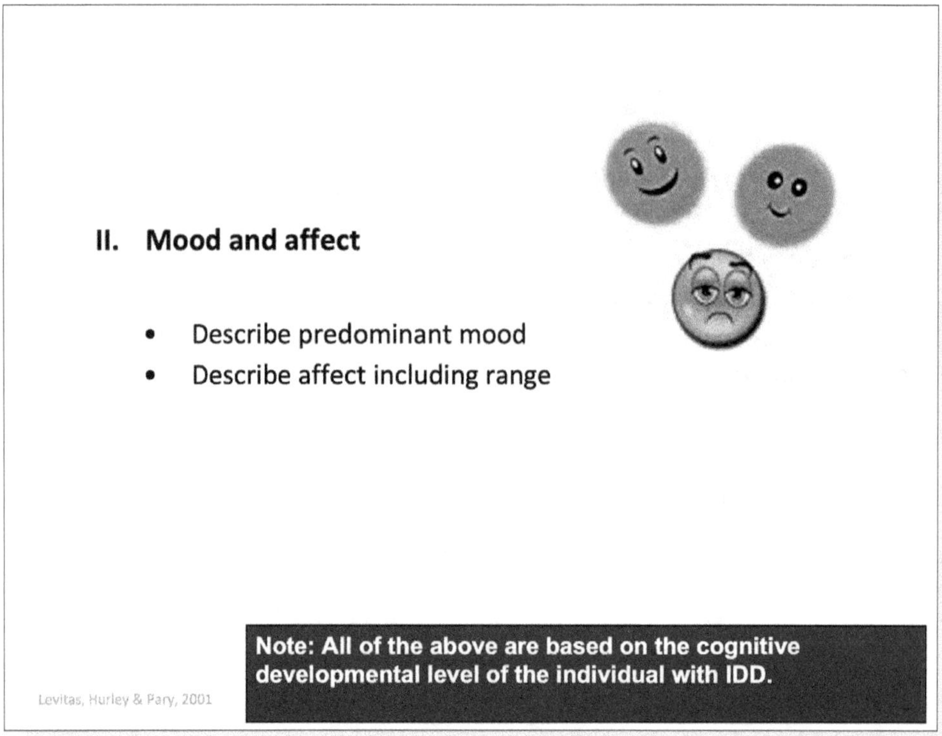

- Describe predominant mood, e.g., neutral, anxious, fearful, elated, euphoric, depressed, angry, irritable.

- Describe affect, including range (e.g., broad, restricted, labile or changes easily); intensity (e.g., blunted, flat, animated); and appropriateness of mood/thought content.

Once again, the direct support professional will need to assist the assessor to understand what typical mood and behavior are for the person and to interpret affect through behavioral expression.

Slide 21

II. Mood and affect (cont.)

- Mood is the prevailing emotional state. Affect is the expression of emotions.
- An examiner can draw faces to help the client identify feeling state.
  - -Ask person to point to face to show how he/she is feeling today.

Happy **Sad** **Mad** **Fearful** **Neutral**

Levitas, Hurley & Pary, 2001

Note: All of the above are based on the cognitive developmental level of the individual with IDD.

Affect, in this context, refers to the observable expression of emotion. Given that many people who have intellectual disability have an affect that can be considered inconsistent with their emotional state, it is critical that the direct support professional provide the assessor with information on the general affect of the person.

For example, a person who has Cornelia de Lange syndrome has difficulty with the facial expression of emotion. In absence of this information, an assessor could inappropriately interpret that the person has a flat affect, when this is the person's typical expression of emotion. Observation of behavior carries more import in this person's case than for someone in the general population.

Slide 22

II. Mood and affect — Ms. Thao

- Ms. Thao exhibited high levels of anxiety throughout the visit. This was her predominant emotional state.
- Her range of emotion displayed included mild euphoria when describing family, pets and gardening.
- Ms. Thao appeared to be quite worried about numerous topics, including street gangs, burglary and graffiti.

Levitas, Hurley & Pary, 2001

High levels of anxiety were consistent with previous reports and psychological assessments.

Care providers reported the mood and affect observed during the MSE were typical for her and they were observed to be generally appropriate and congruous for the setting.

Slide 23

Exercise

II. Mood and affect

- Appropriateness of affect/appropriate or inappropriate to situation. Congruous/incongruous
- Range of affect
- Stability of affect
- Attitude during encounter
- Specific mood or feelings, observed or reported
- Anxiety level rate

Levitas, Hurley & Pary, 2001

Have the participants list examples of possible observations on appearance and behavior.

Slide 24

III. Psychomotor activity and speech

- Assess psychomotor activity and notes
  - Rate of psychomotor activity (e.g., agitated, slowed)
  - Presence of abnormal movements (grimacing, mannerisms, stereotype)
- Assess speech and note amount, volume, rate, organization of speech

Levitas, Hurley & Pary, 2001

Note: All of the above are based on the cognitive developmental level of the individual with IDD.

Slide 25

III. Psychomotor activity and speech (cont.)

- Examiner will need other collateral data in understanding the typical psychomotor activity and speech organization for the person.
  - For example, people who have Fragile X often have difficulty with gross motor coordination, which may lead to assessment as abnormal movements in absence of information about the effect of the syndrome.

Levitas, Hurley & Pary, 2001

Note: All of the above are based on the cognitive developmental level of the individual with IDD.

As with previous sections of the examination, the direct support professional will need to assist the assessor in understanding the typical psychomotor activity and speech organization for the person. Many people who have IDD also have challenges with hyperactivity, challenges with gait, challenges with coordination and challenges with verbal communication.

For example, a person with Williams syndrome frequently experiences emotional immaturity exhibited by overreaction to events and exaggerated displays of fear, excitement, sadness, happiness, etc.

Slide 26

III. Psychomotor activity and speech — Ms. Thao

- Ms. Thao exhibited a high level of motor activity, frequently fidgeting, wringing her hands and adjusting clothing.
- No abnormal movements were observed.
- Ms. Thao's speech was easily understandable.
- Ms. Thao spoke rapidly and in an animated manner no matter what the topic was.
- Ms. Thao made numerous repetitive statements about criminal activity.
- Much of the discussion with Ms. Thao focused on past worrisome events, including a history of cutting.

Levitas, Hurley & Pary, 2001

During the brief observation, Ms. Thao made numerous repetitive statements (e.g., stating, "I don't understand what you are talking about" or "Huh?") which did not seem to be accurately describing what she was really thinking or understanding.

In conversation, topics went from one source of worry to another source of worry, frequently repeating past statements, though speech was generally organized. Care providers reported this as typical.

Slide 27

Exercise

III. Psychomotor behavior

- Gait
- Handshake
- Abnormal movements
- Posture
- Rate of movements
- Coordination

Levitas, Hurley & Pary, 2001

Have the participants list examples of possible observations on psychomotor behavior.

Slide 28

IV. Thought process and content

- Assess thought abnormalities
- Evaluate the content of thought
- Note presence of delusions/hallucinations (if so, note type of hallucinations)

Levitas, Hurley & Pary, 2001

Note: All of the above are based on the cognitive developmental level of the individual with IDD.

Rich fantasy life and self-talk are frequently associated with many types of IDD, especially Down syndrome. There is an extensive clinical history of this being interpreted as delusional behavior leading to misdiagnosis of schizophrenia. In the absence of the knowledge that these traits are "typical" for a person with Down syndrome and the ability to accurately describe their context, assessment on a Mental Status Exam could conclude that these behaviors are abnormal.

Slide 29

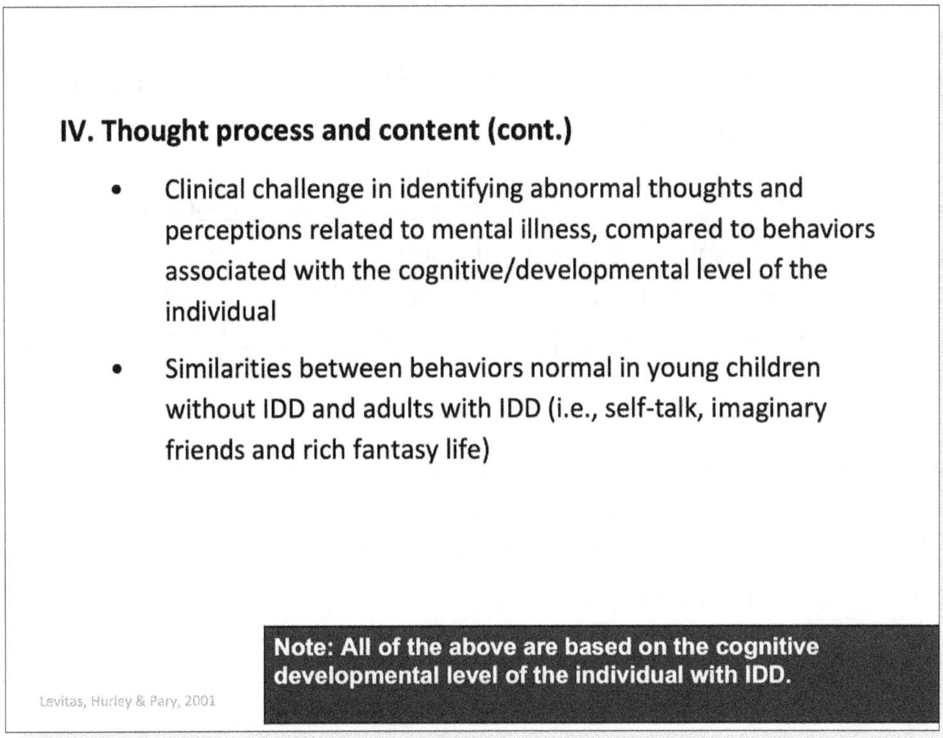

Assess thought abnormalities in logic, organization of words and phrases, association of ideas and comprehensibility.

Evaluate the content of thought, noting presence of ideas of reference, paranoid ideation, delusions (if so, what type of delusions), obsessions, compulsions and phobias. Inquire about suicidal/homicidal ideation. People who have an IDD, particularly those in the moderate to profound ranges, may have difficulty accurately describing thoughts and feelings. In the more severe and profound ranges, they will likely have few verbal communication skills. Lack of meaningful communication complicates assessment of thought processes and content and the presence of delusions and hallucinations. Careful observation of behavior is critical for accurate assessment. The direct support professional will be relied upon to assist in observing and interpreting behavior.

Note presence of delusions or hallucinations, if any. It is extremely difficult, if not impossible, to identify the existence of hallucinations and delusions in persons who have significant impairments in verbal communication. People with mild/moderate levels of IDD can usually express their internal thought process. However, people at the lower end of the IDD range may not be able to communicate their internal states.

Delusions involve false beliefs relating to misinterpretations of perceptions and experiences despite evidence to the contrary. For example, someone may believe they are being followed or "spied on" by interpreting gestures, movements, song lyrics, newspaper articles, etc., as related to them when they are not.

Hallucinations involves perceiving things that aren't really there, i.e., the mind is responding to sensory stimuli that do not exist outside of the mind. An example of a hallucination is a feeling that bugs are crawling on one's skin when, in fact, there are none.

Slide 30

IV. Thought process and content — Ms. Thao

- Ms. Thao's thought process appeared to be clear, though jumping from one source of worry to another and frequently revisiting past topics.
- Ms. Thao displayed directed attention to the interviewer.
- There was no evidence of delusional thinking nor significant fantasy life.
- Ms. Thao had difficulty staying focused on a single topic, though she could be redirected back to a topic of conversation.

Levitas, Hurley & Pary, 2001

During the MSE, there was significant evidence that Ms. Thao does possess theory of mind, understanding that other people may have different thoughts than her own.

Ms. Thao displayed strong attachment to people who had helped her, notably family members and people she knew through her community of faith.

Ms. Thao expressed significant concern and worry about street crime, notably gang activity and graffiti.

Ms. Thao was not able to identify her personal character strengths, though she identified as a good gardener.

Slide 31

Exercise

IV. Thought process and content

- Clarity
- Relevance/logic
- Flow
- Rapidly shifting ideas/thoughts
- Perseveration
- Pressure of speech
- Thoughts/content consistent with reality

Levitas, Hurley & Pary, 2001

Have the participants list examples of possible observations on thought process and content.

Slide 32

V. Cognitive function

- Assess orientations to time, place and persons
- Evaluate attention and concentration
- Assess memory
- Assess intellectual functioning

Note: All of the above are based on the cognitive developmental level of the individual with IDD.

Levitas, Hurley & Pary, 2001

Assess patient's orientations to time, place and persons. Note: A person with IDD may not know how to tell time, but this does not mean there is a cognitive deficit relative to the person's level of IQ with regard to an MSE. A person with IDD should be able to tell you what city they live in, but not necessarily the street address, and this should be considered normative, given the person's developmental level.

Evaluate patient's attention and concentration. Note: Attention and concentration should be evaluated with consideration of the person's developmental level.

Assess patient's memory. Note: Detailed information and chronology of events in the past need to be considered relative to the person's developmental age. Note: The examiner will need to assess intellectual functioning based on estimating the person's level of functioning. For example, a person with an IQ of 68 is below normative range of intellectual functioning. However, an IQ of 68 is at the high end of mild level of intellectual/developmental disability.

Slide 33

V. Cognitive function (cont.)

- Detailed information and chronology of events need to be considered relative to the person's developmental age. For example, they may remember the names of their siblings and know which are older and younger but may not be able to remember the exact age of each sibling.
- The examiner will need to assess intellectual functioning based on estimating the person's level of functioning.

Levitas, Hurley & Pary, 2001

Note: All of the above are based on the cognitive developmental level of the individual with IDD.

A person with IDD may remember events that have importance to them. For example, they may remember that we eat turkey on Thanksgiving.

Slide 34

V. Cognitive function — Ms. Thao

- Ms. Thao understood time, place and persons and also understood the nature of the meeting.
- Ms. Thao successfully gave the observer a tour of her home and understood the roles of her family and people paid to provide her with support.
- Ms. Thao had displayed difficulty with crude recall of facts, although she clearly remembered criminal activity around her neighborhood and described gang signs.

Levitas, Hurley & Pary, 2001

Ms. Thao's cognitive function was appropriate for her general level of intellectual ability as described in prior psychological evaluations. Her attention and ability to focus on topics other than her concerns were challenges but are consistent, as well, with descriptions and diagnoses in prior psychological evaluations.

Slide 35

Exercise

V. Cognitive function

- Attention and concentration
- Memory
- Abstraction concrete thinking
- Orientation

Levitas, Hurley & Pary, 2001

Have the participants list examples of possible observations on cognitive functioning.

Slide 36

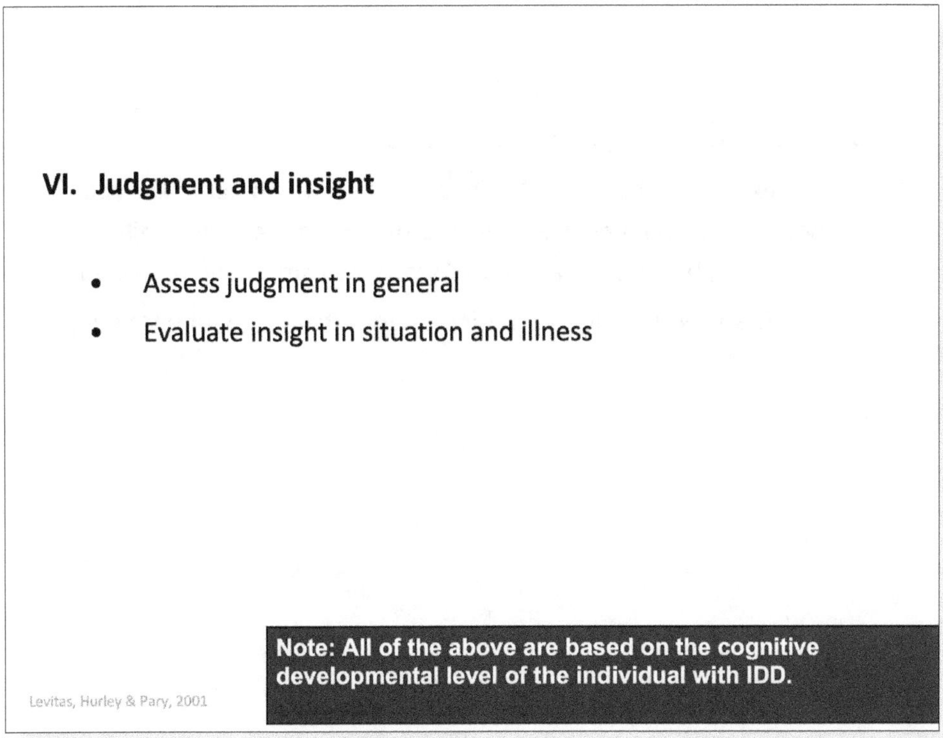

Judgment and insight need to be based on the person's developmental level. The clinician needs to keep in mind a developmental perspective when assessing judgment and insight with regard to a person with IDD.

For example, a 16-year-old adolescent with moderate level of IDD (IQ of 35-55) would not be expected to have a great deal of abilities regarding judgment and would have limited if any insight as to the nature of the problem for which he/she was brought to the clinician's attention.

Slide 37

VI. Judgment and insight — Ms. Thao

- The examiner observed Ms. Thao had insight into her anxiety to the degree that she was aware she worried more than her family members, but felt her additional worry was smart and reasonable.
- Ms. Thao was unable to offer insight into the nature of her worry.

Levitas, Hurley & Pary, 2001

Slide 38

Exercise

VI. Judgment and insight

- Impulsive behavior
- Insight into illness
- Examples

Levitas, Hurley & Pary, 2001

Have the participants list examples of possible observations on judgment and insight.

References: Module IV

Fletcher, R., Barnhill, J., & Copper, S. (Eds.). (2016). *Diagnostic manual – Intellectual disability (DM-ID-2): A textbook of diagnosis of mental disorders in persons with intellectual disability*. Kingston, NY: NADD Press.

Levitas, A., Hurley, A., & Pary, R. (2001). The Mental Status Examination in Patients with Mental Retardation and Developmental Disabilities. *Mental Health Aspects of Developmental Disabilities*, 4, 1-16.

Sovner, R. (1986). Limiting factors in the use of DSM-III criteria with mentally ill/mentally retarded persons. *Psychopharmacology Bulletin*, 22, 1055-1059.

Trzepacz, P. T. & Baker, R. W. (1993). *The Psychiatric Mental Status Examination*. Oxford, UK: Oxford University Press.

Module V

Overview of the Diagnostic Manual for Persons with Intellectual Disability (DM-ID-2)

Slide 2

This module contains information about the DM-ID-2 and how it can assist in the diagnostic process with persons with IDD.

Slide 3

Learning Objectives

- Describe the impact of the DM-ID-2 on the diagnostic process as compared to the DSM-5.
- Articulate the types of adaptations made in the DM-ID-2.
- Describe several adaptations as they compare to the DSM-5 in diagnostic subsets.

Slide 4

Limitations of DSM-5 System

- Diagnostic overshadowing (Reiss et al., 1982)
- Applicability of established diagnostic systems is increasingly suspect as the severity of ID increases (Rush, 2000)
- DSM-5 system relies on self report of signs and symptoms

Up until the development of the DM-ID, clinicians relied on the DSM system to diagnose psychiatric disorders in persons with ID. However, there are significant limitations in using the DSM system for persons who have ID.

The DSM system relies on self report of the client. The person expresses to the clinician their feelings, thoughts and emotions. Many people with ID, especially those with limited verbal skills, are challenged in their ability to give a self report of signs and symptoms.

The DM-ID-2 system relies more on behavioral equivalents than on self reports. This represents a major difference between the DSM and DM-ID.

Also, the concept of "diagnostic overshadowing" makes it difficult for clinicians to identify a mental illness in persons with ID.

Slide 5

DM–ID-2: Two Manuals

Diagnostic Manual—Intellectual Disability: A Textbook of Diagnosis of Mental Disorders in Persons with Intellectual Disability-2

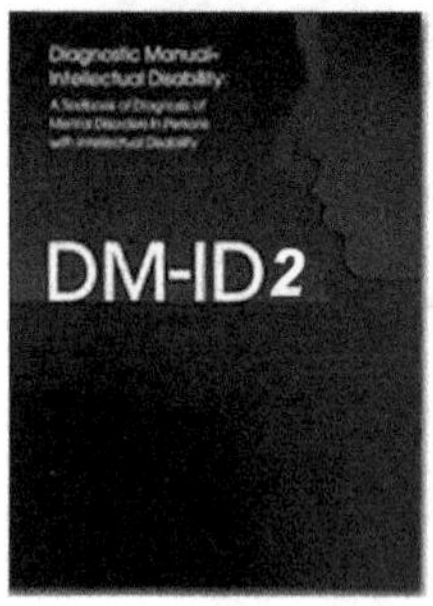

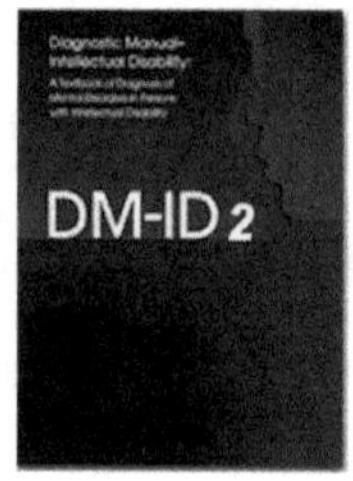

Diagnostic Manual—Intellectual Disability: A Clinical Guide for Diagnosis of Mental Disorders in Persons with Intellectual Disability-2

Actually, two diagnostic manuals were developed: a textbook and a clinical guide. The first version was completed in 2007. The publication of the DSM-5 in 2013 necessitated us to create the DM-ID-2.

The textbook contains a review of the research that is diagnostic-specific, as well as the etiology and pathogenesis of each diagnosis. The textbook contains 686 pages. It is comprehensive with a great deal of background information that is specific to each diagnosis. The clinical guide is an abbreviated version; however, both manuals are useful for diagnosing mental disorders with persons with IDD.

All of the diagnoses, diagnostic subcategories and criteria modifications are identical in both books. Both books can be used to diagnose a specific psychiatric disorder in persons with IDD.

Slide 6

Overview of the DM-ID-2

- An adaptation to the DSM-5
- Designed to facilitate a more accurate psychiatric diagnosis
- Based on expert consensus model
- Covers all major diagnostic categories as defined in DSM-5

DM-ID-2

The DM-ID-2 is a modification or an adaptation to the DSM-5. It uses the same diagnostic categories as the DSM-5. However, there are adaptations to criteria subsets, as warranted.

The DM-ID-2 was designed to facilitate a more accurate psychiatric diagnosis in persons with ID.

It was based on an expert consensus model. Each diagnostic category was developed by a group of experts, represented by between two to eight clinicians and academicians from around the globe. Thus, approximately 100 people were involved in the development of the DM-ID-2.

All of the diagnostic categories that are defined in the DSM-5 are also in the DM-ID-2. Additionally, the codification system, used for insurance purposes, are the same in the DSM-5 as they are in the DM-ID-2.

Slide 7

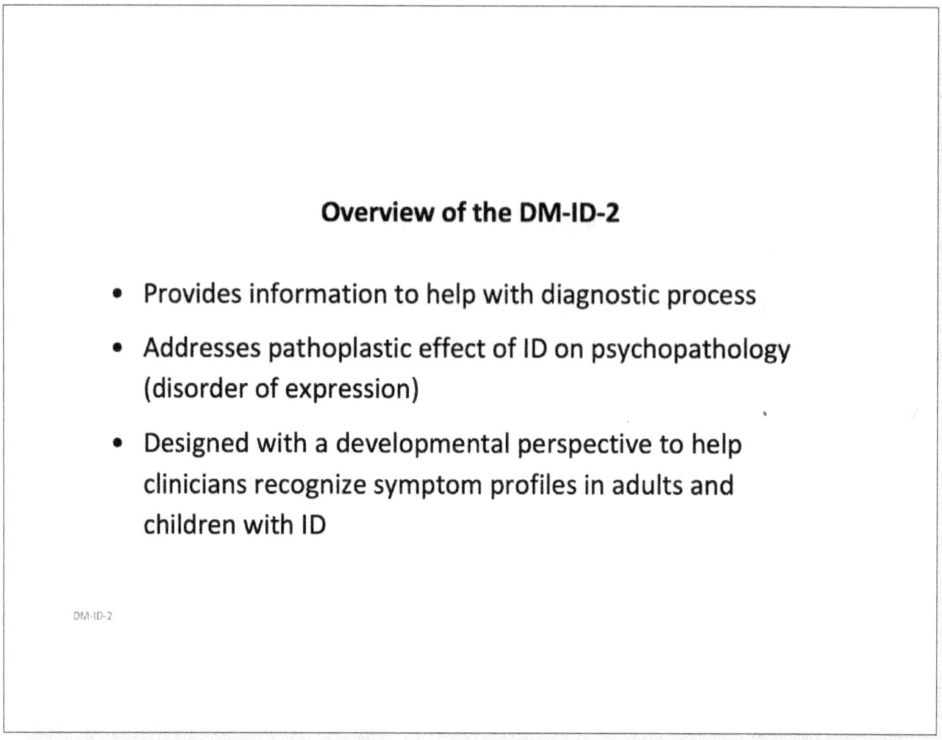

The DM-ID-2 has a wealth of information in each diagnostic category to assist the clinician at arriving at an accurate diagnosis.

Each diagnostic category describes how the psychiatric disorder can be manifested in persons with ID.

A developmental perspective is emphasized throughout the DM-ID-2 to assist the clinician in recognizing psychiatric disorders.

Slide 8

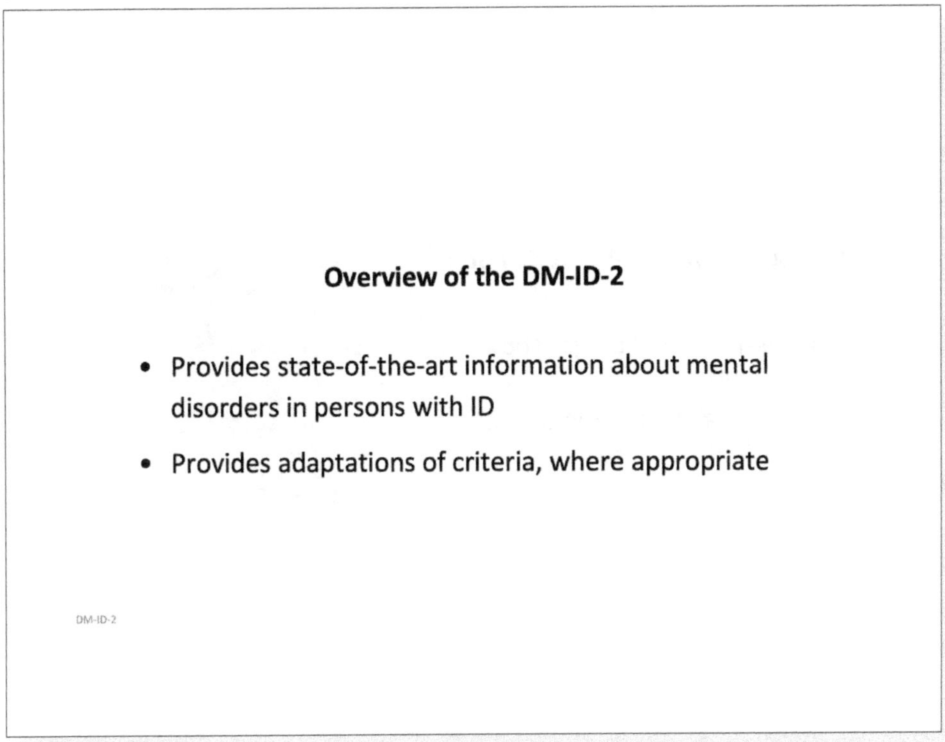

The textbook offers a comprehensive review of the research literature for each diagnostic category.

Both manuals have a wealth of information about how to apply a DSM-5 diagnosis for persons with ID. There is information, for example, on how to differentiate behavioral problems from symptoms associated with a psychiatric disorder.

Slide 9

Two Special Added-Value Chapters

- Assessment and Diagnostic Procedures
- Behavioral Phenotype of Genetic Disorders

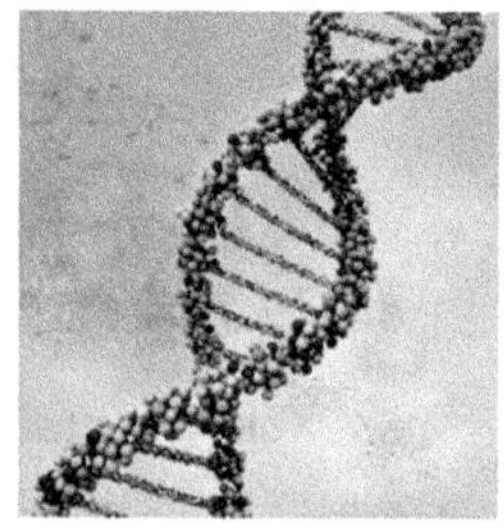

DM-ID-2

The DM-ID-2 offers two chapters that are not part of the DSM-5. One is on assessment and diagnostic procedures, and the other is on behavioral phenotypes of genetic disorders.

The chapter on assessment and diagnostic procedures discusses the types of historical information needed for an effective mental health evaluation.

The chapter on behavioral phenotypes and genetic disorders discusses 12 commonly found genetic disorders and the corresponding behavioral phenotypes associated with each disorder.

Slide 10

Assessment and Diagnostic Procedures

Special Consideration: Language That Is Understandable

- Use simple language
- Create short sentences
- Check back with person for understanding
- Use examples

DM-ID-2

This valuable chapter includes information on how to conduct a mental health assessment in persons with ID. The chapter begins with a section on difficulties in an examination and interpretation of symptoms. There is a section on special considerations for the mental health diagnostic interview for individuals with ID. For example, the chapter discusses how the clinician uses understandable language. There is a section that articulates the information that needs to be gathered in order to conduct an effective mental health evaluation.

Slide 11

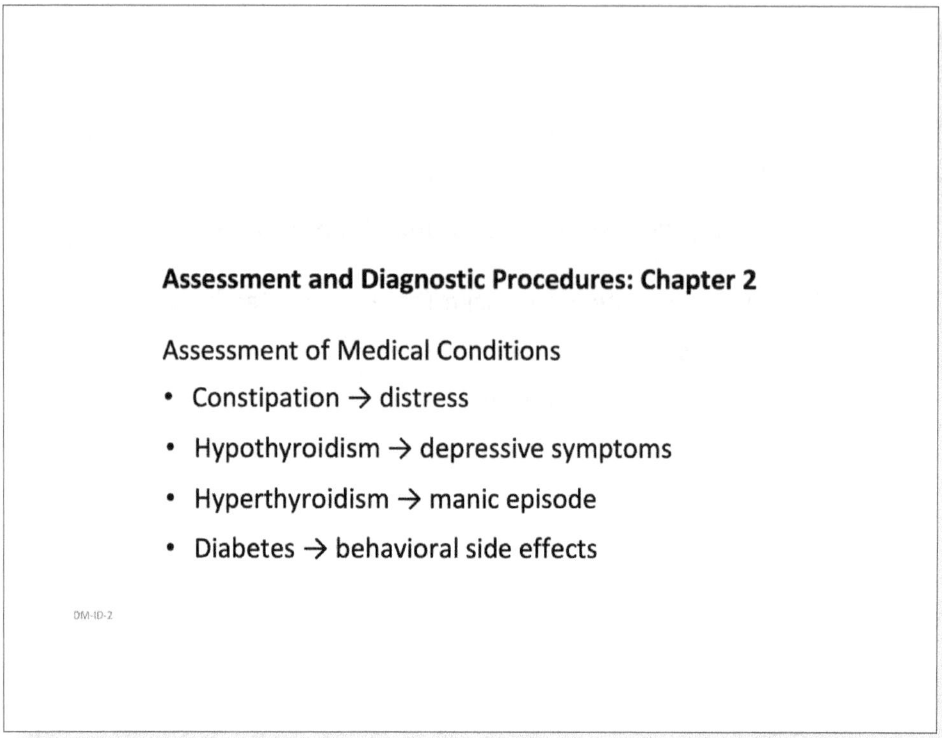

There is a section that discusses medical factors and the need to rule out medical comorbidities. Many medical conditions can look like or mask psychiatric disorders. Additionally, commonly found medical comorbidities, such as seizure disorders, as well as vision and hearing impairments, can cause problems that may be misinterpreted as a mental disorder.

The medical examples, as noted above, can lead to or look like mental health problems.

Slide 12

Behavioral Phenotype of Genetic Disorders: Chapter 3

Angelman syndrome	Prader-Willi syndrome
Cri-du-Chat (5p-) syndrome	Rubinstein-Taybi syndrome
Down syndrome	Smith-Magenis syndrome
Fetal alcohol syndrome	Tuberous sclerosis complex
Fragile X syndrome	Velocardiofacial syndrome
Phenylketonuria	Williams syndrome

DM-ID-2

The phenotype of a genetic syndrome is the set of physical characteristics produced by a genetic abnormality or genotype. The most widely known example is the easily recognized face of a person with Down syndrome.

The phrase "behavioral phenotype" denotes a set of behaviors that are genetically determined and associated with a particular genetic disorder. A behavioral phenotype is the specific and characteristic behavioral repertoire exhibited by persons with a specific genetic disorder.

This chapter lists 12 genetic disorders and their associated behavioral phenotypes. For each of the 12 disorders, there is information on physical findings, diagnosis, cognition and behavioral and associated mental health disorders.

Slide 13

Behavioral Phenotype of Genetic Disorders: Chapter 3

Down syndrome

Phenotype	Small head, mouth; upward slant to eyes; epicanthal folds; broad neck; hypothyroidism; hearing loss; visual impairments; cardiac problems; gastrointestinal; orthopedic and skin disorders; obesity	
Behavioral Phenotype	**Childhood**	Oppositional and defiant; attention-deficit/hyperactivity disorder (ADHD); social, charming personality "stereotype"
	Adulthood	Depressive disorders; obsessive-compulsive disorder; other anxiety disorders; dementia of the Alzheimer's type; mental disorders associated with hypothyroidism

DM-ID-2

This table is an example of a phenotype and behavioral phenotype for Down syndrome. The cluster of characteristic behaviors in a person with Down syndrome is differentiated between childhood behaviors and adult behaviors.

A key value in understanding behavioral phenotypes is that it aids in the diagnostic process. The behavioral phenotypes provide information that, when combined with other sources of information, aids in the diagnostic process.

Combining behavioral phenotypes with other sources of information provides the clinicians with important pieces of the complex diagnostic puzzle.

Slide 14

DM-ID-2
Diagnostic Chapter Structure

- Review of diagnostic criteria
  - General description of the disorder
  - Summary of DSM-5 criteria
- Issues related to diagnosis in people with ID
- Review of literature/research

DM-ID-2

There is a lot of consistency and uniformity throughout the DM-ID. There are categories and subcategories that are listed in each of the 24 diagnostic chapters. For example, each chapter has a section on:

- Review of diagnostic criteria
- Issues related to diagnosis in people with ID
- Review of literature/research (textbook only)

MODULE 5

Slide 15

Application of Diagnostic Criteria to People with ID

- General considerations
- Adults with mild to moderate ID
- Adults with severe or profound ID
- Children and adolescents with ID

DM-ID-2

All of the diagnostic chapters follow a consistent outline of information. The DM-ID-2 has a section for each diagnostic category on the application of diagnostic criteria to people with ID.

In addition to general considerations, this section differentiates adults with mild to moderate levels of ID and addresses the manifestation of a specific disorder for adults who have severe or profound ID. A particular psychiatric disorder can be manifested differently in children and adolescents with ID. Therefore, there is also a subsection for each diagnostic category that articulates the expression of that disorder in children and adolescents with ID.

Slide 16

Etiology and Pathogenesis

- Risk factors
  - Biological factors
  - Psychological factors
  - Genetic syndromes

DM-ID-2

The DM-ID-2 textbook has a section for each diagnostic category concerning etiology and pathogenesis. Under this section, there are subcategories of risk factors including biological, psychosocial and genetic syndromes. This information provides the clinician with a better understanding of the nature and source of the psychiatric disorder. Assembling this information aids in the diagnostic process.

Slide 17

Diagnostic Criteria

DSM-5 Criteria	Criteria Mild-Moderate ID	Criteria Severe-Profound ID

DM-ID-2

At the end of most diagnostic chapters there is a chart with three columns:

- The left column has the DSM-5 criteria and criteria subsets.
- The middle column provides modified diagnostic criteria for persons with mild/moderate levels of ID, where applicable.
- The right column lists modified criteria for persons with severe/profound levels of ID, where applicable.

Slide 18

Adaptation of the DSM-5 Criteria

1. Addition of symptom equivalents
2. Does not apply
3. Changes in symptom count
4. Modification of symptom duration
5. Modification of age requirements
6. Addition of explanatory notes

DM-ID-2

Note to trainer: Each adaptation should be expanded upon based on your experience or knowledge.

The DM-ID has six different adaptations of the DSM-IV-TR criteria.

1. Addition of symptom equivalents: These are observed behaviors that are equivalent to self reports as identified in the DSM system.

2. Does not apply: These are symptoms that do not exist or cannot be identified in persons with ID.

3. Changes in symptom count: This indicates the frequency of a symptom that is required to meet a diagnostic category.

4. Modification of symptom duration: This indicates the length of time a symptom has to be present in order to meet the diagnostic criteria.

5. Modification of age requirements: This indicates a change in the age of a person with regard to a particular criterion of a diagnostic category. This is to take into consideration the developmental perspective of the individual with ID.

6. Addition of explanatory notes: There are many explanatory notes in the context of criteria subsets that are intended to communicate a criteria adaptation. An explanatory note is provided in situations where there was insufficient research data but sufficient clinical expert consensus to explain a change in criteria without an official modification of the criteria subset.

Slide 19

Adaptation of DSM-5 Criteria
Addition of Symptom Equivalent
Social Anxiety Disorder

DSM-5 Criteria	Adapted Criteria for Mild and Moderate ID	Adapted Criteria for Severe and Profound ID
A. Marked fear or anxiety about one or more social situations in which the individual is exposed to possible scrutiny by others. Examples include social interactions (e.g., eating or drinking) and performing in front of others.	No adaptation for mild ID. For moderate ID, anxiety occurs in peer settings.	Fear can be observed rather than subjectively described or expressed by crying, tantrums, freezing, clinging, shrinking, failure to speak in social situations.

Symptom equivalents are observed behaviors that are equivalent to self reports as identified in the DSM system.

Slide 20

Adaptation of DSM-5 Criteria
Symptoms that do not apply
Delusional Disorder

DSM-5 Criteria	Adapted Criteria for Mild & Moderate ID	Adapted Criteria for Severe & Profound ID
A. The presence of one (or more) delusions with a duration of one month or longer.	No adaptation	Does not apply
D. If manic or major depressive episodes have occurred, these have been brief relative to the duration of the delusional periods.	No adaptation	Does not apply

DM-ID-2

Symptoms that do not apply: These are symptoms that do not exist or cannot be identified in persons with ID.

Most criteria subsets to diagnostic categories have an adaptation or no adaptation.

There are a limited number of criteria subsets to diagnostic categories that have a "does not apply" label. Here is an example of the diagnosis of delusional disorder that has the "does not apply" label for severe and profound ID.

Slide 21

Adaptation of DSM-5 Criteria
Change in Count and Symptom Equivalent
Major Depressive Disorder

DSM-5 Criteria	Adapted Criteria for Mild to Profound IDD
A. Five or more of the following symptoms have been present during the same two-week period and represent a change from previous functioning. At least one of the symptoms is either (1) depressed mood or (2) loss of interest or pleasure.	A. Four or more symptoms have been present during the same two-week period and represent a change from previous functioning. At least one of the symptoms is either (1) depressed mood or (2) loss of interest or pleasure or (3) irritable mood.

DM-ID-2

Changes in symptom count: This indicates the frequency of a symptom that is required to meet a diagnostic category.

Major depressive disorder: In this diagnostic category, there are changes in the symptom count as well as changes in symptom equivalence. Specifically, the DM-ID-2 has four or more symptoms, compared to five or more in the DSM-5. This is an example of change in symptom count.

There is also an addition to symptom equivalent, as "irritable mood" was added.

These changes may appear subtle on the surface but have significant importance with regard to the diagnostic process of identifying major depressive disorder in persons with ID.

Slide 22

Adaptation of DSM-5 Criteria
Modification Symptom Duration
Adjustment Disorder

DSM-5 Criteria	Applying Criteria for Mild to moderate ID	Applying Criteria for severe/profound ID
E. Once the stressor or its consequences have terminated, the symptoms do not persist for six (6) additional months.	An adjustment disorder must resolve within six months of the termination of the stressor (or its consequences). However, the symptoms may persist for a longer period (i.e., longer than six months) if they occur in response to a chronic stressor.	An adjustment disorder must resolve within six months of the termination of the stressor (or its consequences). However, the symptoms may persist for a longer period (i.e., longer than six months) if they occur in response to a chronic stressor.

DM-ID-2

Modification of symptom duration indicates the length of time a symptom has to be present in order to meet the diagnostic criteria.

In this example, the symptoms may persist for a period extending six months or longer.

Slide 23

Adaptation of DSM-5 Criteria

Modification of Age Requirement

Antisocial Personality Disorder

DSM-5 Criteria	**Adapted Criteria for Individuals with ID**
A. There is a pervasive pattern of disregard for and violation of the rights of others occurring since age 15 years, as indicated by three (or more) of the following:	A. There is a pervasive pattern of disregard for and violation of the rights of others occurring since age **18** years, as indicated by three (or more) of the following:
B. The individual is at least age 18 years.	B. The individual is at least age **21** years.
C. There is evidence of conduct disorder with the onset before age 15 years.	C. There is evidence of conduct disorder with onset before age **18** years.

DM-ID-2

Modification of age requirements: This indicates a change in the age of a person with regard to particular criteria of a diagnostic category. This is to take into consideration the developmental perspective of the individual with ID.

For antisocial personality disorder, there are changes in modification of age in the three criteria subsets. These changes reflect the cognitive developmental level of the individual with ID.

Slide 24

Adaptation of Criteria
Addition of Explanatory Note
Manic Episode

DSM-IV-TR Criteria	Applying Criteria for Mild to Profound IDD
A. A distinct period of abnormally persistently elevated, expansive or irritable mood, lasting at least one week (or any duration if hospitalization is necessary).	A. No adaptation. Note: Observers may report that the individual with IDD *has loud, inappropriate laughing or singing; is excessively giddy or silly; is intrusive, getting into other's space; and smiles excessively and in ways that are not appropriate to the social context.* Elated mood may be alternating with irritable mood.

DM-ID, 2007

There are many explanatory notes in the context of criteria subsets that are intended to communicate a criteria adaptation. An explanatory note is provided in situations where there was insufficient research data but sufficient clinical expert consensus to explain a change in criteria without an official modification of the criteria subset.

This is an example of the addition of an explanatory note. The explanatory note is similar to an adaptation to the DSM-5 criteria. The difference is that the explanatory note is based on clinical experience rather than research data. The explanatory note communicates to the reader specific behaviors that are characteristic in persons with ID who experience a manic episode.

Slide 25

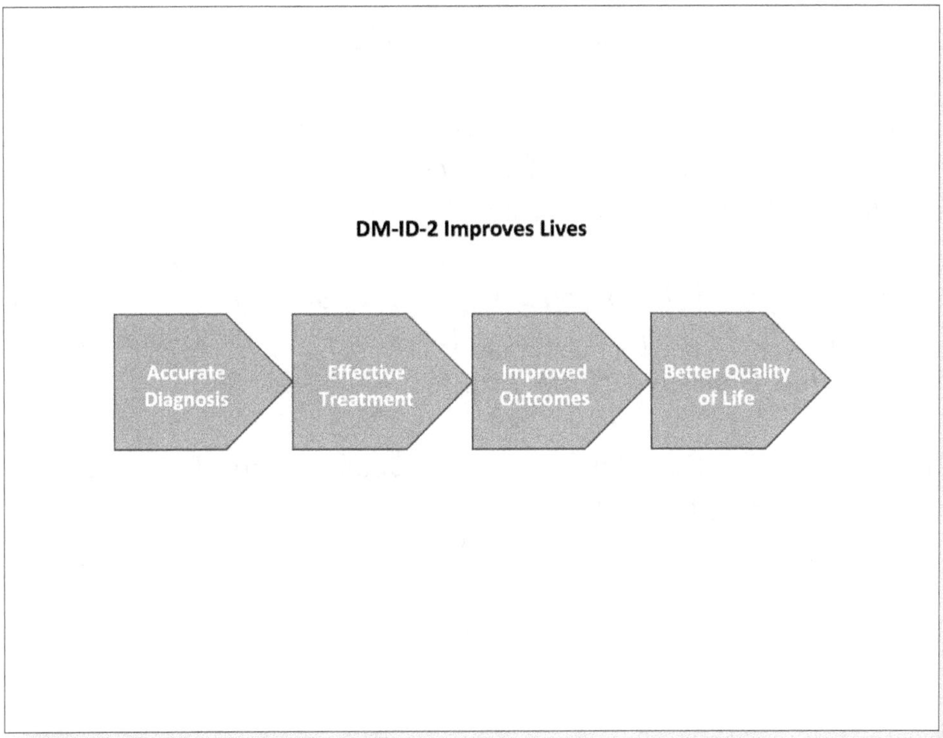

An accurate psychiatric diagnosis is critically important. It will then lead to effective treatment, which leads to improved outcomes, which leads to a better quality of life. The DM-ID-2 is designed to facilitate an accurate diagnosis for individuals with ID.

References for this DM-ID-2 module:

Reiss, S., Levitan, G. W., Szyszko, J. (1982). Emotional disturbance and mental retardation: diagnostic overshadowing. *American Journal of Mental Deficiencies*, 86 (6), 567-74.

Rush, A. J., Frances, A. (Eds.) (2000). Treatment of psychiatric and behavioral problems in mental retardation (Special Issue). *American Journal of Mental Retardation*, 105 (3), 1-71.

References: Module V

Fletcher, R., Barnhill, J., & Cooper, S-A. (2016). *Diagnostic Manual – Intellectual Disability (DM-ID-2): A Textbook of Diagnosis of Mental Disorder in Persons with Intellectual Disability* (2nd ed.). Kingston, NY: NADD Press.

Fletcher, R., Barnhill, J., & Cooper, S-A. (2018). *Diagnostic Manual – Intellectual Disability (DM-ID-2): A Clinical Guide of Diagnosis of Mental Disorder in Persons with Intellectual Disability* (2nd ed.). Kingston, NY: NADD Press.

Diagnostic and Statistical Manual of Mental Disorders (5th ed); DSM-5; American Psychiatric Association, 2013.

Module VI

Signs and Symptoms of Mental Illness

Slide 2

This module includes information regarding signs and symptoms of depressive disorders, bipolar disorder, anxiety disorders, personality disorders and psychosis.

The module highlights the importance of observation of presentation of behavioral equivalents in people with IDD.

Recognizing mental illness in people with IDD can be complicated by a number of factors.

Individuals with IDD may have poor verbal skills. They may communicate their symptoms in other ways. The signs and symptoms of certain psychiatric disorders often present in atypical or unusual ways. Sometimes mental health symptoms are overlooked.

Understanding and ruling out the causes of symptoms can help get a proper diagnosis to guide appropriate mental health treatment and support. Timely and effective treatment requires an accurate psychiatric diagnosis.

Slide 3

Learning Objectives

- Identify signs and symptoms of common mental health disorders
- Recognize presentation of behavioral equivalents mental health diagnoses in people with ID
- Recognize the importance of observation in the assessment process

Sometimes mental health symptoms are overlooked in people with ID. This is particularly common when managing behaviors rather than recognizing symptoms becomes the focus of assessment and treatment.

It can be a challenge to identify and evaluate factors that may contribute to signs and symptoms.

Slide 4

Overview of the
***Diagnostic Manual—Intellectual Disability,* DM-ID-2**

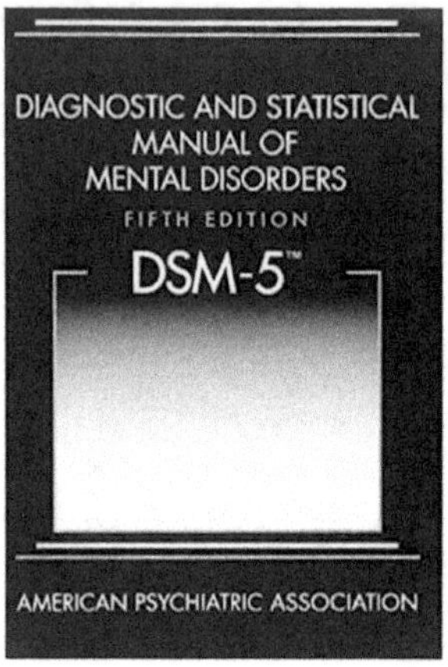

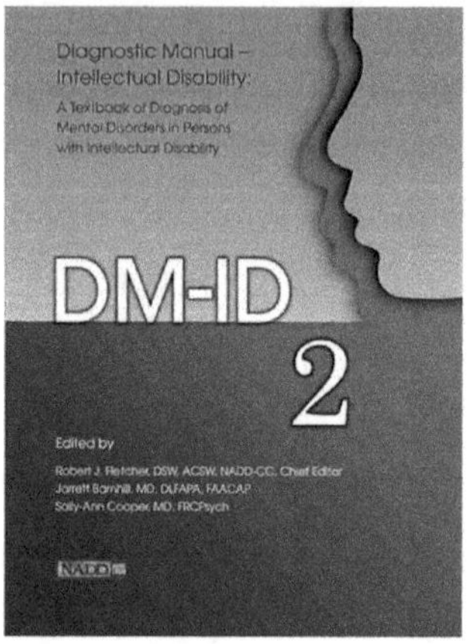

The Diagnostic and Statistical Manual of Mental Disorders (DSM) is the handbook used by health care professionals as the guide to the diagnosis of mental disorders. DSM contains descriptions, symptoms and other criteria for diagnosing mental disorders.

The Diagnostic Manual—Intellectual Disability, DM-ID-2, provides guidance for assessing and diagnosing specific disorders in individuals with IDD by providing information to help recognize signs and symptoms of mental illness. It lists behavior changes that may indicate certain mental health problems that are noticeable.

Slide 5

Diagnostic Challenges

- Communication
- Diagnostic overshadowing
- Acquiescence
- Appearing withdrawn
- Medications
- Behavioral
- Multiple diagnoses

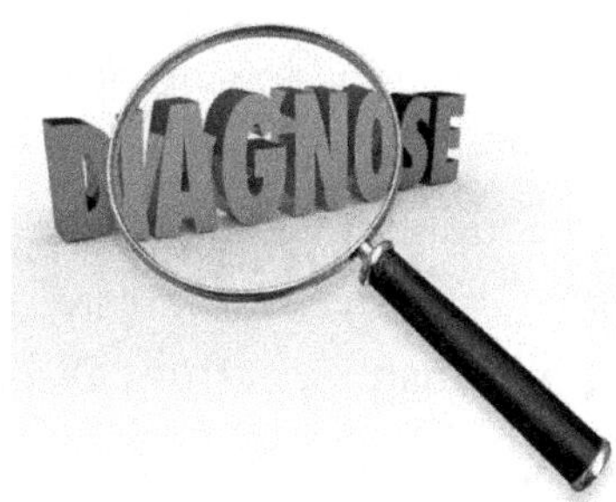

Recognizing mental illness in people with IDD can be complicated by several factors. Obtaining an accurate mental health diagnosis remains very challenging.

These barriers to diagnosis, as well as methods to address them are discussed in the Comprehensive Assessment Practices module (Module III) of this training manual.

Individuals with IDD may have poor verbal skills. They may communicate their symptoms in other ways. Some screening tools rely on self report, which may be difficult for people with IDD who have limited language or self-awareness. Individuals with disabilities may be poor historians and thus unable to provide the necessary details of their current situations or life events (Gentile et al., 2008).

People with disabilities may have difficulty with their behavior, especially if symptoms are affecting how they meet their needs.

The signs and symptoms of certain psychiatric disorders often present in atypical or unusual ways. Sometimes mental health symptoms are overlooked.

Sometimes symptoms of a mental health disorder appear as physical problems, such as abdominal pain, neck or back pain, headaches or other physical discomfort.

Symptoms related to grief and loss, illness, work stress and relating to others are more common in people with IDD.

Diagnostic overshadowing occurs when all symptoms a person is experiencing are attributed to a known diagnosis or disorder, when there may actually be another condition. For example, someone may display repetitive behavior as a sign of Obsessive Compulsive Disorder (OCD) that is overlooked as being a feature of Autism Spectrum Disorder (ASD).

Appearing withdrawn, a lack of observable behaviors or a decrease in functioning may still indicate an overlooked psychiatric condition. Some changes in behavior make providing supports easier.

Caregivers or support staff may tend to bring up problems that make caregiving harder. If something is less noticeable, a family member/staff person they may not think to mention it to a health care professional. For example, they may not mention that a person sleeps 12 hours a day, stopped eating or that their activity level is decreased.

Slide 6

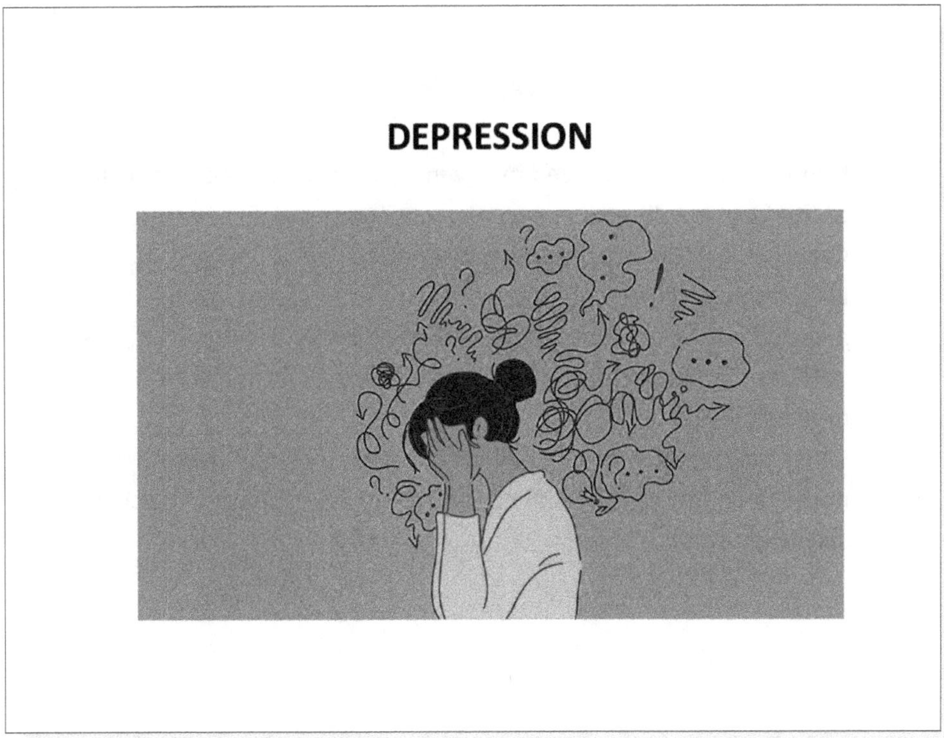

Depression occurs in individuals with intellectual disability and it is likely that this is significantly underdiagnosed as onset tends to be more insidious and changes less dramatic. An individual with ID may have reduced ability to disclose or describe their mood.

Additionally, depression is not diagnosed as quickly for people with ID as for the typical population because change in baseline is not as apparent.

Signs we look for (e.g., loss of relationships, change in recreation levels, sex, dating, etc.) may not be markedly different in a person who did not initially have a lot of these things in life.

Slide 7

Depression

- Depression is characterized by low mood, accompanied by slowing of thinking and difficulty concentrating and sustaining energy.
- Can significantly disrupt school, work, family relationships, social life, hobbies.
- A loss of interest in pleasurable activities can be observed, i.e., the person no longer attending the activities from which he/she derived pleasure.
- Other symptoms include: Feelings of hopelessness or pessimism, appetite and/or weight changes and thoughts of death or suicide; suicide attempts.

People with developmental disabilities are more likely to experience depression than people without developmental disabilities (Walton & Kerr, 2015).

Individuals with ID are often painfully aware of their value in society and often struggle with the limitations and restrictions in their lives as a result of their disability (Gentile et al., 2008).

Contributing variables to depression in persons with ID: lack of social supports, poor coping skills, medications, inability to attribute events, rates of trauma, grief and loss.

Slide 8

Depression

Presentation in Someone with IDD

- Frequent unexplained crying
- Decrease in laughter and smiling
- General irritability and subsequent aggression or self-injury
- Sad facial expression
- No longer participates in favorite activities
- Reinforcers no longer valued
- Increased time spent alone
- Refusals of most work/social activities

DM-ID-2

In the DM-ID, the DSM criteria subsets are listed on the left side and the right side lists the manifestation or presentation in a person with IDD. The right side is a listing of behavioral observations or behavioral equivalents to what is listed in the criteria subsets of the DSM. For more information of the DMI2, visit Module V in this manual, "Overview of the Diagnostic Manual for Persons with Intellectual Disabilities: DM-ID-2."

Note the importance of observation over time for accurate diagnosis of any psychiatric illness.

Slide 9

Depression

Presentation in Someone with IDD

- Measured weight changes
- Increased refusals to come to table to eat
- Unusually disruptive at meal times
- Constant food-seeking behaviors
- Disruptive at bedtime
- Repeatedly gets up at night
- Difficulty falling asleep
- No longer gets up for work/activities
- Early-morning awakening
- Over 12 hours of sleep per day
- Naps frequently

DM-ID-2

Through either self-report for people with mild levels of IDD or through obtaining data from informants, we can identify if there are any changes in weight and sleep patterns. A change in weight or sleep patterns can be a clear indication of depression. Weight gain or loss can also indicate a medical condition and should be monitored to rule out other underlying or contributing causes.

Slide 10

Depression

Presentation in Someone with IDD
• Sits for extended periods • Moves slowly • Takes longer than usual to complete activities • Restless, fidgety, pacing • Increased disruptive behavior

DM-ID-2

Psychomotor agitation can be observed when the person is irritated/restless. On the other hand, psychomotor retardation can be observed when the person's motor activity seems to be slower than baseline behavior. Baseline behavior is the "typical" behavior the person displays before any intervention is started; in other words, behavior that is steady in form, frequency and intensity even before any treatment or intervention is started. There may be a biological cause such a change in neurological functioning, seizure activity or tics. Changes should be discussed with a physician.

Slide 11

Depression

Presentation in Someone with IDD

- Needs frequent breaks to complete simple activity
- Slumped/tired body posture
- Does not complete tasks with multiple steps
- Statements like "I'm dumb," etc.
- Seeming to seek punishment
- Social isolation

DM-ID-2

A person with IDD can express fatigue/loss of energy through difficulty in completing tasks and the fatigue or loss of energy can be observed through body posture.

Feelings of worthlessness can be difficult to elicit in a person with limited verbal skills. However, those with mild/moderate levels of IDD, will often make self-deprecating statements such as "I'm stupid."

Slide 12

Depression

Presentation in Someone with IDD

- Decreased work output
- Does not stay with tasks
- Decrease in IQ upon retesting
- Preoccupation with family member's death
- Talking about committing or attempting suicide
- Fascination with violent movies/television shows

DM-ID-2

Lack of concentration can be observed by one's inability to stay on task and maintain focus.

Thoughts of death are difficult to observe in a person with severe/profound levels of IDD. However, a person with some level of verbal skills may, for example, have a preoccupation with themes of death and dying.

Slide 13

Depression

Treatment Strategies

- Psychotherapy (individual and/or group)
- Regular exercise
- Antidepressant medication
- Engaging in meaningful activities
- Learning stress management strategies
- Social skills
- Positive environment and support strategies

Lack of concentration can be observed by one's inability to stay on task and maintain focus.

Thoughts of death are difficult to observe in a person with severe/profound levels of IDD. However, a person with some level of verbal skills may, for example, have a preoccupation with themes of death and dying.

Slide 14

Wellness Approach to Depression

- Pictures or video sequences
- Relaxation
- Guided Imagery
- Mindfulness
- Employment
- Recreation
- Exercise
- Friendship and dating
- Stress management

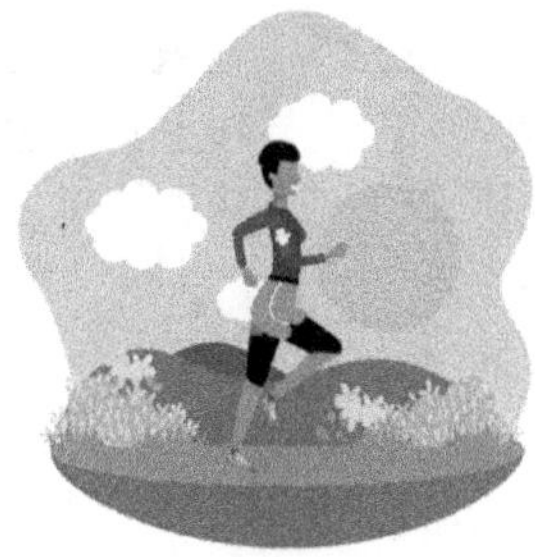

Promoting wellness and relaxation can help an individual self-manage stress, tension, worry, anger, discomfort or other feelings that can interfere with enjoying quality of life. We can encourage deep breathing for individuals who require more structure by using balloons, bubbles, party favors and other instruments. Additionally, everyday activities such as baking bread and gardening will encourage distraction, stimulate muscle involvement and promote mindfulness by engaging other senses.

Knowing the person's interests and being creative alongside them is the best strategy to help through stressful situations as well as build enduring coping skills.

For more information on support approaches and methods, review *Module VII: Positive Support Strategies and Wellness* in this training manual.

Slide 15

What symptoms of depression might look like for a person with IDD

Setup:	Set Off:	So I:	And I get or avoid:
Depression Not interested in previously motivating hobbies.	Prompted regarding "getting ready to leave/go out."	Ignore the cue and become aggressive if prompt is maintained.	Avoid going to out. activities and hobbies previously an incentive, but due to depression, formerly preferred events are no longer preferred.

Activity: Discuss how depression impacts this person's behavior. Use the strategies on the previous slides to design mental health and behavioral approaches to support this individual.

Slide 16

BIPOLAR DISORDER

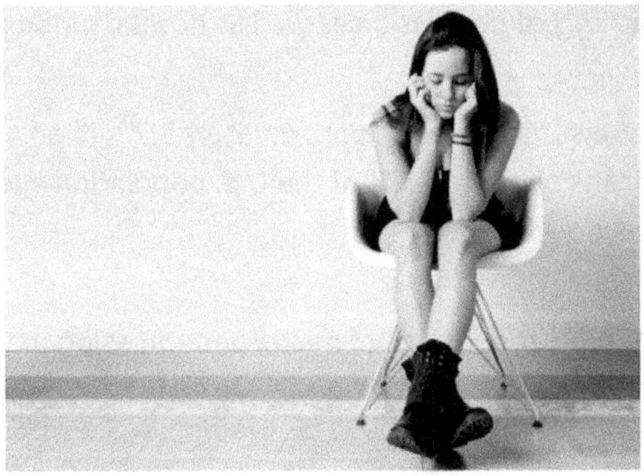

Image: freedigitalphotos.net/nenetus

Bipolar disorder is a mental disorder that causes unusual shifts in mood, energy, activity levels, concentration and the ability to carry out day-to-day tasks. It involves changes in mood, energy and activity levels ranging from periods of extreme elated, irritable or energized behavior (known as manic episodes) to very sad, indifferent or hopeless periods (known as depressive episodes). Less severe manic periods are known as hypomanic episodes.

A person will cycle over the course of weeks or months, not days.

Symptoms of mania can look like psychosis or personality disorders in a person with IDD who does not have typical language or is demonstrating behaviors presented on the following slides.

Slide 17

Bipolar Disorder

- Persons with bipolar disorder may have periods of mania and periods of depression as well as normal moods.
- Bipolar disorder affects approximately 5.7 million adult Americans or about 2.8% of the U.S. population age 18 and older every year.
- Severe bipolar episodes of mania or depression may include psychotic symptoms such as hallucinations or delusions.

National Institute of Mental Health

During an episode of mania, an individual will typically have an oversupply of confidence and energy that may lead to reckless or dangerous behavior. The length of a manic or depressed cycle may last from days to months. Without treatment, bipolar disorder can lead to poor job performance, financial difficulties, problems with family and friends and death from reckless behavior or suicide.

Slide 18

Bipolar Disorder

Presentation in Someone with IDD

- Smiling, hugging or being affectionate with people who previously were not favored by the individual
- Boisterousness
- Over-reactivity to small incidents
- Extreme excitement
- Excessive laughing and giggling
- Self-injury associated with irritability
- Enthusiastic greeting of everyone

DM-ID-2

These are common behaviors associated with mood disorder in people with IDD:

- A lack of motivation or interest may lead to refusal which may be documented as "noncompliance"
- Use behavior to provoke a reaction or create stimulation
- An effort to relieve guilty feelings
- Self-injury to alleviate unpleasant emotions
- To avoid social interaction or activities, meals, unpleasant places or people, etc.
- May engage in food-stealing/sex make oneself feel better

The manifestation of euphoric, elevated or irritable mood in a person with IDD can be observed. Episodic motor overactivity and extreme excitement are common symptoms among people with IDD.

Slide 19

Bipolar Disorder

Presentation in Someone with IDD

- Behavioral challenges when prompted to go to try to sleep
- Constantly getting up at night
- Seems rested after not sleeping (i.e., not irritable due to lack of sleep as is common in depression)

DM-ID-2

People in a manic phase generally have decreased need for sleep. This can be disruptive to others as the manic person may be pacing while others are trying to sleep. Lack of sleep related to mania is a physiological symptom and accommodations need to be made for it as a result.

Slide 20

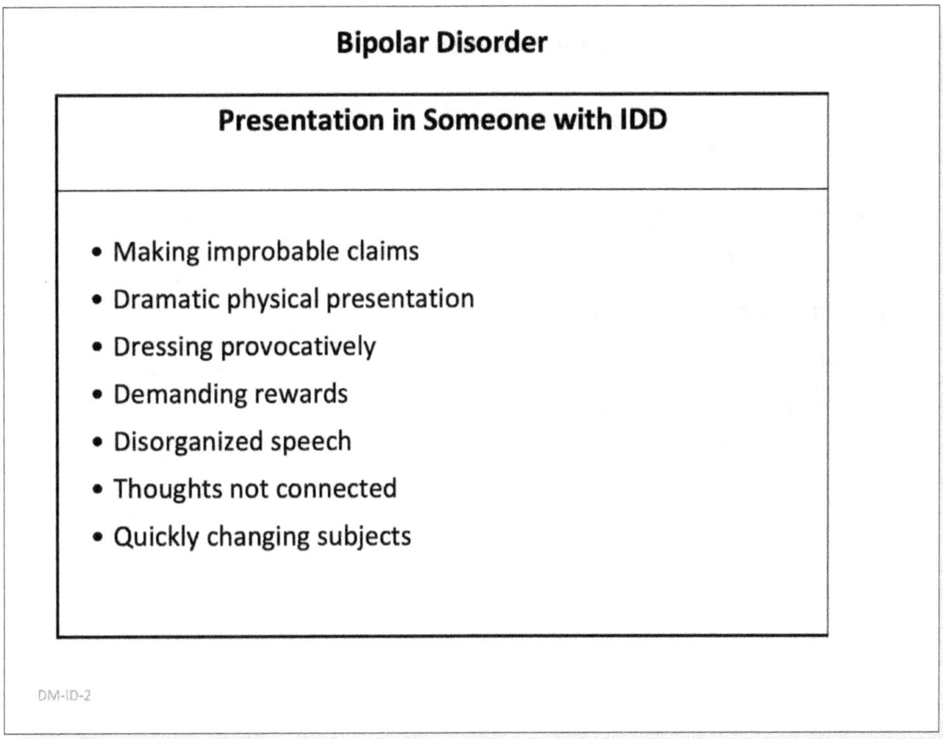

Inflated self esteem/grandiosity: For example, a person with IDD might make claims of having the ability to drive a car or having a profession that is well beyond their current ability.

Flights of ideas are difficult to ascertain in a person with no verbal skills. However, in a person with mild/moderate levels of IDD, a disorganization of speech can occur in a manic stage.

Slide 21

Bipolar Disorder

Presentation in Someone with IDD
• Increased singing • Increased swearing • Perseverative speech • Screaming • Frequent interrupting • Nonverbal communication increases • Increase in vocalizations

DM-ID-2

The presentation of pressured speech in a person with mild/moderate levels of IDD is similar to individuals who do not have IDD.

For people at the severe/profound level of IDD, the presentation of pressured speech may be screaming or an increase in volume, pressure or repetitiveness of the way the person communicates. For example, an increase in grunting sounds. Pressured speech is a tendency to speak rapidly and frenziedly, as if motivated by an urgency not apparent to the listener, it is difficult to interrupt.

Slide 22

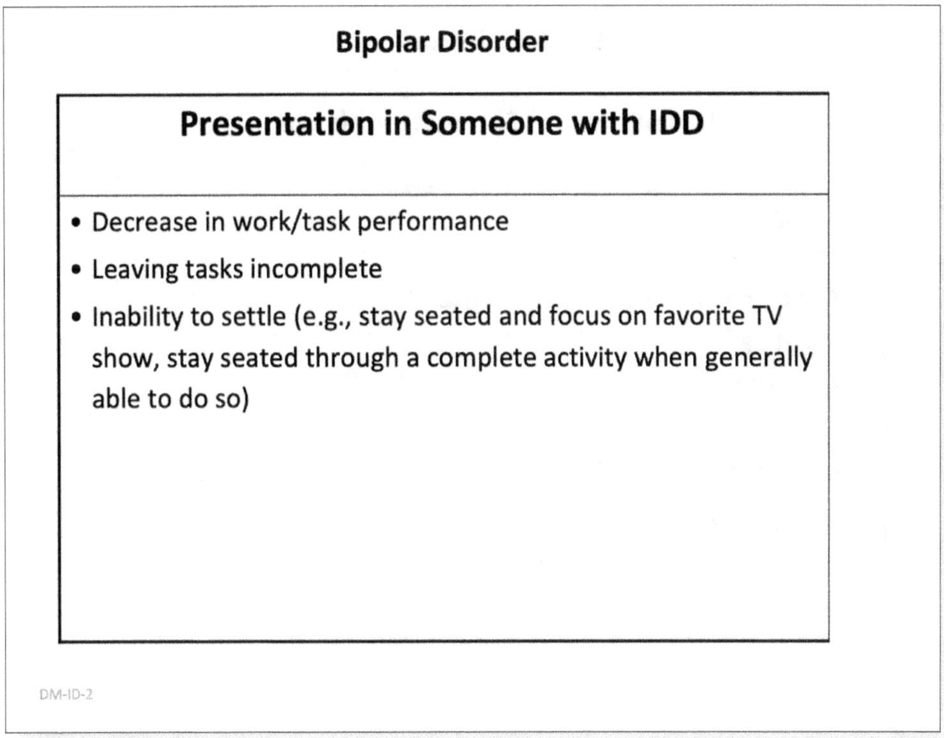

The presentation of distractibility can be observed in a person with IDD. The individual shows reduced productivity at work or a day program. When they are asked to do activities that require concentration, they may have unexplained "skill loss" or may be unable to finish their tasks.

Slide 23

Bipolar Disorder

Presentation in Someone with IDD

- Pacing
- Negativism
- Working on many activities at once
- Fidgeting
- Aggression
- Rarely sits
- Increase in masturbation
- Giving away/spending money

DM-ID-2

Observers may report that the individual with IDD engages in activities in a "sped-up manner," rarely sits down, paces and walks rapidly.

Excessive pleasurable activities may include the individual with IDD engaging in more sexual behavior or talk, reporting more sexual activity or masturbating frequently, increased eating, etc. Symptoms would be more apparent/disruptive in a shared living environment.

Negativism, in this context, refers to resisting suggestions, advice or direction. It is a behavioral attitude common in a variety of disorders including bipolar disorder.

Please note: The lists of symptoms are intended to be representative of the most common symptoms for bipolar disorder. These lists are not intended to be exhaustive or reflective of symptoms of other mood disorders.

Slide 24

Bipolar Disorder

Treatment Strategies

- **Psychotherapy with a focus on understanding and managing the disorder**
- **Environmental and social modification (i.e., increase supervision to ensure safety)**
- **Positive support strategies**
- **Mood stabilizing and antidepressant medication**

DM-ID- 2

A treatment approach needs to be multifaceted and multidisciplinary. The first line of treatment is likely to be medication treatment. This is to assist the individual to become more stable in order to benefit from other treatment and habilitative approaches. Once the person is stabilized then other supports can come into play, such as psychotherapy and positive support strategies, focus on wellness and other supports as needed.

For more information on support approaches and methods, review *Module VII: Positive Support Strategies and Wellness* in this training manual.

Slide 25

What symptoms of bipolar disorder might look like for a person with IDD

Setup:	Set Off:	So I:	And I get or avoid:
Bipolar cycling into manic phase. Not always a good sleeper. Not a lot of friends.	My DSP interrupts the activity I am busy with at 2 a.m. because it is loud (cleaning, laundry, playing guitar, watching TV).	I begin to scream and wake up my housemates.	My DSP allows me to return to activity since it is quieter than my screaming.

Activity: Discuss how bipolar disorder impacts this person's behavior. Work together to develop team-based mental and behavioral health strategies to support this person to have a better life.

Alternate Activity: Ask the group to think of another example following the format above where having information about an underlying mental health condition provides a better understanding of behavior and treatment approaches.

Slide 26

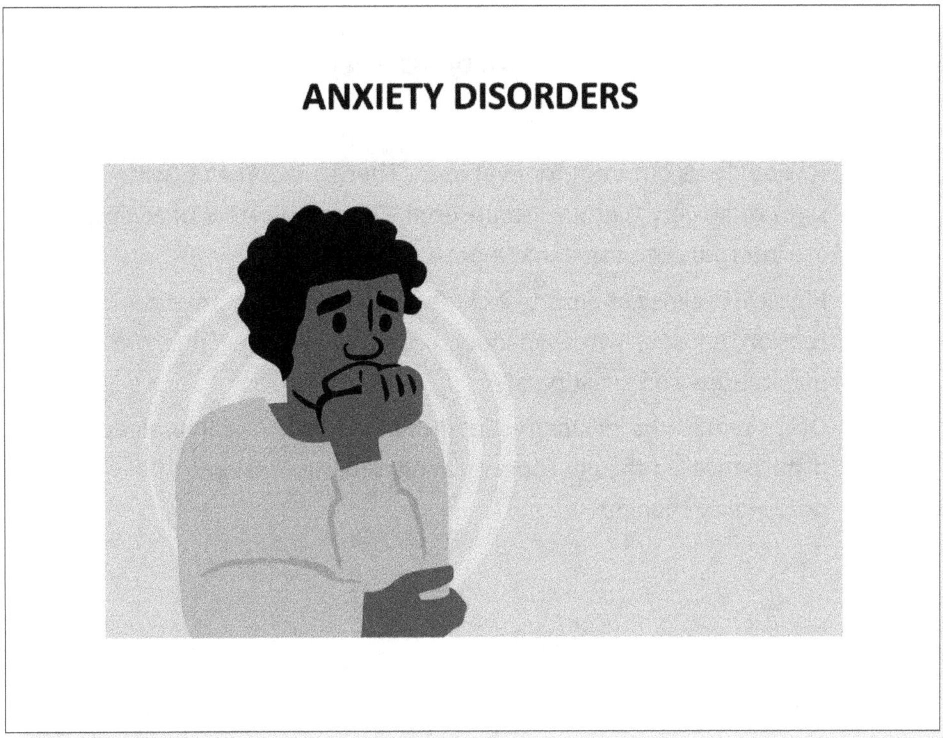

Anxiety disorders are the most common mental health concern in the United States. An estimated 40 million adults in the U.S., 18% have an anxiety disorder (NAMI, 2018). Higher rates of anxiety disorders have been reported for individuals with Intellectual and Developmental Disabilities (IDD) (Agarwal, Guanci & Appareddy, 2013).

Slide 27

Anxiety Disorders

- Anxiety feels different for everyone. There are some outward signs of anxiety that we can observe. Other indicators of anxiety are internal symptoms that a person feels.
- Physical feelings of anxiety include rapid breathing, muscle tension, nausea, increased blood pressure, sweating, heart palpitations and chest pain.
- Other symptoms include restlessness, fatigue, irritability, sleep disturbances, difficulty concentrating, muscle tension, personality changes.

People with IDD may be more likely to experience an anxiety disorder due to social and communication differences, varying sensory needs, limited experiences, trauma history, limited coping skills and increased grief and loss.

Slide 28

Anxiety Disorders

Among the anxiety disorders listed in the DSM-5 are:

- **Generalized anxiety disorder:** This disorder involves excessive, anxiety or worry occurring more days than not for at least six months, about a number of events or activities.
- **Specific phobias:** Marked fear or anxiety about specific objects or situations, such as snakes, heights, flying, etc.
- **Social anxiety disorder:** Marked fear or anxiety about one or more social situations in which the person is exposed to possible scrutiny by others.
- **Panic disorder:** Recurrent, unexpected panic attacks.

APA, 2013

Anxiety is the body's reaction to stress; it includes emotions like feeling nervous, afraid or uneasy and physical signs such as rapid heart rapid, headache, upset stomach or sweating. Most anxiety comes from worry/fear about upcoming events, it is worse when person feels a lack of control over those events. It causes changes in our emotions (feeling scared, nervous, worried) and in our body (nausea, headache, fast heartbeat).

An anxiety disorder is a medical condition that develops when worry or fear is too much to manage or control and interferes with having a happy, healthy life. An anxiety disorder is diagnosed if the person's response is not appropriate for the situation, if the person cannot control the response or if the anxiety interferes with normal functioning.

Slide 29

Anxiety Disorders

Presentation in Someone with IDD

- Restlessness
- Easily fatigued
- Difficulty concentrating
- Irritability
- Muscle tension
- Sleep disturbances
- Fear
- Avoidance

DM-ID-2

Someone may communicate discomfort, anxiety or worry through changes in behavior.

Diagnostic criteria that rely on subjective descriptions of symptoms are difficult to apply or detect in those with communication/cognitive problems. Therefore, incorporating behavioral equivalents within the context of cognitive, developmental and adaptive functioning, are proposed to facilitate accurate diagnosis. Excessive worry and difficulty controlling the worry may present in persons with oral communication skills as perseverative talk about the topic or issue creating the worry (self-talk or to others).

Difficulty concentrating or mind going blank are very difficult to apply in persons with severe IDD and inapplicable for persons with profound IDD. However, anxiety can be observed as self-injury (skin-picking, pinching, etc.), pacing, inability to settle (restlessness), muscle rigidity (tension) and changes in sleep patterns, hyperarousal, exaggerated startle responses, etc.

A person with IDD and anxiety may experience anxiety as a loss of skills that had been acquired, particularly for tasks with several steps in the sequence of completion like doing laundry, meal preparation, personal hygiene, etc.

Please note: The lists of symptoms are intended to be representative of the most common symptoms for generalized anxiety disorders. These lists are not intended to be exhaustive or reflective of symptoms of other types of mood disorders.

Slide 30

Anxiety Disorders

Anxiety and Repetitive Behavior

- Some anxiety disorders are accompanied by behaviors which are common in autism spectrum disorder (ASD) and other disorders.
- Many people, including individuals with ASD, engage in repetitive behaviors to help feel organized or comfortable.
- Compulsions are time-consuming and unhelpful behaviors. They interfere with other important and enjoyable areas of life. Behaviors are no longer functional or helpful if they cause distress rather than provide comfort.

Sometimes anxiety can look and feel like other conditions such as ADHD (Attention-Deficit/Hyperactivity Disorder), autism or mood disorders. Many people with an anxiety disorder also have a physical illness, which can make their symptoms worse and delay diagnosis. PTSD and OCD are closely related to anxiety and can overlap.

Repetitive behavior is a common coping mechanism used by persons who experience ASD and others to help with focus, with narrowing interests and to maintain comfort. Some repetitive behaviors are preferred activities (provide structure, order and predictability and help people cope with the uncertainties of daily life).

Obsessive Compulsive Disorder (OCD) is a type of mental illness that includes strong and powerful, ongoing thoughts called "obsessions" and repetitive, unhelpful behaviors or compulsions.

Obsessions are persistent, unwanted images or thoughts that become intrusive (unwelcome). They come from anxiety and cause more anxiety and distress. Compulsions are time-consuming and unhelpful behaviors. They interfere with other important and enjoyable areas of life. Sometimes a compulsion (behavior) can relieve or calm anxiety, but the obsession returns and a ritual (procedure or habit) of behavior develops.

Many people have behaviors they repeat to keep them feel organized or comfortable. For a person with OCD, the compulsion (behavior) is not helpful because it does not eliminate the obsession (thought). An ongoing, unhealthy pattern develops and the anxiety gets worse for the person.

Consider interventions based on level of risk and interference with daily living. Compulsions that can lead to injury (e.g., skin-picking) need to be addressed intensely and quickly. Provide a sensory-rich environment and opportunities to address anxiety related to obsessions and compulsions (e.g., teach relaxation skills, develop self-awareness).

Offer alternatives: Help the person identify preferred items or incongruent activities that block compulsive behavior (hand massages, clay sculptures) or change the setting or environment to minimize discomfort.

Slide 31

Anxiety Disorders

Treatment Strategies

- Psychotherapy with a focus on understanding and managing the disorder
- Environmental and social modification
- Social skill training
- Regular exercise
- Wellness-based approaches
- Learning stress management strategies
- Anti-anxiety medication

Hughes, 2006

A multidisciplinary treatment approach is recommended for generalized anxiety disorder. Generalized anxiety, when caught early, can be more easily treated successfully. This can include medication as well as non-psychopharmacological approaches. Once the person is stabilized then other supports can come into play, such as psychotherapy and positive environmental adaptations and other positive supports as needed. Modifications for treatments are found in Module IX: Adapting Therapy Practices.

Relaxation strategies are also effective in distracting the person from the cause of the potential anxiety and focusing them on an alternative activity or behavior. For example, if someone is very stressed about being in an elevator, they can participate in a relaxation exercise involving a combination of deep breathing and counting while closing their eyes and visualizing a calming setting for the duration of the elevator ride.

Other approaches for supporting individuals with anxiety include:

- Increase the amount of structure in the environment to add predictability and clarify expectations for individuals.
- Provide visual cues and gestural prompts can be more effective than verbal instruction when communicating.
- Provide opportunities for stress management, including exercise and preferred recreational activities.
- Support individuals in building and accessing coping strategies and social supports that address anxiety (desensitization, relaxation, journaling).

For more information on support approaches and methods, review *Module VII: Positive Support Strategies and Wellness* in this training manual.

Slide 32

What symptoms of anxiety might look like for a person with IDD

Setup:	Set Off:	So I:	And I get or avoid:
"I experience an anxiety disorder and autism." Low tolerance for "things out of place." Sensitive to noise and crowds. Poor verbal skills.	Sees item "out of place" (e.g. thread on clothing, jars on a shelf, store display).	Charge at items or person to "fix" or rearrange, knocking down things in the process.	I fix the item out of place. I feel relief and control over my environment.

Activity: Discuss how this person's anxiety impacts their behavior. What other factors are contributing to observable signs of anxiety?

Slide 33

PERSONALITY DISORDERS

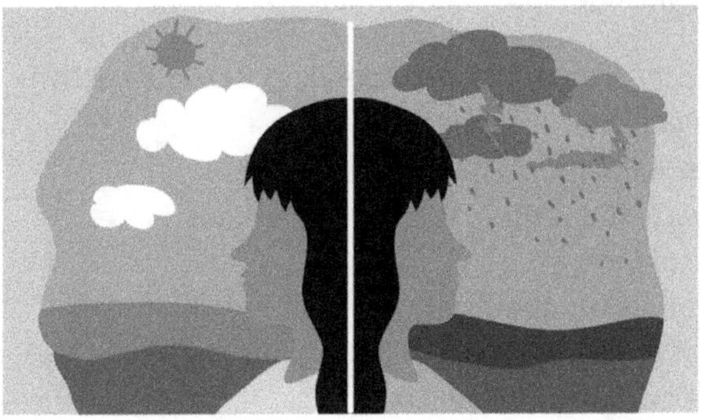

Personality disorders cause difficulty perceiving and relating to situations and people, including self.

Borderline personality disorder, the most common, is adapted in the DM-ID 2 and has overlapping symptoms with mania (bipolar disorder), anxiety, depression and the experiences of disability, including grief, loss and trauma.

Slide 34

Personality Disorders

Personality disorders are mental health disorders characterized by inflexible and unhealthy patterns of thinking, feeling and behaving.

Symptoms include:

- Impulsivity with risk taking, spending, sexuality activity
- Overreliance on caregivers
- Mood swings
- Volatile relationship
- Social isolation
- Need for instant gratification
- Mistrust of others (especially strangers)
- Intense anxiety or irritability
- Poor impulse control

Observation and documentation of symptoms in persons with IDD is important since the challenge of staff turnover can limit diagnostic information. Additionally, consistency (or lack of) in taking medications can change presentation of symptoms.

Slide 35

Personality Disorders

Among the different types of personality disorders listed in the DSM-5 are:

- **General Personality Disorder:** Enduring pattern of inner thoughts or behavior that deviates markedly from the expectations of the individual's culture.
- **Paranoid Personality Disorder:** Pervasive distrust or suspiciousness of others such that their behavior is interpreted as malevolent.
- **Dependent Personality Disorder:** Pervasive and excessive need to be taken care of that leads to submissive and clinging behavior and fear of separation.

APA, 2013

People with personality disorders experience patterns of behavior, mood, impulsiveness and social interaction that can interfere with relationships with other people in their lives and create distress in those relationships. The symptoms of different personality disorders vary depending on type.

Slide 36

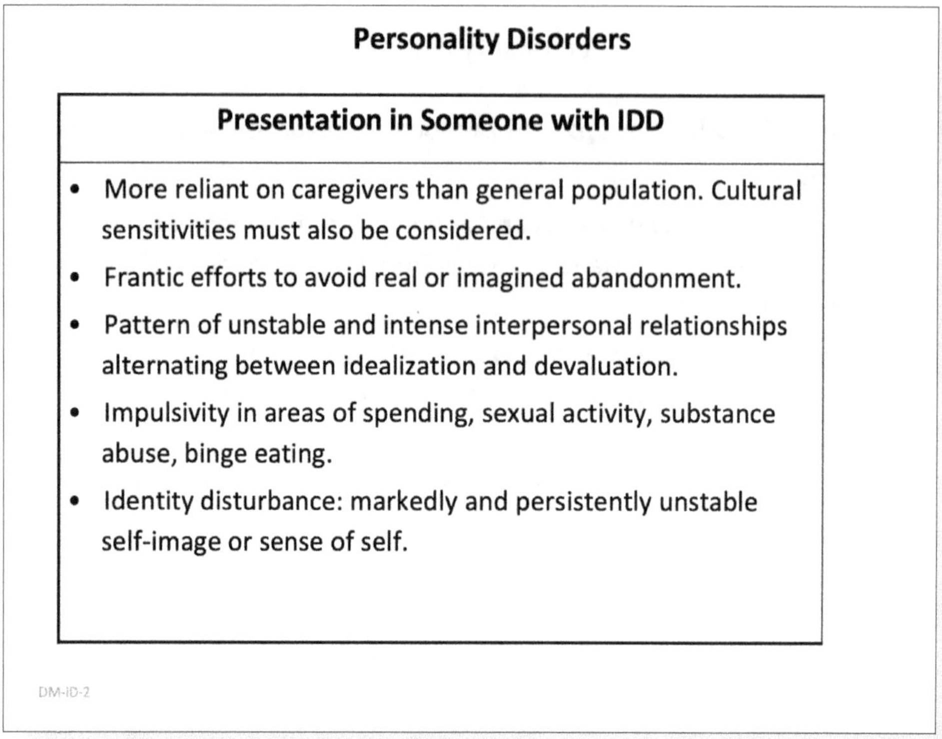

Fear of abandonment can present as acts designed to "get rid of" others, unreasonable demands of staff at times, repeatedly calling family members on the phone, dramatic acts intended to keep the person from leaving.

Patterns of unstable relationships can often be observed in the relationships between the person and their support staff, when applicable. The person may alternately choose one staff as a particular "favorite" on one occasion and adamantly refuse their involvement on other occasions.

People who have IDD can display identity disturbances by stating they are someone other than who they are.

Slide 37

Personality Disorders

Presentation in Someone with IDD
• Recurrent suicidal behavior, gestures, threats or self-mutilating behavior. Note: Self-injury can be a frequent problem for people with IDD and can be attributed to different causes. • Irritability, intense episodic dysphoria/feeling of unease, anxiety usually lasting only a few hours. • Chronic feelings of emptiness which may be difficult to express.

DM-ID-2

Mood reactivity presents as extreme changes in mood due to minor or nonexistent issues.

Personality disorders cause difficulty perceiving and relating to situations and people, including self. Borderline personality disorder, the most common, is adapted in the DM-ID-2 and has overlapping symptoms with mania (bipolar disorder), anxiety, depression and the experiences of disability including grief, loss and trauma.

Slide 38

Personality Disorders

Treatment Strategies

- Individual or group therapy—cognitive and dialectical behavior therapy are most effective
- Environmental and social modification
- Social skill training
- Regular exercise
- Positive behavioral supports
- Psychotropic medication can be helpful for primary presenting symptoms
- Emotional regulation
- Learning stress management strategies/stress tolerance
- Positive identity development

Therapies should focus on helping the person understand their illness; developing skills to control impulsivity; identifying ways to recognize and change negative thinking.

For more information on support approaches and methods, review *Module VII: Positive Support Strategies and Wellness* and *Module IX: Adapting Therapy Practices* in this training manual.

Slide 39

What symptoms of borderline personality disorder might look like for a person with IDD

Setup:	Set Off:	So I:	And I get or avoid:
Borderline personality disorder. Lots of staff turnover. Live with roommates who are not good peer match, prefer company and role of staff. New manager creates conflict on the team.	Staff are arguing back and forth.	Make the divide between staff bigger escalating their argument.	I get to watch the conflict and drama that result. I am in the "starring role."

Often, traditional approaches may focus on the pattern of behaviors or symptoms without recognizing how setting events, such as diagnosis, can impact how a person interacts with others/the environment.

Reliable and valid assessment of behaviors is essential in empirically verifying prevention and intervention for individuals with intellectual or developmental disabilities (Rojhan and Schroder, 2013).

When we understand the underlying causes of behavior and symptoms, we can address them in a more meaningful way.

Activity: How can we address the "setup" of this behavior pattern while addressing the mental health diagnosis?

MODULE 6

Slide 40

SCHIZOPHRENIA AND OTHER PSYCHOSIS

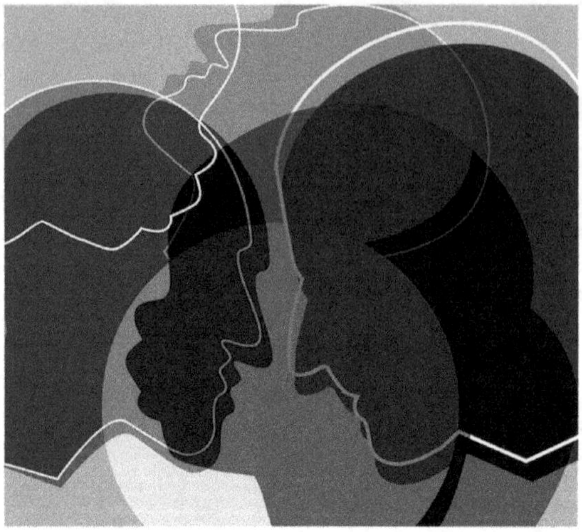

Slide 41

Psychosis

- The defining characteristics of psychosis are delusions, hallucinations and disorganized speech or behavior.
- Clinicians should be aware that any significant change in behavior can signify the possibility of psychosis (e.g., increase in self-injury, aggressive behavior or atypical behavior for the person).

DM-ID, 2007

Schizophrenia is characterized by thoughts or experiences that seem incongruent with reality, disorganized speech or behavior and decreased participation in daily activities.

There is evidence that current diagnostic criteria from DSM-5 can be used reliably for people with IDD, but behavioral disturbances seem more significant for people with severe to profound IDD than with mild IDD. This has been noted in the area of self-injury (Rojhan, 2002).

Slide 42

Psychosis

Among the psychotic disorders listed in the DSM-5 are:

- Schizoaffective disorder
- Delusional disorder
- Schizophreniform disorder
- Substance/medication-induced psychotic disorder

APA, 2013

Psychotic disorders are characterized by abnormal thinking and perceptions and loss of touch with reality. The main symptoms are hallucinations and delusions. Hallucinations are false perceptions (e.g., seeing something that isn't there, hearing a voice that isn't there). Delusions are false beliefs, such as believing one has superhuman strength when one does not.

Slide 43

Psychosis

Presentation in Someone with IDD

- Delusions
- Hallucinations
- Disorganized speech
- Grossly disorganized behavior
- Negative symptoms (i.e., affect flattening, newly evidenced inability to speak, general lack of motivation or desire to pursue meaningful goals)

NOTE: Developmentally appropriate self-talk, imaginary friends, fantasy play and beliefs based on faulty learning can be confused with hallucinations and delusions.

DM-ID-2

Schizoaffective disorder is largely a disorder of mood and thought. Common symptoms are auditory hallucinations, paranoid thinking, and disorganized speech and thinking.

Symptoms of depressive bipolar disorder include irritability, guilt, unpredictable mood swings, restlessness, slowed speech and movement, and increased sleep. It also involves an increased tendency to lose contact with reality (psychosis).

Slide 44

Psychosis

Treatment Strategies

- Structure and consistency
- Social skills and stress management teaching
- Vocational training
- Positive support strategies
- Education regarding schizophrenia
- Recreation therapy
- Antipsychotic medication

There is evidence to indicate that psycho-social or cognitive therapy, and peer support groups can be effective in conjunction with medications.

External structure can be helpful to people who lack internal structure. Provide organization that should be flexible to allow for change if a person feels uncomfortable or unsafe.

- Provide validation and active listening.
- Avoid joking about delusions or beliefs.
- Add structure.
- Be consistent.
- Use a calm, direct tone of voice.
- Reduce stress or stimulation.

For more information on support approaches and methods, review *Module VII: Positive Support Strategies and Wellness* and *Module IX: Adapting Therapy Practices* in this training manual.

Slide 45

What symptoms of psychosis might look like for a person with IDD...

Setup:	Set Off:	So I:	And I get or avoid:
Psychosis Lives with three other people with IDD.	Auditory hallucination at breakfast.	Yell back to "the voice."	Roommates take their coffee out to the porch.

Activity: How can we address the "setup" of this behavior pattern while addressing the mental health diagnosis?

Consider what the person gets or avoids as a result of behaviors.

Slide 46

Indicators of a Mental Health Condition

- There is rapid onset, increase or change in behavior or symptoms
- There are changes in sleep or eating patterns
- There is a decrease in living skills or change in appearance or hygiene
- There is evidence of purposeful self-harm
- There are signs of hallucination or delusion
- There is co-occurring substance abuse
- The behavior/symptoms occurs across all environments, not just one specific setting

Understanding behavior is an important part of the assessment process. However, consider behavior as a possible sign of an underlying mental health condition to prevent psychiatric disorders from being misidentified or overlooked entirely. For example, if someone's performance is declining at work, it is an opportunity to check in with them or consider other symptoms of a possible mental health concern.

If moving to a different location eliminates or reduces the challenge, it suggests the cause was likely due to the environment. For instance, a person may be distracted and unfocused in a noisy, crowded work setting but concentrate better in a less stimulating space. They were responding to a temporary challenge in the environment.

Medical or health symptoms that are unrelated to injury will be more insidious (develop slowly)—ulcers and arthritis don't happen overnight.

There are changes in sleep or eating patterns related to mood and affect, less so around discomfort, pain, acid reflux, dental issues (rule out these things or they have been addressed).

For more information, visit *Module III: Comprehensive Assessment Practices* in this manual.

MODULE 6

References: Module VI

American Psychiatric Association. (2013). *Diagnostic and statistical manual of mental disorders* (5th ed.). Washington, DC.

Agarwal, R., Guanci, N., & Appareddy, V. L. (2013). Issues in treating patients with intellectual disabilities. *Psychiatric Times.*

Brown, J. (2015). *The Emotion Regulation Skills System for Cognitively Challenged Clients: A DBT-Informed Approach.* New York: Guilford Press.

Deb, S., Thomas, M. & Bright, C. (2001). Mental disorder in adults with intellectual disability: prevalence of functional psychiatric illness among a community-based population aged between 16 and 64 years. *Journal of Intellectual Disability Research*, 45, 495–505.

Fletcher, R., Loschen, E., Stavrakaki, C., & First, M. (Eds.). (2007). *Diagnostic Manual – Intellectual Disability (DM-ID): A Clinical Guide for Diagnosis of Mental Disorders in Persons with Intellectual Disability.* Kingston, NY: NADD Press.

Gentile, J. P. & Jackson, C. S. (2008). Supportive psychotherapy with the dual diagnosis patient co-occurring mental illness/intellectual disabilities. *Psychiatry*, Vol. 5, pp. 49-57. PMCID: PMC2710105.

Hemmings, C. P. (2006). Schizophrenia spectrum disorders in people with intellectual disabilities. *Current Opinion in Psychiatry*, 19, 470-4.

McGilvery, Sharon and Sweetland, Darlene. (2011). *Intellectual Disability and Mental Health: A Training Manual in Dual Diagnosis.*

Matson, J. L., Barrett, R., & Helsel, W. J. (1988). Depression in mentally retarded children. *Research in Developmental Disabilities*, 9, 39-46.

Reid, K. A., Smiley, E. and Cooper, S-A. 2, (2011). Prevalence of anxiety disorders in adults with intellectual disabilities. *Journal of Intellectual Disability*

Research, Vol. 55, pp. 172-81.

Rojahn, J., Matson, J., Lott D. J., Esbensen, A. (2002). The Behavior Problems Inventory: An Instrument for the Assessment of Self-Injury, Stereotyped Behavior, and Aggression/Destruction in Individuals with Developmental Disabilities. *Journal of Autism and Developmental Disorders* 31(6):577-88.

Rojahn, J., Schroder S., Mayo-Ortega, L., Oyama-Ganiko, R., LeBlanc, J., Marques, J., and Berke, E. (2013). Validity and Reliability of the Behavior Problems Inventory, the Aberrant Behavior Checklist, and the Repetitive Behavior Scale. *Research in Developmental Disabilities* Volume 34, Issue 5.

National Institute of Mental Health. Depression Basics. National Institute of Mental Health. Washington, D.C. [Online] n.d. https://www.nimh.nih.gov/health/publications/depression/index.shtml.

Shooshtari, S., Martens, P. J., Burchill, C. A., Dik, N. & Naghipur, S. (201). Prevalence of depression and dementia among adults with developmental disabilities in Manitoba, Canada. *International Journal of Family Medicine*, Vol. 319574. doi:10.1155/2011/319574.

Walton & Kerr. (2015). Severe intellectual disability: Systematic review of the prevalence and nature of presentation of unipolar depression. Walton, C. & Kerr, M. 29, s.l.: *Journal of Applied Research in Intellectual Disabilities.*

Module VII

Positive Support Strategies and Wellness

Slide 2

Learning Objectives

- Discuss five principles for achieving a therapeutic relationship.
- Name three special considerations when conducting therapy with people who have IDD/MI.
- Describe the main characteristics and components of positive behavior supports.

Slide 3

In this module, we will discuss the following advanced support strategies:

1. Positive behavior supports
2. Communication tone
3. Environmental
4. Choice and self-determination
5. Relaxation techniques
6. Verbal strategies

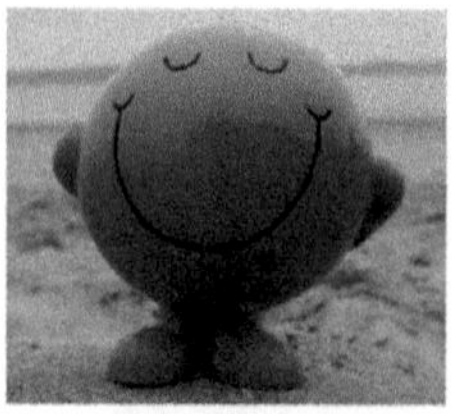

Slide 4

Positive Behavior Support

Positive Behavior Support (PBS) involves the changing situations and events that people with problem behaviors experience in order to reduce the likelihood of their occurrence and increase social, personal and professional quality in their lives.

Carr & Sidener, 2002

Positive behavior support (PBS) is an approach to behavior intervention largely derived from applied behavior analysis (ABA) that uses a system to understand what maintains an individual's challenging behaviors and a holistic, person-centered approach to addressing them. People's inappropriate behaviors are difficult to change because they are functional: they serve a purpose for the person. These behaviors are supported by reinforcement in the environment.

Positive behavior support (PBS) developed in the 1980s and 1990s as an approach to enhance quality of life and minimize challenging behavior (Carr & Sidener, 2002). PBS might require a "whatever it takes" approach for people with IDD/MI (Klaehn, 2019).

Slide 5

What Does PBS Consider?

- Values about the rights and dignity of people who have disabilities and self-determination
- Practical science about how learning and behavior change occur
- Biomedical concerns
- Lifestyle concerns
- Changes in systems of support
- Team-based approaches

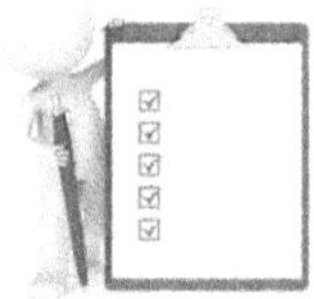

Carr & Sidener, 2002

Carr & Sidener (2002) described PBS as "an applied science that uses educational methods to expand an individual's behavior repertoire and systems change methods to redesign an individual's living environment to first enhance the individual's quality of life and, second, to minimize their problem behavior." It was developed out of an identified need to eliminate aversive (unpleasant or punitive) consequences with people who have intellectual/developmental disabilities.

Human rights are in the forefront of considering how to address problem behaviors. Many problem behaviors are learned, and as such, teaching new skills is often the most important intervention. Other problem behaviors are caused by physical problems, such as dental pain. Idle hands are the devil's work tools, and bored people might seek entertainment with actions we consider problems.

Slide 6

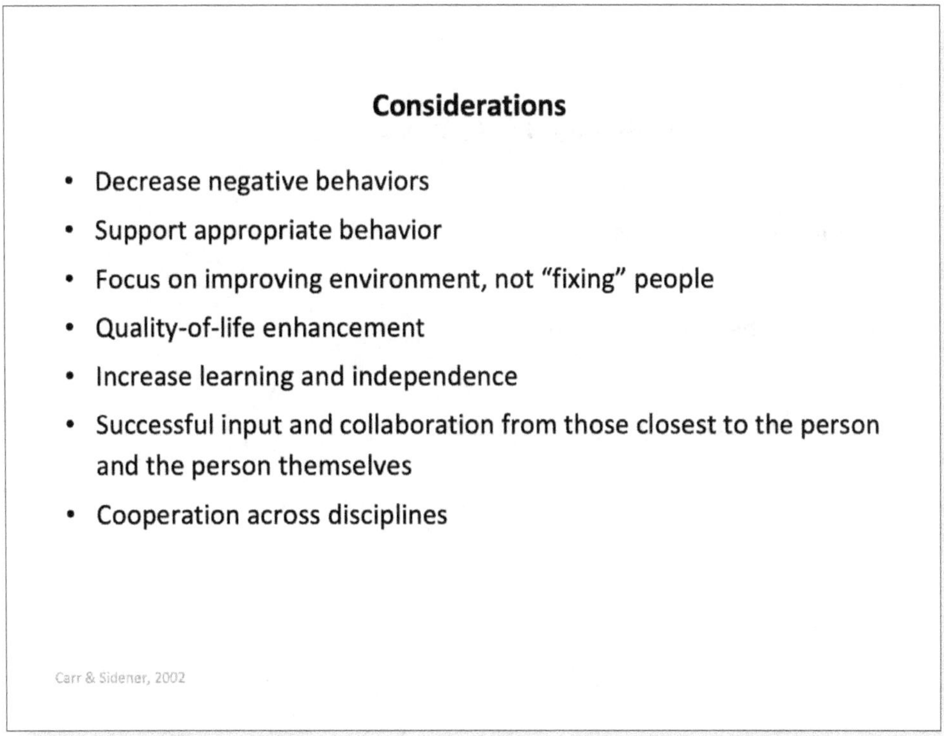

PBS values include commitments to respect for the individual, meaningful outcomes, dignity, normalization, inclusion in the community, person-centered planning, self-determination and stakeholder participation, among others.

Slide 7

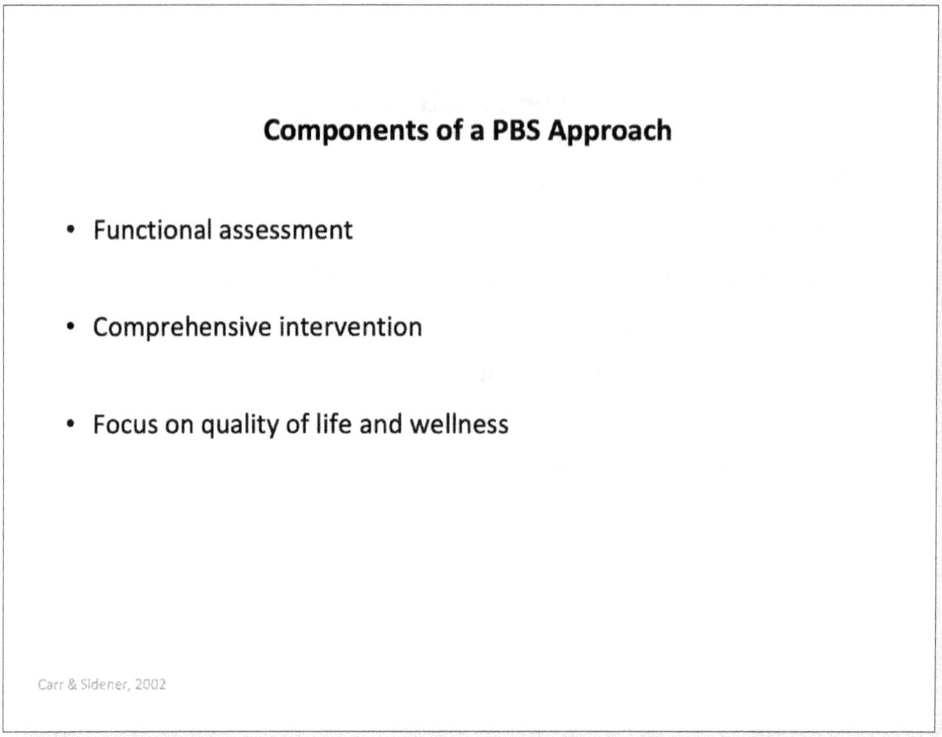

Components of a functional assessment include:

- A clear description of the problem behaviors
- Events, times and situations that predict when behaviors will and will not occur (i.e., setting events)
- Consequences that maintain the problem behaviors (the function)
- Summary statements or hypotheses
- Direct observation data to support the hypotheses

Interventions include:

1. Proactive strategies for changing the environment so triggering events are removed,

2. Teaching new skills that replace problem behaviors,

3. Eliminating or minimizing natural reinforcement for problem behavior and

4. Maximizing clear reinforcement for appropriate behavior.

The underlying focus is overall enhancement of the quality of life of the person with a meaningful life, meaningful activities and relationships, and addressing the underlying causes for problem behaviors.

Slide 8

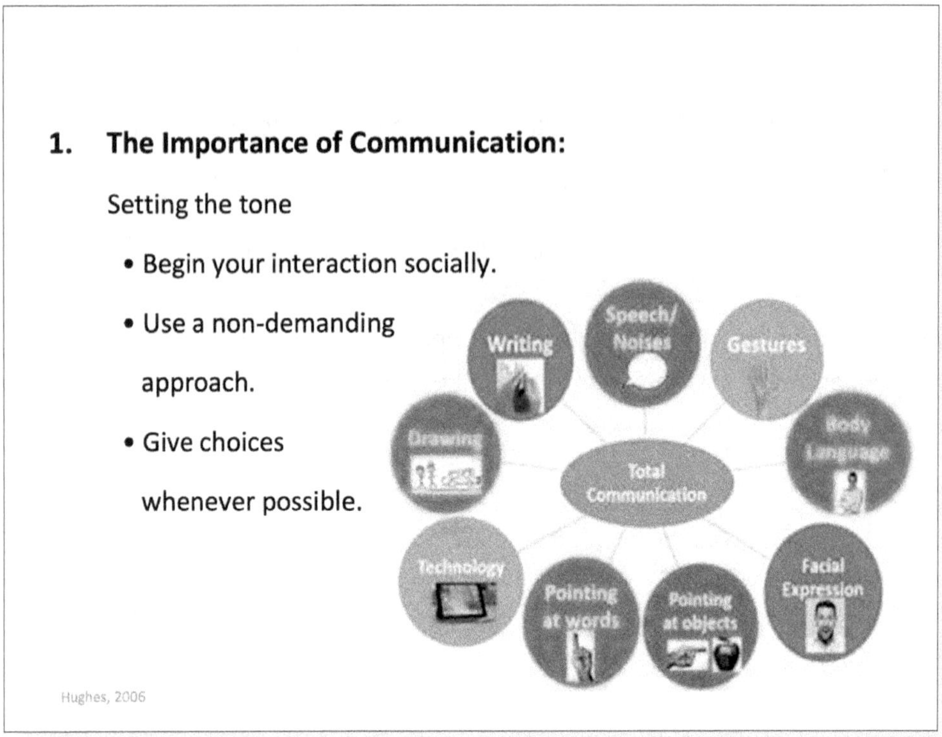

The manner in which we approach others can have a significant impact on their feelings and behavior. If we are tense or anxious, the person we are interacting with is likely to become tense or anxious. Since tension or anxiety can serve as contributing events for problem behavior, we must try to ensure our actions do not create these feelings in others. On the other hand, if our actions contribute to positive emotions, these emotions can serve as contributing events for appropriate behavior.

Slide 9

2. Environmental Contributors to Problem Behaviors

- Important to evaluate the environment
- Look for things that might be contributing to, or triggering, problem behaviors

NOTE: Important to look at environment from the person's perspective.

Griffiths, Gardner & Nugent, 19998

Before implementing treatment strategies for problem behavior, the places in which the behavior occurs should be assessed. When we evaluate the environment in which the problem behavior is occurring, we are looking for things that might be contributing to, or triggering, these difficulties. Features of the environment that may serve as triggers or contributing events include:

- Noise
- Uncomfortable temperatures
- Poor lighting
- Uncomfortable clothes
- Lack of privacy, visual overstimulation, limited space

It is important to look at the environment from the individual's perspective. For example, a room that seems perfectly quiet and calm for one person, may be experienced as overstimulating by a person with autism.

Slide 10

Exercise

Activity: Consider environmental contributors and solutions for the following behaviors:

- Eduardo has been removing his clothes in the classroom. This only occurs in the winter months when he is often wearing sweaters.
- Laura will scream and bite her hand at the kitchen table during meal times.
- Angel bangs his head against the window on the school bus. Recently, the bus changed routes, so this changed the order of his pick-up and the location of his seat on the bus.

Slide 11

3. Providing Choice and Self-Determination

Guiding Principle: Choice has positive benefits:

- Increases community integration
- Increases adaptive behavior
- Improves overall quality of life
- Decreases problem behavior

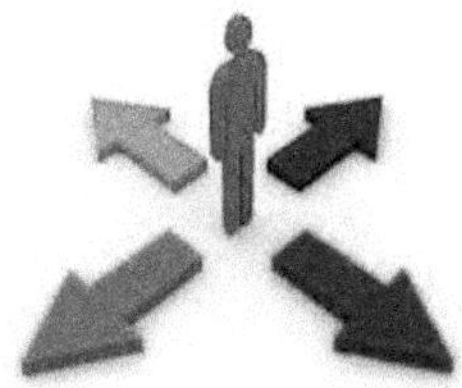

Providing individuals with choice and control over their lives is a founding principle in person-centered planning, self-determination and many other positive initiatives undertaken by families, self-advocates and professionals over the past 10 to 20 years. The promotion of choice and control is based on the belief that individuals prefer to have choices and that making choices for oneself has positive benefits.

Research on this topic suggests that when individuals with an intellectual/developmental disability have choice and control in their lives they experience increased community integration, as well as increases in adaptive behavior (Kern et al., 1998). This makes a good deal of sense when we think about it. After all, if an individual has, for example, a choice in what they are going to eat for dinner, it seems logical they would be more interested in learning to prepare the meal.

Slide 12

4. Relaxation Techniques

The purpose is to help the individual self manage and reduce stress, tension and/or angry feelings.

Relaxation strategies distract the person from the source of the stress and place focus on appropriate behavior.

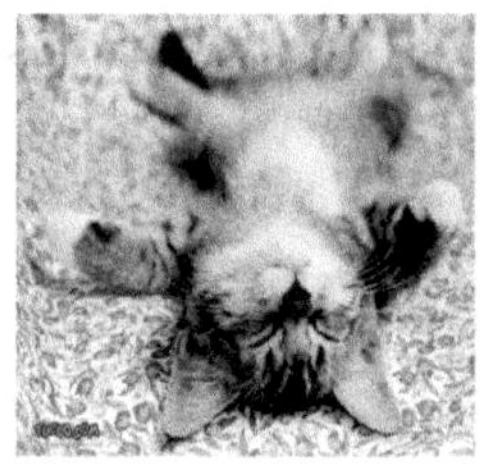

Hughes, 2006

The use of calming or relaxation techniques is an often-overlooked strategy in helping to prevent problem behavior. The teaching of calming strategies really serves one purpose. That purpose is to help the individual self-manage stress, tension or anger, all of which may serve as contributing or triggering events for problem behavior. Relaxation strategies are also effective because they distract the person from the source of the stress and focus the person on an appropriate behavior. There are many types of relaxation, but we give the most common and simplest strategy here as an example.

Deep Breathing:

1. Sit or lie down
2. Breathe in slowly through the nose and try to ensure the stomach rises
3. Slowly exhale while counting or saying "relax"
4. Repeat 10 times

Slide 13

Let's Practice Together
PMR: Progressive Muscle Relaxation

Sit in a relaxed position.
Focus on yourself and on achieving relaxation in specific body muscles.
Tune out all other thoughts.
Squeeze fists together tightly. Slowly count to five and release.
Shrug your shoulders up to your ears for five seconds. Relax.
Arch your back off the floor for five seconds. Relax.
Squeeze legs tightly and slowly count to five and release.
Repeat for other body parts that are tense.
Avoid body parts that are sore or uncomfortable.

Guide the participants in progressive muscle relaxation (PMR), cautioning attendees to avoid sleep. Ask the attendees what their experiences were in practicing PMR.

Slide 14

What Do You Find Relaxing?

Activity: Think of an activity that you find relaxing:

- Playing an instrument? Listening to music? Attending concert?
- Taking a walk or hiking?
- Word puzzles or board games?
- Dancing, aerobics, jogging or other exercise?
- Watching TV? Going to the movies?
- Cooking, reading, sewing, scrapbooking?

Using your interest and familiarity, design an activity for an individual or group in the setting where you work that promotes proactive relaxation opportunities. Build the most successful ideas into your regular routine!

Slide 15

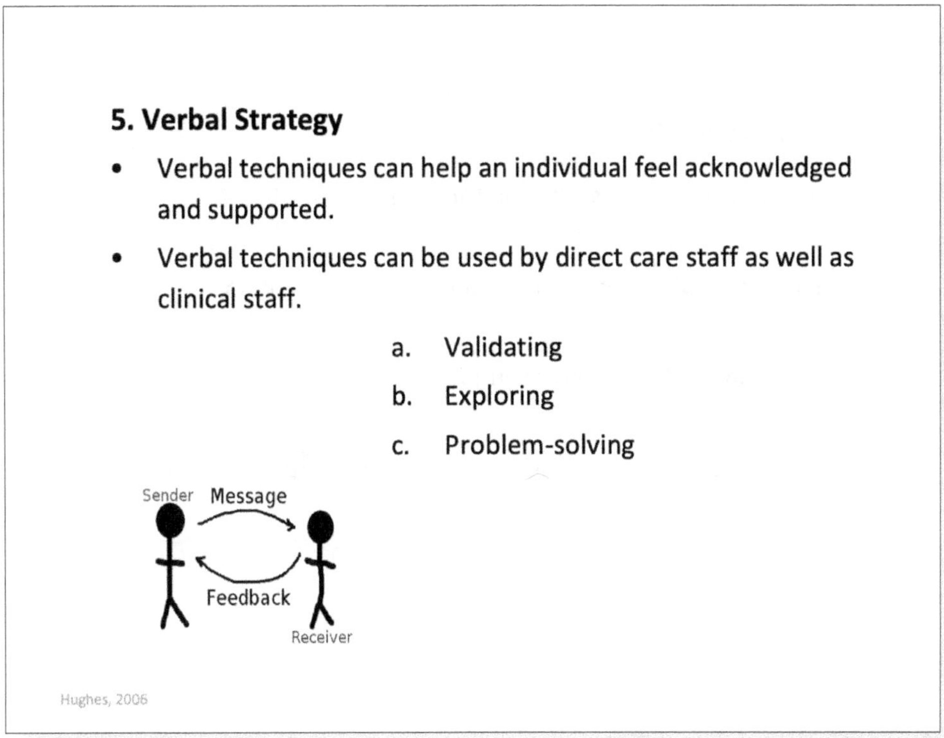

How we use our words can have a significant impact on whether an angry or agitated individual will engage in problem behavior. By using simple verbal strategies, we can communicate that we are sincerely interested in the person, are concerned about the person's problems and are willing to help. When we communicate feelings such as these, we can often prevent problem behavior from occurring.

Exploring, validating and problem-solving can help develop a therapeutic relationship and thereby help prevent problem behavior.

Chaplin, E., Craig, T., McCarthy, J., & Bouras, N. (2017). The SAINT: A guided self-help approach for people with intellectual disabilities. *Journal of Mental Health Research in Intellectual Disabilities*, 11, 237-252.

Slide 16

5. a) Validating

Validating involves confirming the person's emotions.

An example of this is shown in the following scenario:

Jack: "Everybody around here hates me!"

Staff: "It sounds as though you are pretty angry."

Hughes, 2006

In the example above the staff did not challenge Jack's feelings or beliefs by telling Jack everyone likes him. Rather, the staff validated Jack's feeling and attempted to encourage Jack to further explain what made him feel this way. Challenging Jack's feelings (e.g., "No, Jack, everybody likes you.") would probably have led to more frustration (contributing event) and increased the chances for problem behavior. Correcting people's perceptions can feel dismissive or like the staff does not really understand the issue.

The author most associated with this is Naomi Feil, who works primarily with persons experiencing dementia, but her strategies translate perfectly for persons with IDD and MI (Feil, 1993). She also encourages questioning the person and asking him/her to describe more of his/her feelings and thoughts as a means of de-escalation.

Slide 17

5. b) Validating and Exploring

Validating and exploring can be combined and involve encouraging the individual to further explain whatever it is the individual is trying to communicate.

An example of this is shown in the following scenario:

Jack: "Everybody around here hates me!"

Staff: "It sounds like you are pretty angry. Can you tell me what you are so mad about?"

Hughes, 2006

Exploration provides an opportunity for the staff to be an active listener and for the client to have an opportunity to discuss issues and concerns. The combination of using both validating and exploring strategies can be effective techniques in helping individuals to decrease tension and stress. The staff must evaluate the person's readiness to move forward to exploring strategies. Delivering information before people are ready to move forward can be overwhelming and counterproductive.

Slide 18

5. c) Problem-Solving

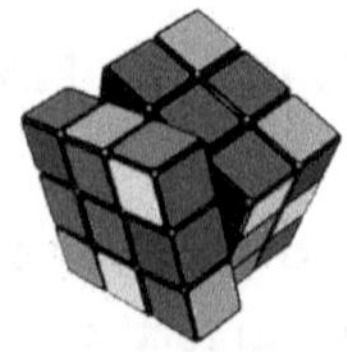

- **Identify the nature of the problem from the client's point of view.**
- **Explore alternative solutions to the problem.**
- **Implement the best alternative solution.**

Hughes, 2006

Problem-solving can be a strategy used informally by DSPs or in a more formal way by clinicians. For DSPs, problem-solving approaches are appropriate for working with the client in his/her environment when the client is calm and ready to move forward. Staff must be cautious to avoid moving too quickly from validating to exploring and then problem-solving. This could be, for example, in a residential environment. It is a here-and-now "in-vivo" approach to problem-solving. A problem-solving approach can also be used by mental health clinicians in an office environment. This is different than an "in-vivo" approach, as it requires a great deal more time and is significantly more methodical in its application.

Slide 19

Exercise: Verbal Strategies

You are working with a woman named Lorraine who believes that one of her staff or roommates steals her clothes from the laundry room. As a result she will no longer wash her clothes, wearing the same soiled outfits to work every day. When you approach Lorraine about this, she screams and yells about people stealing and not trusting anyone to help her.

Activity: Consider the three verbal strategies reviewed on the prior slides to help Lorraine feel acknowledged and supported in reaching a productive and positive outcome.

Slide 20

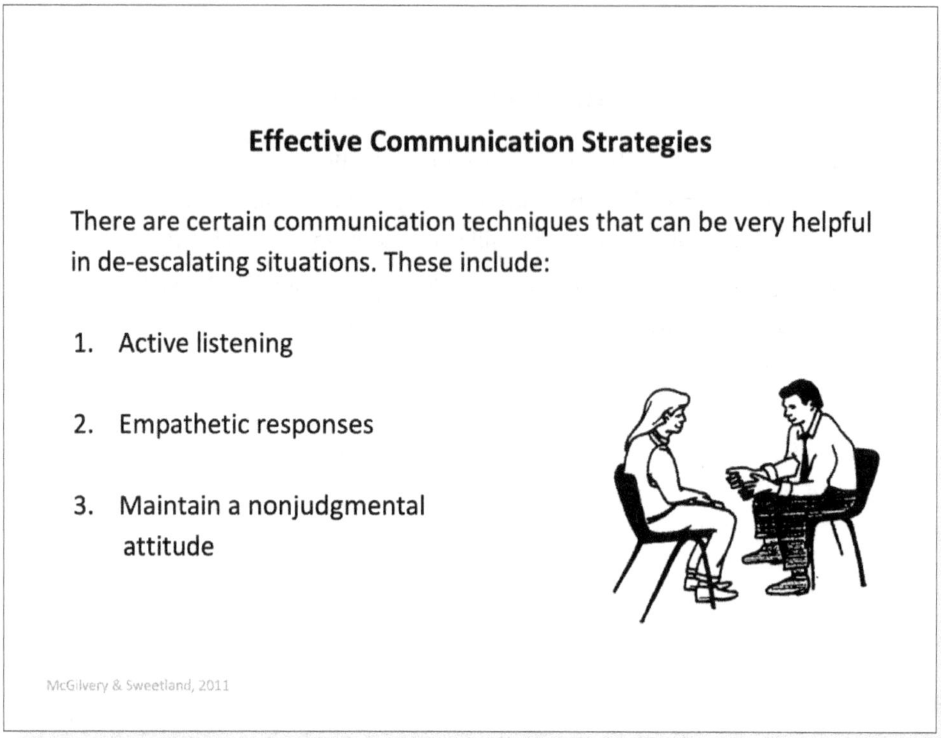

1. **Active listening** — This involves reflecting to the person what you have heard them say.

2. **Empathetic responses** — There is a difference between sympathy and empathy. Giving a sympathetic response is a response reflecting your feelings. Empathy is the ability to understand another person's feelings and to understand how the person views a situation.

3. **Maintain a nonjudgmental attitude** — This conveys an attitude that you accept the person and you are not critical. This does not mean that you are necessarily accepting the behavior, just understanding it is important to the person. It is important to maintain a calm, matter-of-fact and neutral voice. Aggression leads to aggression, i.e., if care providers are verbally aggressive or hostile, it is more likely that the person will react in kind.

Slide 21

Effective Communication Strategies

4. Recognize and avoid power struggles
5. Watch your posture and body language
6. Validate feelings
7. Put the choices back to the person

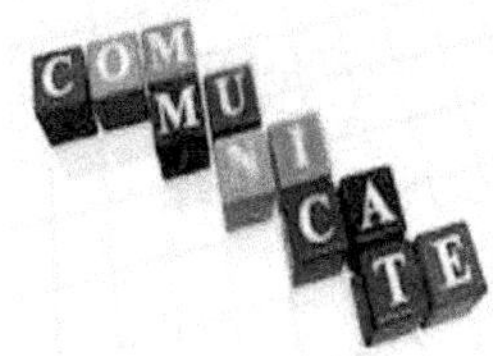

McGilvery & Sweetland, 2011

4. **Avoid power struggles** — It is important in interacting with the people that you work with that you do not get into arguments with them. Avoid being confrontational and avoid arguing with them. Avoid trying to control things that are not essential for safety or structure.

5. **Watch your posture and body language** — Avoid any physical stance or posture that can be viewed as challenging.

6. **Validate how they are feeling** — You can validate the person's feelings without agreeing with the person.

7. **Put the choices back to the person** — If someone's behavior is escalating you can say, "You have a decision to make. You can hit someone or you can... " Put it back on the person and remind the person of the more productive and effective choices that can be made.

Slide 22

Crisis Prevention and Planning

By addressing environmental, biological, psychological and social factors that may contribute to problem behavior, staff may be able to assist the person to cope, maintain control of his/her own behavior and learn positive, productive ways that address the function of the behavior.

Some of the prevention strategy considerations to be aware of for people who have a dual diagnosis:

- Know internal triggers related to past history, health, psychiatric conditions a person may experience, effects of medications, etc.
- Support the person to develop positive relationships.
- Reduce the stress around transitions.
- Maintain an appropriate activity/interest level for the person's needs.
- Be aware of external environmental triggers—room temperature, noises, people, disorganization, if they need things done in a certain way, disappointments, etc.

Identifying the factors that contribute to problem behavior is a component of a functional assessment as discussed in *Module III: Comprehensive Assessment Practices.*

Slide 23

Nonverbal De-Escalation Strategies

1. Monitor your body position and body language.
2. Avoid physically putting yourself in harm's way.
3. Maintain a demeanor of calmness, neutrality and confidence.

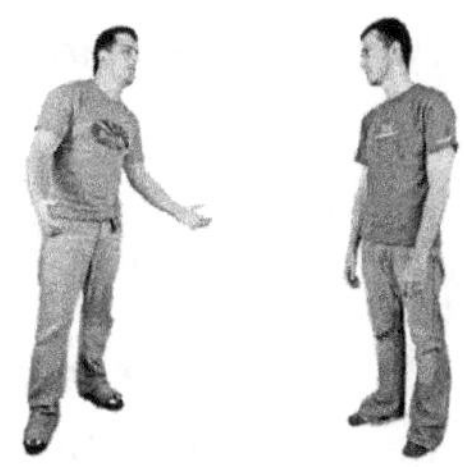

McGilvery & Sweetland, 2011

1. **Monitor your body position and body language** — Do not engage in any posturing that can be construed as aggressive or intimidating. For example, don't get in the person's space, point a finger at the person or give body language cues that signal hostility.

2. **Avoid physically putting yourself in harm's way** — For example, avoid directly facing an agitated person and putting yourself directly in front of that person. This would make the front of your body fully vulnerable to getting hit. Keep a safe distance of at least three to four arm's lengths away. This will decrease the likelihood of the person grabbing, punching, pulling or lunging at you.

3. **Maintain a demeanor of calmness, neutrality and confidence** — You want to present with a nonjudgmental demeanor but one that indicates you are also attentive. If the person is feeling out of control, they need to know someone around them is going to take control if needed. This gives the person a sense of security.

Slide 24

Verbal De-Escalation Strategies

1. Use a calm tone of voice.
2. Use reflective listening.
3. Avoid threatening punishment.
4. Avoid power struggles.
5. Do not ignore escalations of behaviors that could lead to severe behaviors.

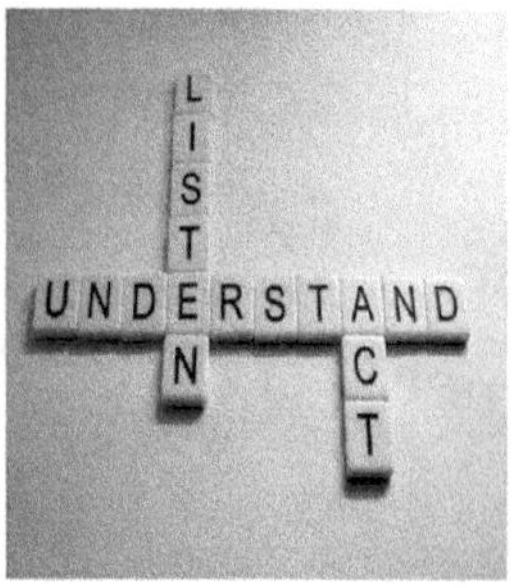

McGilvery & Sweetland, 2011

1. **Use a calm tone of voice** — Avoid showing any strong emotional reaction to the person.

2. **Use reflective listening** — Reflect the feelings you think you are hearing and seeing. For example, "I know that must have really upset you."

3. **Avoid threatening punishment** — You can remind the person of the possible consequences of their actions without threatening punishment. For example, you can say "Now remember, you are working toward that weekend pass."

4. **Avoid power struggles** — It is important the person feels their views are important and valid. Getting into a conversation about who is "right" can cause a power struggle, so avoid those conversations.

5. **Do not ignore escalations of behaviors that could lead to severe behaviors** — Intervene as early in the stages of escalation as possible.

Slide 25

Verbal De-Escalation Strategies

6. Change staffing if necessary.
7. Affirm that you understand.
8. Change the subject if it appears to agitate the person more to talk about it (e.g., offer a drink of water, bring up an topic that interests him or her such as sporting event or TV program).

McGilvery & Sweetland, 2011

6. **Change staffing if necessary** — If the individual is very angry at you, it would not be helpful to continue to try and deal with that person. Have another staff member take over. Otherwise the person is likely to continue staying agitated in your presence. Also, if you feel you can no longer deal with a person effectively on that shift because of your own emotional reactions, ask another staff member to assist or take over. We are only human. Another staff member can intervene to redirect the individual to another activity or let them vent appropriately.

7. **Affirm that you understand** — You do not need to communicate that you agree with the person's perspective, simply that you understand that whatever happened was upsetting from that person's perspective.

8. **Change the subject if it appears to agitate the person more to talk about it** — Help the individual focus on something else. If they keep ruminating about the issue that caused the anger, the agitation will continue. An effective example is offering the person a drink of water or

some other tangible item. It is both supportive for the person who is agitated and offers a distraction/change of topic from the subject which is causing the agitation.

Slide 26

Verbal De-Escalation Strategies

9. Change aspects of the environment.
10. Set limits by reminding the person of the choices and outcomes but do so in a firm, fair manner and with a non-emotional tone of voice.
11. Remind the individual of the desirable consequences of choosing a positive behavior as opposed to a problem behavior. Then remind the persons of the undesirable consequences that can occur if they engage in the problem behavior.

McGilvery & Sweetland, 2011

9. **Change aspects of the environment** — For example, decrease stimulation in the environment in order to produce a more calming and peaceful environment. Simply turning off a TV or moving people out of the room can have a calming effect.

10. **Be limit-setting by reminding the person of the rules but do so in a firm, fair manner and with a non-emotional tone of voice** — For example, if a client is yelling and screaming at another person in the living environment, the staff could inform the client that this behavior is not acceptable.

11. **Remind the individual of the desirable consequence if he/she chooses a more acceptable/appropriate behavior and the undesirable consequences that can occur if they engage in the behavior** — For example, a client is yelling and screaming in the home as mentioned above, and the person does not stop the behavior; the staff should remind the client that discontinuing the behavior will result in being able to go out as planned

but the continuation of his behavior will result in the consequence of not going out with the other residents that evening (consequence articulated in the client's service plan). By leading with the desirable consequence, the staff is refocusing on the positive outcomes, which has greater potential to positively influence the choices the person makes.

Slide 27

Promoting Mental Wellness:
What Is Mental Wellness?

- Sometimes we miss asking whether people are "well."
- Are we thinking about how to support the person in engaging in a healthy lifestyle that will promote mental wellness and having a good life?

When we start to think about wellness, we start to look at a person's overall life and whether the person has a life that promotes wellness.

Slide 28

Promoting Mental Wellness:
How Do We Often Look at Supports?

- When we think about how to support people with Intellectual or Developmental Disabilities (IDD) who are having a difficult time, we think about how the disability impacts the person's life or we look at what support to use to make things better.
- For people with challenging behavior (also referred to as *interfering* behavior), we often consider why the person has difficulties. In other words, we are often focused on what is "wrong" with a person's life.

Supports for people with IDD often focus on fixing problems. This is especially true when we consider a person with IDD who is having a difficult time, especially when the person presents problem behaviors.

Slide 29

Promoting Mental Wellness:
How Do We Promote Wellness?

- **There are day-to-day factors that make up what we call *wellness.* Think about this in our own lives; when we are not feeling ourselves or feeling stressed, we may have many ways of coping.**
- **We also have our own ways of living a life that is meaningful to us.**
- **We can take actions such as: taking a new and better job, having the ability to be spontaneous and splurge, take a day for ourselves, enjoy a relaxing bath, hit the gym or get lost in in our favorite hobby.**

This is how we take care of our own mental wellness, but we tend to forget this important dimension when we start planning, especially in the area of behavior support.

Slide 30

Promoting Wellness as Part of Supporting a Person with IDD?

- **Mental wellness is an important part of a positive supports framework.**
- **JoAnn Cannon offers an evidence-based way to think about wellness (Cannon, 2005)**

We will consider the research-based framework of wellness developed by JoAnn Cannon, Ph.D. Her research is described in her book *Embracing the Good* (Seaside, CA: Inward Bound Ventures, 2005). With help from a MacArthur Genius Grant, Dr. Cannon did an exhaustive study of over 600 people on all continents except for Antarctica with good, successful lives, and she found that these 15 factors were traits often seen in this group. Below each one of these wellness factors, we added a number of different ideas for how somebody's wellness in that area could be improved.

Note: When we use the word "you" below, it refers to the person with IDD.

Slide 31

Promoting Mental Wellness
How Do We Promote Wellness?

JoAnn Cannon's 15 Factors Related to Wellness
(*Enhancing the Good,* 2005)

Contact with nature	Experienced creativity
Optimism	Balanced nutrition
Work satisfaction	Goal accomplishment
Economic essentials	Intellectual stimulation
Coping with stress	Rest and sleep
Spirit awareness	Time and space alone
Positive self-image	Physical prowess
Fulfilling relationships	

Review this list. If there is time and interest, ask the participants to rate themselves a thumbs-up or thumbs-down on each factor. Then have the participant think of a person with IDD whom they support and ask them to rate again for each wellness factor. Discuss the differences in the number of thumbs-ups. Keilson (2019) notes the impact loneliness has on the lives of people with IDD and sees supporting social connection as a moral imperative.

Slide 32

Exercise

Pick one of the wellness areas identified by Dr. Cannon and identify three different things you could do to assist a person with IDD to have a better life in that area.

This can be done individually or in groups.

For example, if you pick "Coping with Stress," identify three things that could help a person cope better with stress. After completion of this exercise, have all groups or attendees share their ideas and list them.

Slide 33

Are Wellness Factors Included in Your Support Plans?

- Where would they fit?
  - Behavior support plan?
  - General support planning document?
- What data would you collect?

Guide a discussion on this topic area. These may be important factors to consider, but we often don't include them in annual planning efforts.

Slide 34

How Might Wellness Be Considered?

- Consider the "15 Factors of Wellness" when creating support plans.
  - Does the person have a chance to engage in each of these factors?
  - Can we provide assistance in working to better the person's life with respect to these factors?
- If somebody is having challenging behaviors, look at wellness as part of the assessment process.
- If a team of care providers looks at that list and doesn't know how the person is doing on them, the first step is to learn more about how the person sees his or her life.
- Support wellness to ensure that you are not only meeting the person's immediate needs, but also the things that will increase the quality of life.

Assessment of wellness can occur as part of an intake or functional behavior assessment. The simplest strategy is to use a thumbs-up or -down, but JoAnn Cannon's assessment of wellness cited earlier offers a more thorough way to consider each factor.

Slide 35

RATIONAL APPROACH TO PSYCHOPHARMACOLOGY

Slide 36

MYTH: MEDICATION TREATMENT IS USED TO CONTROL MALADAPTIVE BEHAVIORS

Premise:

Medication-based therapies directly affect behavior.

Reality:

Behaviors such as self-injury and aggression are too nonspecific to be considered as direct targets for drug therapy.

Treatment implications:

The appropriate targets for medication therapy are the changes in neurophysiological function that mediate behavior associated with psychiatric disorders.

A rational approach to using medication is to target the underlying psychiatric disorder. For example, using an antidepressant medication for persons who are diagnosed with major depression.

Another example is using an antipsychotic medication for persons who are diagnosed with schizophrenia.

A third example is using an antianxiety medication for people who are diagnosed with an anxiety disorder.

The take-home message is to use medication treatment associated with a specific psychiatric disorder.

Slide 37

Medication Treatment

Pharmacotherapy is therapeutic and may be the first choice treatment for some psychiatric disorders:

- Major depression
- Mania states
- Schizophrenia

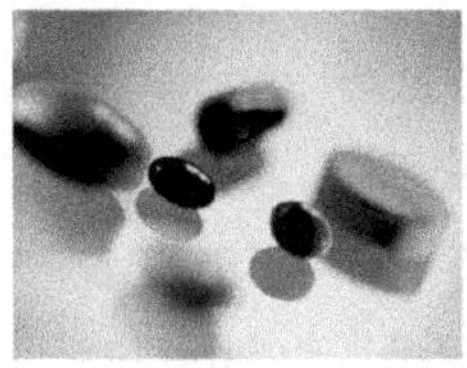

Medication treatment should be diagnostically related to a DSM-5 diagnostic and treatment guideline or the DM-ID.

Medication treatment is often used as the first choice of treatment for mental health issues and/or problem behavior. This is the case when medication treatment is needed to stabilize the individual's mental health or assist to calm someone who is physically and emotionally struggling for control. Once the person has been reasonably stabilized, then other supportive approaches can be applied.

Please note that referral for medication therapy can often take a significant period of time. Concurrent positive supports, environmental adaptation (when possible) and supportive responses by caregivers are necessary while awaiting consultation and for mediation therapy to reach efficacy levels.

Psychotropic medication use can be therapeutic for long-term stabilization of serious mental illness and should be considered as part of a comprehensive treatment plan when appropriate.

Slide 38

General Best Practices in Psychopharmacology

- An assessment of mental illness should guide intervention and findings should be shared.
- Medication and non-medication intervention should be used together.
- A written treatment plan should be developed and shared.
- Generally, one medication at a time should be prescribed.

Highlight for the attendees that written treatment plans and sharing of information by all parties is crucial.

Slide 39

Necessary Communication

- The prescriber should share all relevant information about the medication in understandable language.
- The prescriber should dictate what information is needed back to make good decisions about medication management.
- Side effects monitoring should be established.

Highlight for the attendees that written treatment plans and sharing of information by all parties is crucial.

Slide 40

PRN Medication

- Some medications can be offered as needed, which is termed "pro re nata" or PRN.
- The prescriber should give detailed information about when PRNs should be given and monitor how much they are used.
- Be aware that there might be rules about PRN medication in some areas.

It is important to note that PRN medication usage is often either overdone, with the PRN medication being used very frequently in response to potential challenging behavior. This is a poor use of PRN medication. PRN medication treats symptoms, not behaviors. As a result, some areas discourage PRN medication use. That is also a mistake, as PRN medications can be very effective when used properly and infrequently. PRM medications are used in the general public. Solid guidelines for use should be developed.

Slide 41

Putting It All Together

Activity: Develop a blueprint wellness plan for someone you support. Consider the support strategies reviewed in this chapter that would apply to him/her.

Tips:

- Identity the person's strengths and interests.
- Consider the person's diagnosis and mental health needs.
- Promote relaxation opportunities.
- Anticipate challenges and be prepared with de-escalation and validation strategies.
- Build in ways to help the person feel good about him/herself and develop positive identify.
- Monitor behavior and medication information.

References: Module VII

Carr, J. E., & Sidener, T. M. (2002). On the relation between applied behavior analysis and positive behavioral support. *The Behavior Analyst*, 25, 245-253.

Cannon, J. (2005). *Embracing the Good.* Seaside, CA: Inward Bound Ventures.

Chaplin, E., Craig, T., McCarthy, J., & Bouras, N. (2017). The SAINT: A guided self-help approach for people with intellectual disabilities. *Journal of Mental Health Research in Intellectual Disabilities*, 11, 237-252.

Feil, N. (1993). *The Validation Breakthrough.* Baltimore, MD: Health Professions Press.

Griffiths, D. M., Gardner, W. I., Nugent, J. A., (1999). *Behavioral Supports: Individual Centered Interventions: A Multimodal Functional Approach: A Clinical Manual for Practitioners in Dual Diagnosis (Developmental Disabilities and Mental Health Needs).* Kingston, NY: NADD Press.

Hughes, R. B. (2006). Achieving Effective Health Promotion for Women with Disabilities. *Family & Community Health* 29(1) Supplement: Promoting Health in Persons with Chronic and Disabling Conditions, 44S-51S.

Kern, L., Vorndran, C. M., Hilt, A., Ringdahl, J. E., Adelman, B. E., & Dunlap, G. (1998). Choice as an intervention to improve behavior: A review of the literature. *Journal of Behavioral Education*, 8, 151–169.

Keilson, J. (2019). A moral imperative: Invest in eradicating loneliness. *The NADD Bulletin*, 22, 12-14.

Klaehn, B. (2019). Community-based approaches to treatment of persons with a dual diagnosis. *The NADD Bulletin*, 22, 10.

McGilvery, S., Sweetland, D. (2011). *Intellectual Disability and Mental Health: A Training Manual in Dual Diagnosis.* Kingston, NY: NADD Press.

Module VIII

Crisis Prevention and Intervention: Reducing Risk

Slide 2

Learning Objectives

- Recognize why people with IDD/MI are more likely to experience conditions that can lead to a crisis.
- Recognize how unmet mental health needs can contribute to a crisis.
- Identify components of safe, effective crisis prevention and intervention strategies.

Slide 3

What Is a Crisis?

- Crisis is defined as a situation when support needs for a person are greater than what the setting can offer.
- Crises might occur when a person's level of behavioral health challenges overwhelm a home or job site.
- Instability in a home setting may reduce supports available.
- Support needs include health care.

Slide 4

Crisis Intervention and Prevention

A crisis occurs when a person is feeling threatened, suffers sudden loss or change or cannot access skills or resources.

Behavior is an attempt to meet a need; it has meaning for the person. Repeated problem behavior should not be looked at as a crisis. Inadequate or improper supports contribute to ongoing unmet needs.

We often identify a crisis when there is an immediate threat to a person's health or safety or when their behavior has escalated to a dangerous or unmanageable level.

These occurrences and other triggers can lead to more long-term crises: the person losing their home or job, loss of participation in activities and community involvement, loss of relationships, criminal justice involvement, or inappropriate treatment, medication or supports.

Slide 5

Impact of Crisis

- Consider the risk factors (history of behaviors) and protective factors (social supports, community) that determine how severe a crisis can become.
- Strengthening these protective factors for a person prior to a potential crisis is a crucial prevention step.
- Trauma can trigger or exacerbate a crisis.

Factors to consider that can affect the impact of a potential crisis or trigger: Lifestyle: Is this person engaged in the community? To what degree does this person have an active role in choice-making? What skills can they use at this juncture? Who can help this person? When is the best time to get help?

Slide 6

Being Proactive

- Use behavior and health information to help prevent or prepare for a crisis.
- Describe how to recognize patterns of escalating behaviors or symptoms and ways to intervene as early as possible.

Always be mindful of health factors that could lead to a behavioral crisis, such as a urinary tract infection or a toothache (SAMHSA, 2020).

Slide 7

Crisis Identification

- What does crisis mean to you?
- Who's really having the crisis?
- Ongoing monitoring and observation
- The earlier we recognize the problem, the better.
- It helps to know the person well, what his/her needs are, patterns of behavior, identify precursors of escalation, recognize and document response strategies.

At this point, discuss the nature of crisis with the trainees. What are their experiences? Have they identified patterns that indicate a crisis? How do our own experiences impact how we interpret and respond to a crisis?

Slide 8

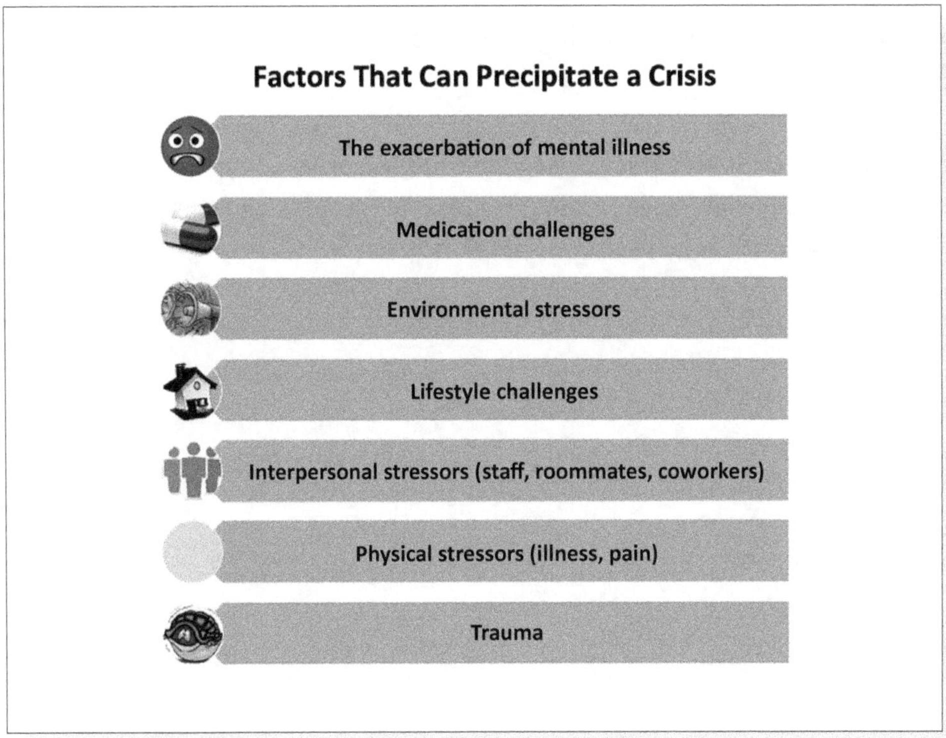

When certain conditions are present, people are more vulnerable to a crisis. Consider the examples on this slide: How can these examples make people feel more anxious? If someone has a mood disorder or other diagnosis, how does a risk factor become greater?

Risks in the environment or lifestyle: unstable staff or staff burnout; decision-makers/team do not support the person; access to health care, doctors, therapists, medications, finances.

These challenges can lead to larger crises: loss of job, loss of home, loss of participation in activities/community, loss of relationships or criminal justice involvement.

We need to start in the early stages where we can make the most difference and/or add more supports/connect to other resources.

Protective factors: Lifestyle measures can also protect against a crisis or prevent a behavior from escalating — relationships, routine, relaxation, visual aids.

Questions to ask: Is this person engaged in the community? To what degree does this person make meaningful choices? What skills can they use? Who can help? Do they know how to ask for help?

Slide 9

More Factors That Can Precipitate a Crisis

- Inadequate behavior supports
- Grief and loss
- Effects of medication
- Transition
- Loss or change in services
- Diagnosis
- Unemployment
- Poverty

Cheplic, 2016

Be sensitive to the impact of psychotropic meds on the person, including their ability to process information, as well as effects on memory, energy level and ability to concentrate.

Slide 10

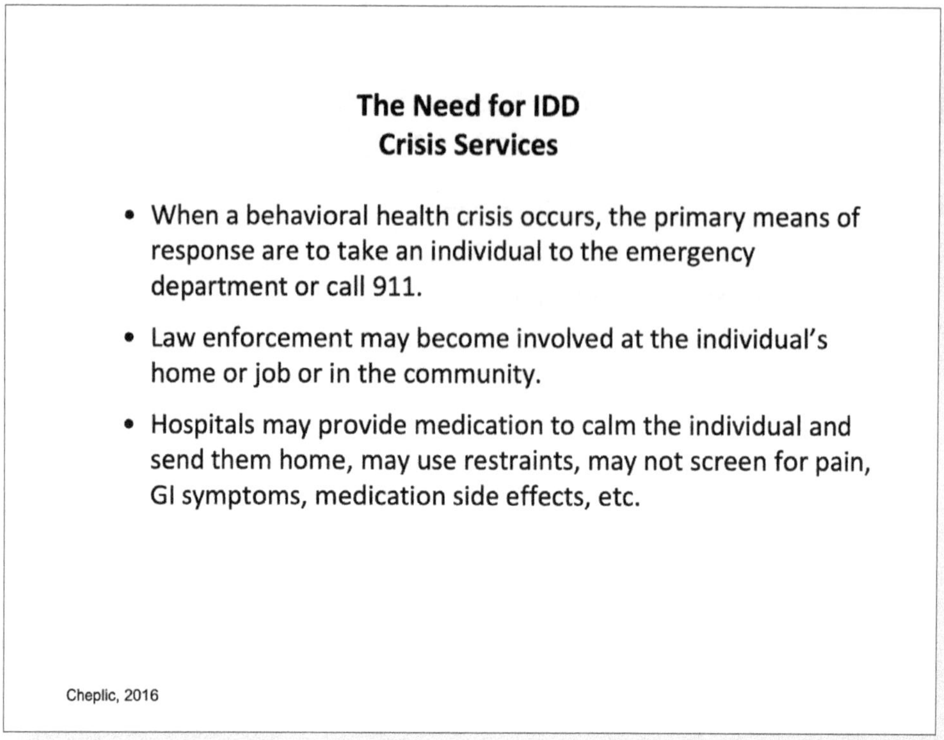

Emergency departments and law enforcement are often not able to offer the holistic types of support a person might need.

By "managing" a situation, we miss the opportunity to support the person as a whole and address underlying unmet needs.

Slide 11

Understanding Behavior

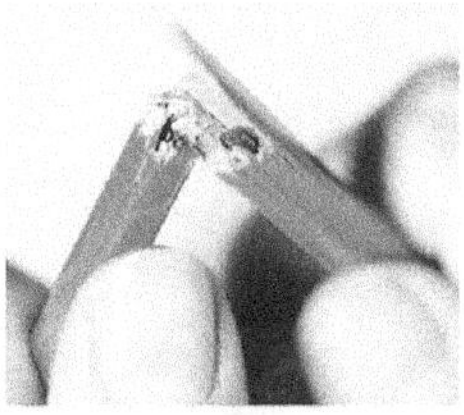

- Repeated problem behavior should not be seen as a crisis.
- By addressing environmental, biological, psychological and social factors that contribute to problem behavior, crises can be prevented or interrupted.
- The continued need to consider emergency/crisis services is an indicator that behavior or treatment plans aren't working.

Many people with IDD/MI have trouble with challenging behavior. A behavioral crisis is a situation in which the person's behavior puts them or others at risk of immediate and serious physical harm or death.

"Crisis," by definition, should not be a regular event. If we are continuing to experience the same events and approach them the same the way with no improvement, that is a failure of our approach.

Behavioral/mental health risk factors include: aggression/self-injury; rapid cycling or changes in mood; fire-setting; destruction to property; inappropriate sexual behavior in the community; drug and alcohol problems; history of trauma; suicidal ideation, threats or attempts; previous history of inpatient or psychiatric hospitalization.

Behavior may appear to come out of nowhere. It may seem like someone snaps or there is no reason for the behavior. But knowing these things (via FBA, documentation, team process), we can learn how to prevent them.

Staff can assist the person to cope, maintain control of their own behavior and learn positive, productive ways to address the function of the behavior.

Slide 12

Recognizing Signs and Providing Supports

The following example is an illustration of a scenario that, when handled poorly, resulted in a crisis:

Kyle was fired from his job yesterday. At breakfast, he tells his roommate he is going to get even with his boss when the time is right.

What are your next steps?

Adjust daily support and expectations in order to prevent crisis when there are signs of increased needs of individuals at risk for crisis. Consider immediate as well as long-term outcomes for the person in choosing responses.

Alternate discussions:

- After Dwight's mom died, the family sold Dwight's home. Sometimes Dwight will take a bus to his old neighborhood, but he gets lost and ends up very far from his group home.
- When Connie gets on the crowded bus to go to work, she will sometimes repeat the same phrases over and over when she is anxious. If someone bumps into her, she can get into verbal or physical altercations. Today, the bus is very crowded and she is telling the driver, "Make room, make room, make room."
- Tom forgot to renew his prescription and he has been without his SSRI for four days. He decides to take a double dose once he picks up his new pills from the pharmacy.

Slide 13

Crisis Intervention and Prevention

- What immediate steps should be taken to ensure safety?
- What factors contributed to this incident?
- How could this crisis have been prevented?
- What could each of the players have done differently?
- What are the next steps in planning Bill's behavior supports?

Bill, a 35-year-old man with ID and an anxiety disorder, works at a consignment shop.

Bill is waiting for a delivery that usually arrives around 3 p.m. It's his job to sort the items and prepare them for sale.

Bill keeps asking what time it is, stares at the clock and is looking visibly agitated. (It is 3:15.)

Bill begins to pace and press his face to the door.

"Nothing yet?" asks a staff person who manages the store. "Leave me alone," replies Bill, who then kicks the door and causes the shade to fall down.
Bill's coworker Aaron yells, "Stop that, Bill!"

The manager tells Bill, "Yeah, knock it off and go sit down."

Bill then picks up the shade and heads toward Aaron, who is on the other side of the store.

The manager runs toward Bill, grabs the shade from his hand, and Bill falls to the floor.

Aaron continues to yell at Bill to stop as he struggles with the manager. Bill's coworker Louise runs out from the stockroom, sees the struggle and calls 911.

Bill is bleeding from his ear. Louise is crying.

The store manager is yelling to Aaron and Bill to calm down and wait for the ambulance.

A customer who was shopping in the store quickly exits.

When the EMTs arrive, the manager accompanies Bill to the ER so when the delivery truck arrives, it is sent away by Louise, who has closed the store early.

Slide 14

Crisis Response

- Provide visual aids and include individuals in planning to help reduce uncertainty and anxiety.
- Recognize that repeating questions or ruminating on a topic may be a coping strategy for the person.
- Setting clear expectations in advance helps support respectful communication and recognize a problem as early as possible.

It is important to deliver information to people when they are calm and ready to listen. A person may have processing challenges that impact their ability to understand information or instructions. When individuals are escalating, our responses should be supportive and person-centered. Remember the person's risk factors (diagnosis, lack of coping skills, communication challenges) and let that information guide your choice of engagement and interaction.

Slide 15

The Big Picture: Reducing Crises

- Establish environments that reduce/prevent crisis.
- View behaviors as indicators of where assistance is needed.
- Support ongoing wellness and relaxation opportunities for all individuals, with extra emphasis on mental health supports for those with a psychiatric diagnosis.
- Make activities engaging, supportive, interactive, person-centered, choice-driven and safe.
- Provide immediate crisis prevention and response services in the community.

Crisis management and intervention is a response-driven support to an acute or temporary situation that is often caused by more long-standing factors (mental health, relationship issues, unemployment, lack of coping skills, other unmet needs.)

We look for overall ways to reduce the likelihood of a crisis by supporting people to feel happy, included, valued and safe in smaller, everyday ways on an ongoing basis.

In other words, we reduce crises by focusing on protective factors as well as risk factors.

For individuals with intellectual and developmental disabilities and mental health needs, crisis stabilization resources are needed, including after hours. Importantly, gainful employment conveys benefits for community stabilization (Kalb, L. G., Beasley, J., Caoili A., McLaren, J., & Barnhill, J. [2020]).

Slide 16

Challenges with Current System

- Community has a lack of psychiatric services for both adults and children with IDD/MI.
- Overutilization of community emergency resources due to lack of community crisis programs.
- Potential loss of residence or employment when an individual is admitted to a hospital or goes to jail.

Crisis behavior often develops due to lack of understanding the best way to support individuals.

Need for training on interacting with individuals in an appropriate manner, including crisis prevention and response.

Slide 17

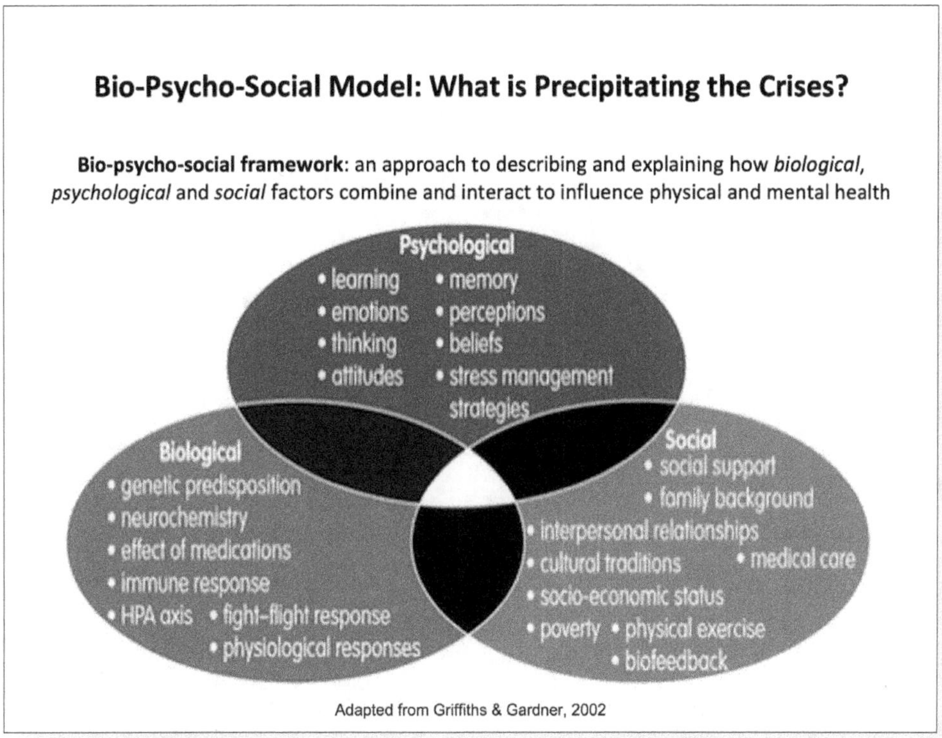

The bio-psycho-social framework provides an integrated model of assessment. If we limit ourselves to a single way to try to understand the challenges posed in supporting a person with IDD/MI, we will miss the mark in most cases and fail to understand the true complex nature of needs. One of the philosophical difficulties we encounter in supporting this population is that many professionals only consider their specific discipline and professional training and, as such, don't consider other ways to view the challenges of the person.

Exacerbating this is the fact that many assessment tools are based on the practices of a specific discipline. For example, a behavior analytic assessment tool may primarily ask questions leading to a functional assessment of behavior, considering setting events, discriminative stimuli and maintaining consequences, but not delving into physiological events or asking why certain events have such a degree of salience. Similarly, a mental health assessment may fail to account for the explanatory power of a person's culture. The bio-psycho-social assessment is an effort to address these types of problems by creating an assessment model that includes and embraces multiple disciplinary perspectives.

Slide 18

Crisis Prevention and Management Plan

Slide 19

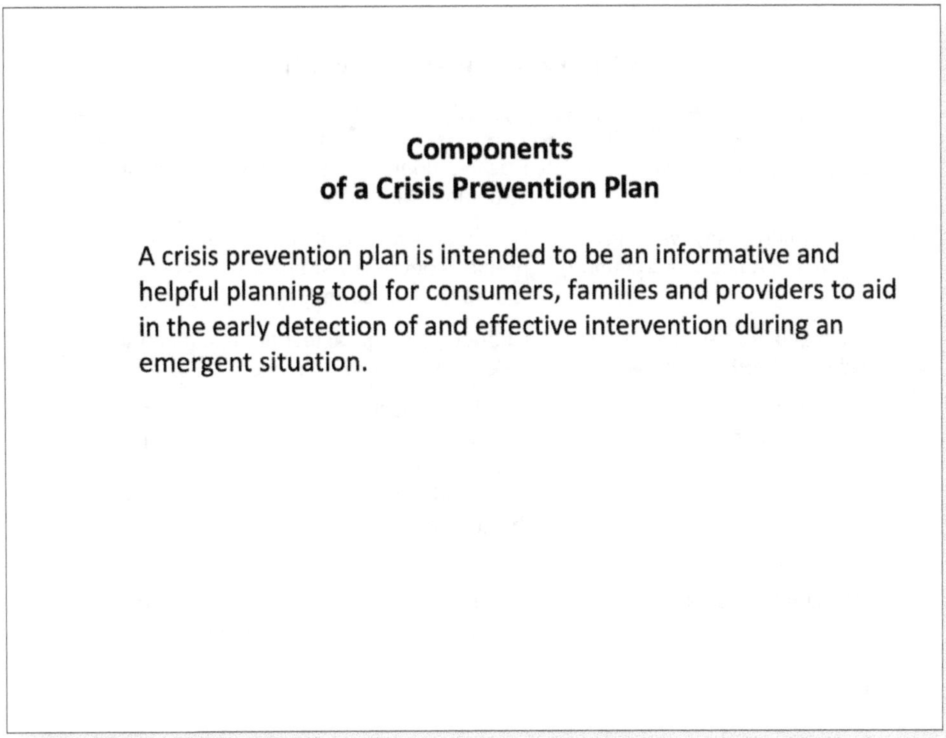

Planning for support to avoid crises is a critical component of supports for many people. The crisis prevention steps can easily be included in other types of plans, such as annual service plans. Use whatever strategy is most helpful to the person and the team.

Slide 20

Crisis Intervention and Prevention

Stage of Behavior	Response
Baseline: Normal, calm	Positive approaches: clear communication, structure, routine, sensory needs
Prevention (early warning signs, i.e. anxiety or agitation)	Be supportive, modify environment to meet needs & decrease stressors (de-escalation strategies)
Escalation (defensive or resistant, verbal threats)	Reduce risk, verbal techniques, maintain safety, distraction, validation
Crisis (aggression, risk of harm to self or others)	Continue positive interaction, safe response strategies, i.e., remind the patient with DD of pre-established boundaries; remind him/her about outcomes and next steps without threatening
Resolution and calming	Re-establish routines and re-establish rapport; prevent future escalation

porticonetwork.ca CAMH

Slide 21

Components of a Crisis Prevention Plan

- Presenting problem
- Early warning signs (precipitants)
- What has helped in the past?
- What action is helpful?
- What action is not helpful?
- Summary

This slide and the next slide illustrate common components of crisis plans.

Slide 22

Components
of a Crisis Prevention Plan

- What needs does the behavior seem to meet?
- List known antecedents/triggers
- List protective factors: What is valuable and important to him/her?
- Communication skills: Describe the primary methods used by this person to communicate (vocal speech, signs, gestures, communication books, electronic devices or behavior etc.).

The elements on the slide reflect more behavioral and person-centered considerations.

Slide 23

Components of a Crisis Prevention Plan

- It identifies a person's response patterns to manage a crisis when it occurs.
- The crisis prevention and management plan is best developed by a team.

First Response to Victims of Crime, 2008

Whenever possible, get the perspective of the person on what helps avoid crises and what helps to resolve crises.

Slide 24

Components of a Crisis Prevention Plan

- Outlines safe and effective crisis intervention strategies when necessary.
- Describes how to recognize patterns of escalating behaviors.

Ensure the plan includes a description of what a crisis is for the specific person. Include triggers and possible precursors.

Outline the appropriate actions to address the issues at the earliest possible stage of crisis unfolding.

The plan should also include appropriate intervention strategies that are effective when dealing with problem behavior.

- What is the function of the behavior?
- What may help the person calm down?
- What should the team avoid?
- Can we recognize the earliest triggers?

Slide 25

Components of a Crisis Prevention Plan

- Purpose is to help prevent or prepare for a crisis.
- Includes specific needs and triggers of individuals supported.

First Response to Victims of Crime, 2008

Sometimes when incidents do occur, they can escalate quickly when we are not prepared, so it's important to have some practical strategies to respond.

- Provide visual aids to help reduce uncertainty and anxiety.
- Use positive and respectful verbal techniques.
- Learn and utilize the person's protective factors.
- Support opportunities for relaxation.

Slide 26

Components of a Crisis Prevention Plan

Describe the behavior in operational terms (specify how the behavior is performed):

Behavior	Operational Description

Ask the trainees to assist in designing operational definitions of crisis-type behaviors they have encountered. "Aggression" to others or "self-injury" are frequently seen as crisis-type behaviors, but it is important to have a clear, nonjudgmental, unbiased description of behavior in order to provide a person-centered response.

Someone may be demonstrating early signs of an illness or pain.

Slide 27

Crisis Prevention and Management Plan

Stage of Observed Behavior	Recommended Caregiver Responses
Stage 1: Normal, calm behavior	Use positive approaches, encourage usual routines.
Stage 2: Prevention (Identify early warning signs that signal increasing stress or anxiety.)	Be supportive, modify environment to meet needs (Identify de-escalation strategies that are helpful for this person with DD).
Stage 3: Escalation (Identify signs that the person is escalating to a possible behavior crisis.)	Be directive (use verbal direction & modeling), continue to modify environment to meet needs, ensure safety.
Stage 4: Crisis (Risk of harm to self, others or environment or seriously disruptive behavior, e.g., acting out.)	Use safety and crisis response strategies.
Stage 5: Post-crisis resolution and calming	Re-establish routines and re-establish rapport.

Surrey Place Centre, 2011

Become familiar with verbal techniques and identify which are useful with the individual — some people respond to humor, others require reassurance, while others need some distraction from the topic or setting entirely.

We often hear words like “redirection,” “de-escalation” and “distraction” without particulars or details. Planning includes specific strategies that consider the person’s interests and preferences.

Slide 28

Risk Assessment Tool for Behavioral Crisis

Utilize risk assessments applicable to the general population. Take into account how the person's developmental disabilities affect both risks and protective factors. Note whether recent changes have occurred in any risk or protective factors.

Flag all areas where there are risk issues. Also consider factors that may protect from harm.

Adapted from Surrey Place Centre, 2011

Assessment of risk has become a more common feature of supports for people with disabilities and is performed on admission to a service setting at times. The key consideration in a risk assessment is determining the nature and severity of risk so safeguards can be wisely utilized.

Slide 29

Risk Assessment Tool for Behavioral Crisis

Risk Area	Person – Risk Factors	Caregivers / Environment Assessment
Harm to self	Is the person verbalizing suicidal thoughts or intent? Is there evidence of suicidal behaviors, poor judgment or mental illness? Is there a history of suicidal or para-suicidal behavior? Is the patient unable to identify reasons to keep on living? Is the patient engaging in, or is there evidence of, self-harm? Is the patient verbalizing intent to self-harm? Does the person have a history of self-harm? Is the person unable to care for self? Is the person unwilling to accept support from others? Is there evidence of neglect & behaviors that put the patient at risk?	Is a means available for the person to commit suicide? Are means available for individual to harm self? Are caregivers able to supervise and protect the person? Are others available and able to assist in the person's care?

Adapted from Surrey Place Centre, 2011

Slide 30

Risk Assessment Tool for Behavioral Crisis

Risk Area	Person – Risk Factors	Caregivers / Environment Assessment
Victimization or exploitation	Is the patient being victimized or exploited? Has the person been victimized or exploited in the past? Is the person unable to protect self? Does the person lack insight into possible dangers of the situation? Has the patient failed to show evidence that he/she would ask for help? Has the person been unable to get help or protection from others in the past?	Are caregivers able to supervise and protect the person?

Adapted from Surrey Place Centre, 2011

Review the risk-assessment slides with the trainees. Do they understand the nature of the risk? What other caregiver/environment considerations can the trainees generate?

Slide 31

Risk Assessment Tool for Behavioral Crisis

Risk Area	Person – Risk Factors	Caregivers / Environment Assessment
Harm to others	Is the person verbalizing intent to harm others? Is the person making physical gestures about hurting others? Has the person caused physical harm to others? Does the person have sufficient mobility and strength to potentially harm others? Does the patient's aggression/harmful behavior tend to escalate quickly and/or unpredictably?	Are there vulnerable individuals in the setting who cannot protect themselves? Can caregivers recognize cues and intervene safely? Can the person be supervised safely in current setting without caregivers being at risk of harm while trying to prevent harm to others?

Adapted from Surrey Place Centre, 2011

Slide 32

Risk Assessment Tool for Behavioral Crisis

Risk Area	Person—Risk Factors	Caregivers / Environment Assessment
Risk to environment	Has the person damaged or attempted to damage property in recent past? If yes, what was the nature and extent of damage? Does the person have sufficient mobility and strength to be able to cause damage? Does the patient escalate rapidly and/or unpredictably?	Are caregivers able to recognize the escalation and intervene effectively? Do caregivers feel comfortable about being able to predict and prevent it?

Adapted from Surrey Place Centre, 2011

Slide 33

Components
of a Comprehensive Crisis System

1. Crisis Prevention Services
2. Crisis Telephone Services
3. Mobile Crisis Outreach Services
4. Crisis Residential Service
5. Cross-Systems Collaboration

Adapted from Dept of Health & Human Services, nd

Developing a comprehensive crisis system requires a variety of different types of service. Special attention is required to how collaboration occurs across systems, as different parts of the service system often must work together. A common area of collaboration is the intellectual or developmental disability service system and the mental health service system.

Slide 34

Components of a Comprehensive Crisis System

1. Crisis Prevention Services
   a) Proactive, comprehensive, individualized
   b) Designed to avoid a crisis
   c) Accomplished through consultation and education
      - Trained staff
      - Skilled staff
      - Competent staff
   d) Through the development of a crisis prevention plan

Adapted from Dept of Health & Human Services, nd

Preventing crises is always better than responding to crises. Crisis prevention services can proactively help improve the capacity to support a person presenting challenges. Often this can take the form of training in intervention strategies and mentoring care providers.

Slide 35

Components of a Comprehensive Crisis System

2. Crisis Telephone Services
   a) Often the first point of contact
      - Initial triage point
      - Able to reach a wide geographical area
      - Accessible 24 hours a day
   b) Services provided include
      - Supportive communication
      - Consultation
      - Problem-solving
      - Information and referral

Adapted from Dept of Health & Human Services, nd

Crisis telephone services could be generic crisis lines all people can use or dedicated telephone services for people with intellectual or developmental disabilities.

Explore adding a website or text-messaging communication system to support people with IDD/MI access resources during a crisis.

Slide 36

Components of a Comprehensive Crisis System

3. Mobile Crisis Outreach Services
   a) Provided where the crisis occurs
      - Most feasible
   b) Outreach could occur at
      - Home
      - Work
      - Group home
      - Day services
      - Anywhere in the community

Adapted from Dept of Health & Human Services, nd

Mobile crisis services go directly to where people are. Depending on the service, the assistance could be delivered with a short wait, or there could be a longer wait for the mobile crisis workers to arrive.

Outreach can also be done via telehealth or other virtual connection.

Slide 37

Components of a Comprehensive Crisis System

4. Crisis Residential Service
    a) Very short-term, highly supervised and supportive residential setting
        - Staffing 24 hours a day
        - Crisis stabilization
        - Trained staff
        - Crisis planning
        - Monitor medications, if needed
        - Linkages to community resources

Adapted from Dept of Health & Human Services, nd

Crisis residential services refers to a setting where a person can go and live during a crisis time. Crisis residential services staff are typically highly trained. One problem with crisis residential services is that they are often full, and difficulties can be encountered in moving people from crisis homes back to their prior settings or into new settings. Crisis residential settings are not a replacement for capacity of the general system.

Slide 38

Components of a Comprehensive Crisis System

4. Crisis Residential Service
    b) Crisis residential settings are:
        - Less restrictive
        - Less disruptive
        - Less costly compared to inpatient programs

Adapted from Dept of Health & Human Services, nd

Crisis residential settings are typically a fraction of the cost of inpatient settings and offer a more typical setting where care providers can learn what kind of community supports are most effective.

Slide 39

Components of a Comprehensive Crisis System

5. Cross-Systems Collaboration
   a) Establishment of collaboration among key systems and stakeholders
      - IDD system
      - MH system
      - Education system
      - Forensic system

Adapted from Dept of Health & Human Services, nd

What other systems should be considered in cross-system collaboration? How can resources be blended, shared or braided across different service systems?

Slide 40

Components of a Comprehensive Crisis System

5. Cross-Systems Collaboration (cont.)
   b) Collaboration is based on the idea that:
      - Negative outcomes result from faulty systems, rather than ineffective people
   c) A dual diagnosis task force:
      - Review high-risk individuals
      - Make recommendations

Adapted from Dept of Health & Human Services, nd

How can we promote further collaboration? We recognize that it is very easy for people to fall between the cracks, especially when they have a variety of co-occurring conditions. The dual diagnoses of intellectual or developmental disabilities and a mental health disorder represent a unique challenge, as knowledge is needed from both systems at times. Dual diagnosis task forces often can identify key needs and suggest resources and interventions.

References: Module VIII

Baker, D. J., Albin, R. W., Craven, K., & Wieseler, N. (2002). Training and technical assistance strategies to prevent and respond to behavior-related crises. In N. Wieseler and K. C. Lakin (Eds.), *Crisis: Alternative Community Behavioral Support and Crisis Response Programs* (pp. 165-198). Washington, DC: AAMR.

Beasley, J., Kalb, L. G., & Klein A. (2018). Improving mental health outcomes for individuals with intellectual disability through the Iowa START (I-START) program. *Journal of Mental Health Research in Intellectual Disabilities*, 11 (4), 287-300.

CAMH Health Promotion Resource Centre (CAMH HPRC), 2017.

Griffiths, D. M., & Gardner, W. I. (2002). The integrated biopsychosocial approach to challenging behaviours. In D. M. Griffiths, C. Stavrakaki, & J. Summers (Eds.), *Dual Diagnosis: An introduction to the mental health needs of persons with developmental disabilities.*

Horner, R., Dunlap, G., Beasley, J., et al. (2005). Positive Support for Behavioral, Mental Health, Communication and Crisis Needs. In K. C. Lakin and A. Turnbull (Eds.) *National Goals and Research for People with Intellectual and Developmental Disabilities*. The ARC of the United States & AAMR.

Kalb, L. G., Beasley, J., Klein, A., Hinton, J., & Charlot, L. (2016). Psychiatric hospitalisation among individuals with intellectual disability referred to the START crisis intervention and prevention program. *Journal of Intellectual Disability Research*, 60 (12), 1153-1164.

Kalb L. G., Beasley J., Caoili A., McLaren J., & Barnhill J. (2020). Predictors of mental health crisis among individuals with intellectual and developmental disabilities enrolled in the START program. *Psychiatric Services*.

SAMHSA (2020). National Guidelines for Behavioral Health Crisis Care Best Practice Toolkit.

United States Department of Justice (2018). First Response to Victims of Crime.
Surrey Place Centre (2011). Communicating Effectively with People with Developmental Disabilities.

United States Department of Health & Human Services (2017, 2019). Components of a Comprehensive Crisis System.

Module IX

Adapting Therapy Practices

Slide 2

This module introduces concepts in adapting therapy to make it more useful for persons with IDD.

Slide 3

Learning Objectives

- List therapy guidelines
- Describe ways to adapt psychotherapy practices
- Describe therapeutic models

Slide 4

Myths About Psychotherapy

Myth: Persons with IDD are not appropriate for psychotherapy.

Premise: Impairments in cognitive abilities and language skills make psychotherapy ineffective.

Reality: Level of intelligence is not a sole indicator for appropriateness of therapy.

Treatment Applications: Psychotherapy approaches need to be adapted to the expressive and receptive language skills of the person.

Fletcher et al. 2015

There is an increasing acceptance of the use of psychotherapy for people with IDD. The issue is no longer whether people with IDD are entitled to psychotherapy or can benefit from it, but how the psychotherapy techniques can be adapted to meet the needs of people who have limitations in expressive and receptive language skills.

Slide 5

Facts

- Individuals with ID are at high risk for mental health problems (Summers, Fletcher & Bradley, 2017).
- Significant mental health problems occur in 30-50 percent of people with ID (Fletcher et al., 2016).
- In recent years, research on psychotherapy with persons with ID has advanced (Prout, Brooke, Browning, 2011).
- There is a burgeoning acceptance of the efficacy of psychotherapy with persons with ID and the adaptations that are needed (Shankland & Dagnan, 2015).

Slide 6

Definition of Psychotherapy

- Relationship between a client and a therapist/counselor
- Engaged in a therapeutic relationship
- To achieve a change in emotions, thoughts or behavior

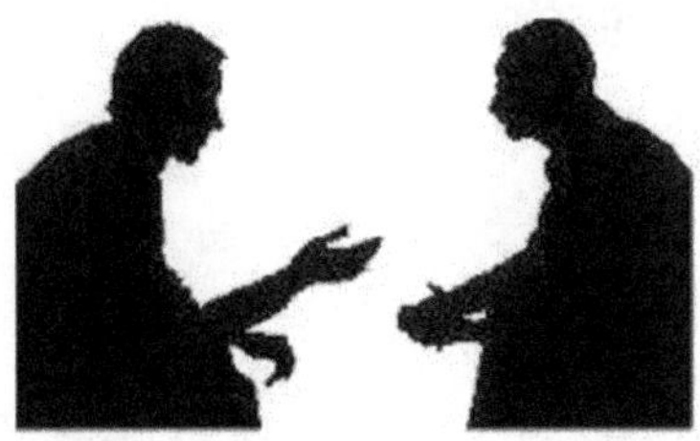

The purpose of psychotherapy is no different than the purpose used for the general population. How we define psychotherapy is also the same.

Slide 7

Adapted Therapies

Many typical therapy sessions start with this question: "Have you been feeling better since last time I saw you?"

- Must remember feelings from last visit
- Must know current feelings
- Must be able to compare
- Must know what the therapist is really asking

And so on and so on...

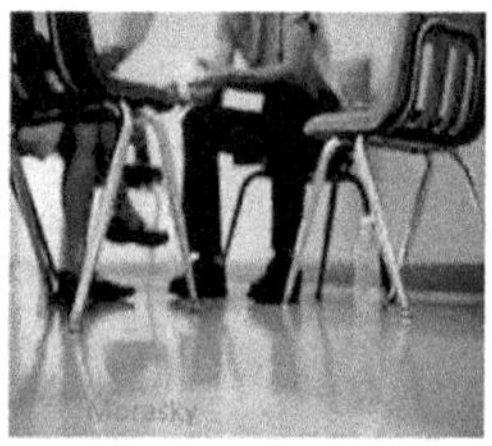

Traditional, non-adapted therapy models require significant memory retention and self-awareness that may exceed the cognitive ability of a person who has a dual diagnosis (questions that require high cognitive load to process and respond). Morasky (2007) also suggests that to help figure out what needs to be adapted, the therapist must first ask what makes the intellectual activity difficult for the person. This is the area for which adaptation is required.

Slide 8

Helping People Cope with Their Daily Problems

A Problem-Solving Model

Slide 9

Why Do People with IDD Need Therapy?

- People with IDD often experience difficulties in coping with daily problems.
- People with IDD have a history of being devalued, leading to feelings of defeat and inadequacy.
- Coping requires self-awareness and a plan for coping in challenging situations.
- People with IDD experience a host of bio-psycho-social vulnerabilities.

Adults with IDD are susceptible to the bio-psycho-social vulnerabilities associated with mental health problems. These problems can include negative life events, bullying, abuse and neglect.

Slide 10

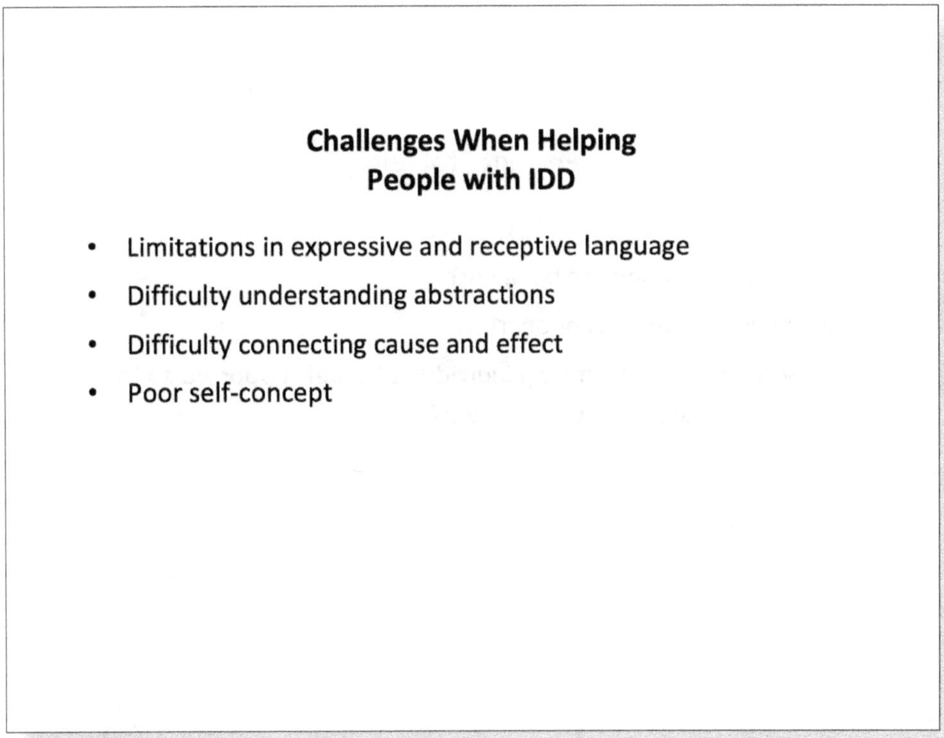

These issues are often experienced by people with IDD. These are characteristic of people with IDD. The therapist needs to understand how each of these characteristics impacts their clients.

Slide 11

Present Problem

- What is the immediate behavior?
- Is the person anxious or angry?
- How can the therapist help individuals to feel supported so they can better cope with the problem?

This reflects a "here-and-now" approach to helping a person cope with their day-to-day problems.

Slide 12

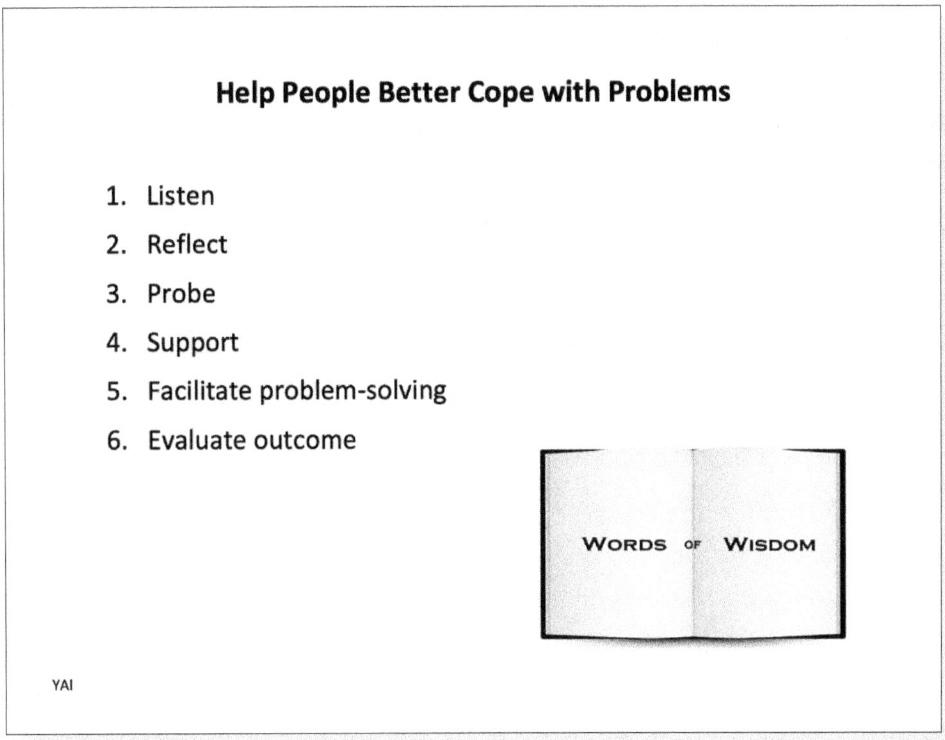

Providing therapy for people with a dual diagnosis is not significantly different than providing therapy for people in the general population. The principles of therapy remain the same, but the approach to therapy is modified. Approaches to therapy are adapted according to the expressive and receptive language skills of the individual.

The model described here is appropriate for persons who have IDD co-occurring with MI. This model can be used for either short-term or long-term therapy. It is rather simplistic in nature but contains the essential components needed to realize positive outcomes.

This model is intended to be used either in formal psychotherapy or as a here-and-now model that can be used by DSPs.

The model is designed to support staff (DSPs, other staff) in being more helpful and supportive when working with people who function in the mild/moderate levels of intellectual/developmental disabilities (IDD) and who have mental health issues — even not conducting formal therapy.

It is a therapeutic, positive interaction we can use to be supportive on a daily basis.

Slide 13

Therapy Model

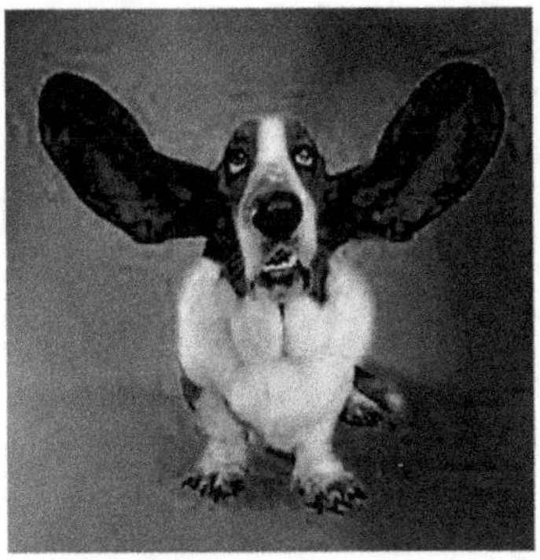

Active Listening

- Attentive
- Interested

Active Listening – It is important for the therapist to demonstrate active listening skills. Good eye contact and body posture are two ways in which we can communicate to the individual our interest. With permission from the client, a tap on the shoulder at the beginning of the session can indicate a caring message, which can set the positive tone and demonstrate interest in the client.

Slide 14

Exercise

Pair up and practice active listening. Each person gets to be the client and the listener. Make sure to use the active listening strategies described on the previous slides.

Slide 15

Therapy Model

Reflect

- Repeat a few words.
- Reflection demonstrates active listening.

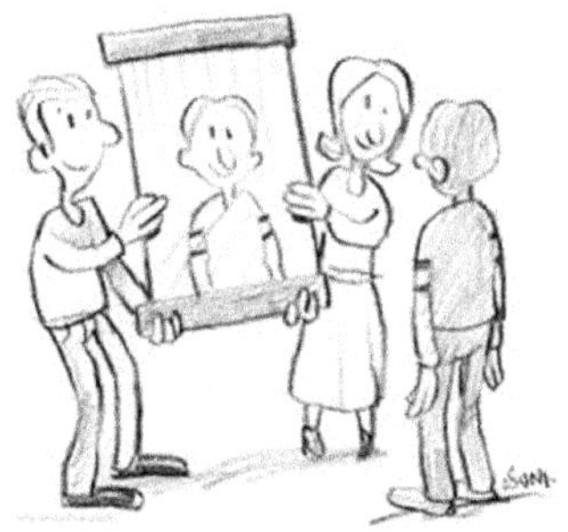

Reflect – Using a reflective technique can be very valuable in "checking out" whether the client and clinician understood what is being communicated. The client statements are restated or rephrased to the client so as to emphasize their emotional significance.

Slide 16

Therapy Model

Probe

- Ask direct questions.
- Avoid interrogation.
- *How* and *what* questions are usually easier to answer than *why* questions.

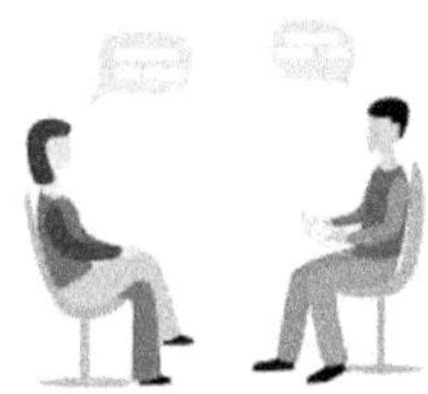

Probe – It is generally useful for the therapist to take an active role in the therapy process. At times it may be difficult for a person with IDD to have a back-and-forth conversation in the absence of the therapist taking an active role. It is difficult for individuals with IDD to answer questions that begin with "why." This is because "why" questions generally require the client to think abstractly. Questions should be relevant to the person's language skills. Asking an individual to describe a situation can be a useful method of probing.

Slide 17

Therapy Model

Support

- Supportive statements indicate understanding.
- Express that you care.
- Acknowledge having been in a similar situation.

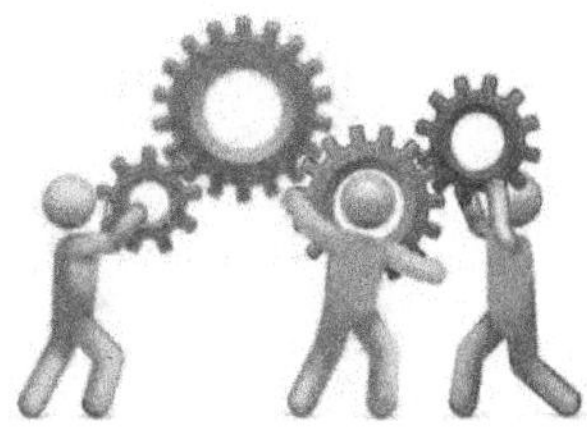

Support – Providing support during the course of the therapy process is important. It acknowledges the value of the individual and conveys an expression of concern and caring. It can normalize the individual's feelings and responses. Try to start and end each session on a positive note.

Slide 18

Therapy Model

Facilitate problem-solving

- Explore alternative options.
- Support acceptable solutions.

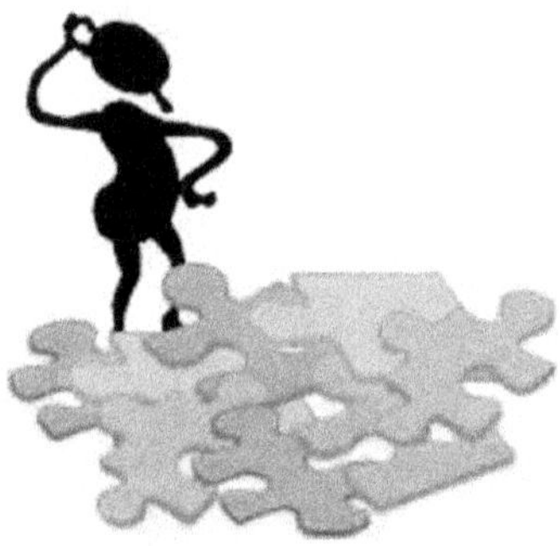

Facilitate Problem-Solving – Facilitating problem-solving can be considered the meat and potatoes of therapy. Once the problem has been clearly identified by both the therapist and the individual, the therapist will work with the client to identify two or three alternate ways to solve the problem.

It can be useful to have the problem written on a piece of paper along with the alternative solutions to the problem. Then, the client and therapist can analyze the alternative solutions by identifying the pros and cons of each alternative solution. This, too, can be written on paper as a visual. Lastly, an acceptable alternative option can be selected and supported by both the client and therapist.

The therapist can give the client a "homework assignment" related to the problem and solution. This is a concrete tool to help the client stay on track and maintain continuity from one session to another. The therapist can also develop a self-monitoring tool to enable the client to self-monitor work conducted outside the therapy session and to measure progress.

Slide 19

Therapy Model

Evaluate Outcome

- Was the outcome acceptable?
- Was it positive?
- What was learned?

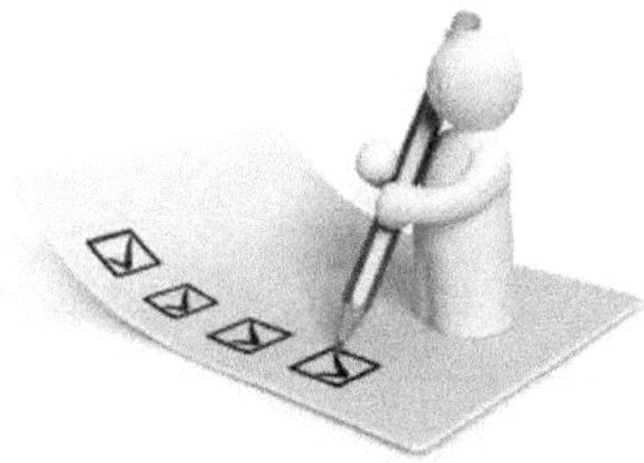

Fletcher, 2007

Evaluate Outcome —There are several ways in which the outcome of therapy can be evaluated. One way is for the client to use a self-monitoring tool to measure progress. Another way to evaluate is through the client's self report of progress, which can be obtained during the therapy session. A third way is to obtain information from parents and other care providers regarding the individual's change in behavior as it relates to the therapeutic goal.

Slide 20

Encouraging Hope: Guiding Principles

- Use language that promotes hope.
- Raise expectations of what people are capable of accomplishing.
- Stay focused on strengths.

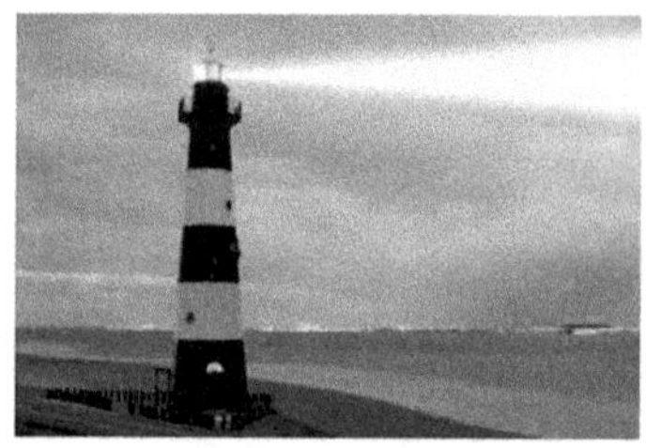

Guiding Principles — There are guiding principles for promoting mental wellness that can be used by staff at all levels. These principles come from the recovery model employed in the mental health field. The focus is strength-based and with an emphasis on success.

Slide 21

Encouraging Hope: Guiding Principles

- Build everyone's hope.
- Instill a source of hope whenever possible.
- Feeling a sense of hope for the future can be transformative.

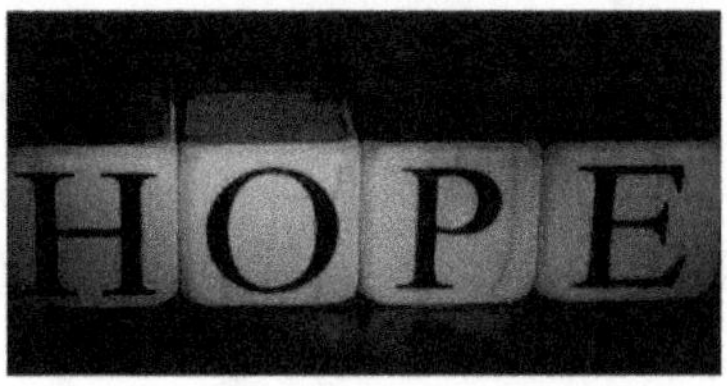

Guiding Principles — The recovery model embraces the concept of hope. The role of the therapist, therefore, is to instill hope in the client. This is particularly poignant with individuals who have a dual diagnosis, because they often have histories of abuse, neglect and despair.

Slide 22

Encouraging Hope: Guiding Principles

- Celebrate accomplishments.
- Find ways to listen to the people you serve.

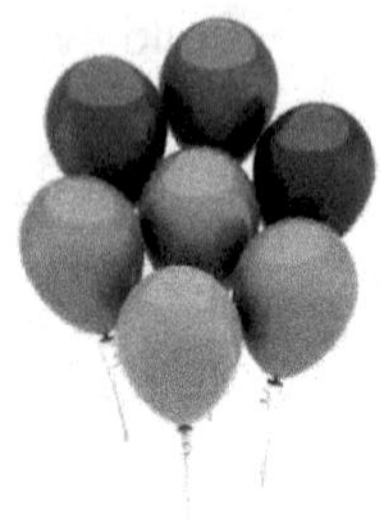

Guiding Principles — Celebrating accomplishments can be done in incremental ways. It is a way to express support for the individual. Celebrating accomplishments can be expressed when a person has acted in some positive manner. Frequent expression of accomplishments represents value for the individual and hope for the future.

Slide 23

Clinician Characteristics

Warmth: Ability to be encouraging and offer positive reinforcement where appropriate while utilizing an empathic approach coupled with an informal and friendly attitude toward the individual. This improves response and motivation to engage in therapy.

Genuineness: Being honest without being too harsh or judgmental. Avoid the misinterpretation of directness as criticism, hostility or rejection.

Ability to develop rapport: Fostering security and trust to counter possible previous experiences of distorted ideas and representations of therapists or authority figures in general. Overcoming this hurdle is essential to effective treatment.

Fletcher et al., 2011

These characteristics, along with unconditional positive regard, were identified by Carl Rogers in the well-researched humanistic approach to person-centered therapy.

Slide 24

Therapy Guidelines

Intellectual disability affects many aspects of the person's day-to-day life.

People with an intellectual disability usually have some difficulty:

- communicating
- remembering things
- understanding social rules
- understanding cause and effect for everyday events
- solving problems and thinking logically
- reacting and interacting in ways that are characteristic for their age

Fletcher et al., 2011

People with IDD may have specific profiles, as listed in this slide. This necessitates the therapist both understanding these characteristics and adapting therapeutic practices in order to accommodate these characteristics.

Slide 25

Therapy Guidelines

- Use appropriate language
- Speak clearly and slowly.
- Speak in a calm, quiet voice.
- Use simple, short statements or questions.
- Avoid using abstract ideas and jargon.
- Be specific.
- Use a normal tone; don't shout or raise your voice.
- Use non-threatening language (including body language).

Fletcher et al., 2011

These guidelines are universal in how to convey your message.

But keep in mind that the therapist should use words that are appropriate to the receptive and expressive skills of the client.

Slide 26

Therapy Guidelines

- **Ask one question or make one request at a time.** Keep the conversation simple.
- **Avoid using leading questions.** People with intellectual disability are often suggestible and will tell you what they think you want to hear or what they think is the "right" answer.
- **Use open questions** where possible, e.g., "How are you feeling?" or "Tell me about …." Closed questions may be useful to clarify something; however, be careful they are not leading questions.

Morasky (2007)

It is essential for the therapist to be a good listener.

Slide 27

Therapy Guidelines

- **Check the person's understanding from time to time.** If you are not sure they have understood, ask them to explain to you in their own words what you have just asked or said.
- **Do not assume** the person's ability to express themselves is an indication of how much they understand.
- **Be patient**; give the person time to respond.
- **Don't assume** the person with an intellectual disability is able to generalize skills learned in one context or situation automatically to another.
- **Don't pretend to understand.** Use checking questions or paraphrasing to assist your understanding. Ask them to repeat what they have said in another way if they can.

Morasky, 2007

It is important to check with the person to ensure they have an understanding of the nature of the conversation. In fact, assumptions in either direction can be problematic. Frequently people with ID may play to one's lower expectations even when they have greater intellect and abilities.

Slide 28

Therapy Guidelines

- Ensure the privacy of the person within the boundaries of confidentiality.
- Be prepared to repeat information more than once if necessary.
- Listen to the person. Don't be judgmental, critical or sarcastic in your response.
- Appear calm, relaxed and confident and provide respect and dignity.
- Keep an upbeat attitude, reassure the person and let them know you are available and supportive.
- Do not make any promises that cannot be kept.
- If the person is alone, ask whether they want family or a support professional involved in therapy. They may have contact details on them.

Morasky, 2007

We can't stress enough that trust, rapport and mutual respect are the building blocks of successful psychotherapy.

Slide 29

Multimodal Assessment Considerations

- Medical history
- Medication history
- Developmental history
- Etiology and type of developmental disability
- Trauma/abuse history
- Known problems in other family members
- Forensic history
- Ability level
- Residential history
- Educational history
- Vocational history
- Communication style and ability
- Substance use history

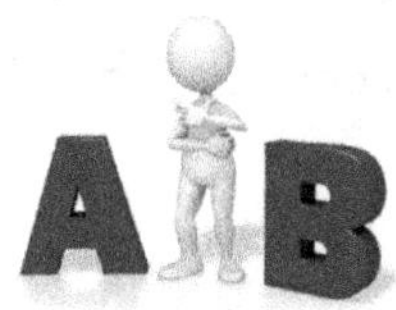

DM-ID 2

It is important to have an understanding of the depth of the person's past assessments.

Slide 30

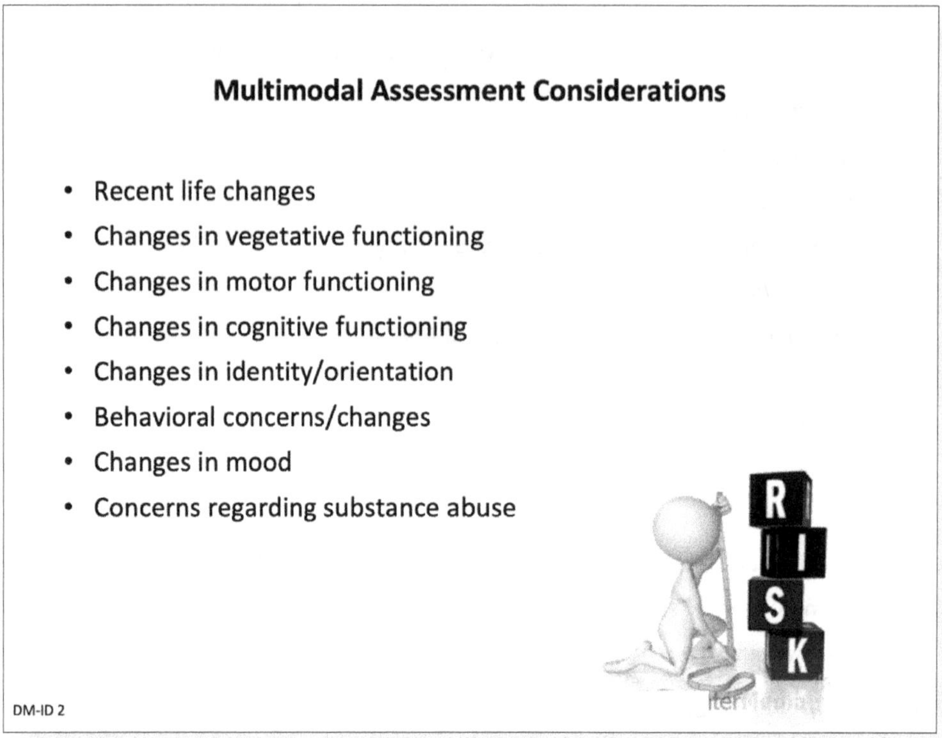

The last slide looked at a person's history. In this slide, we are ascertaining changes that have occurred recently.

Slide 31

Therapeutic Principles

- Empathetic understanding
- Respect and acceptance of people we support
- Concreteness
- Confidentiality
- Draw the person out
- Express genuine interest
- Be aware of your own feelings

Fletcher, et al. (Eds.), 2015

Principles of achieving a therapeutic relationship are relevant to a psychotherapist.

Empathetic understanding — Trying to understand the "inner world" of the individual. What would it be like to be in his/her shoes?

Respect for and acceptance of the client — This is a fundamental principle that is essential in developing a therapeutic relationship. It is analogous to Carl Rogers' concept of "unconditional regard."

Concreteness — Using language that is understood by the person with IDD. Avoid analogies and use language appropriate to the language skills of the person you're working with.

Therapeutic genuineness — This implies being yourself in a real and authentic way.

Accept the client's life circumstances — Many of the individuals we serve have horrendous backgrounds. Regardless of the nature or extent of "background baggage" they carry, it is important that we accept the individual. The life circumstances of the individuals we serve should not have a negative influence on how we value the individual.

Confidentiality — This is an essential concept in therapy. This principle should be understood to include other significant people in the life of the person.

Draw the client out — There may be situations and circumstances that may warrant the therapist to spend time outside the office with the person as means to develop a trusting relationship — for example, taking a walk.

Be aware of your own feelings — It is not necessary to like each and every person, but it is important to be aware of our feelings toward the person (transference).

Slide 32

Confidentiality

- Nothing discussed in therapy will be released without the person's permission.
- With the client's permission, the therapist will work collaboratively other care providers.

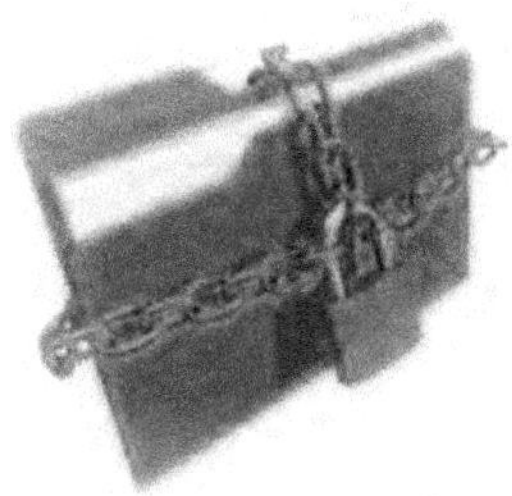

Fletcher, et al. (Eds), 2015

Confidentiality traditionally means there is an expectation of both the therapist and the client that what happens between them is private in that the information revealed during their interactions will not be divulged to others under ordinary circumstances. "What is said in the session, stays in the session."

However, when conducting therapy with a person who has IDD/MI, it is important for the therapist to communicate with family members and other care providers involved in the person's life. This communication is done only after the client has given both verbal and written permission. If the client is under age 18 or has a legal guardian, the permission may also involve the parent or legal guardian.

In essence, the therapist should not work in isolation. Rather, the therapist works as part of the person's treatment or habilitative team. The communication from the therapist should be around conceptual issues and not details of what was discussed in therapy (Fletcher, Baker, Cheplic, 2015).

Slide 33

Cognitive Load of Therapy and Intervention

Cognitive load refers to the amount of information and interactions processed simultaneously (or) thinking and reasoning required for people to build on what they already understand.

- Many of the typical ways we provide therapy are complex and require significant cognitive functioning to work.
- Typical practices may not work for a person with IDD.

Many different types of therapy have been found to be effective in treating people with IDD. Treatment providers need a strategy for adaptation so language, goals, strategies and tasks can be adapted to the intellectual/developmental abilities of the client.

Slide 34

Cognitive Processes

- Typical therapy might require inductive reasoning.
  - Therapists help see patterns across multiple incidents.
  - This requires a person to make connections from multiple examples.
- Typical therapy might require deductive reasoning.
  - Therapists help to figure out how to handle certain situations using general rules.
- Typical therapy might require self-awareness to report on feelings and insights about actions and situations.
- These can be difficult for a person with IDD.

Baker, 2011

All of these are components of typical verbal therapy and may challenge a person's cognition. That is why adaptation is required for many typical verbal therapy activities. This module presents many strategies for adaptation.

Slide 35

Ten Adaptations of Therapy

1. Language
2. Frequency of sessions
3. Shorter sessions
4. Duration of therapy
5. Utilize a more structured and directive approach
6. Communication with collaterals
7. Modify complexity of interventions
8. Therapist needs to be supportive
9. Therapist needs to be flexible
10. Use of visual supports

Therapy for a person with IDD or IDD/MI requires a strategy of adaptations.

- Adaptations may be necessary before and during the course of therapy.
- Adaptations are needed to consider the developmental perspective.
- Adaptations can be referred to as "developmental adaptations."
- These adaptations may include, for example, a change in modification of language, goals, strategies and tasks (Robert Morasky, 2007).

Slide 36

It is important for the therapist to use language that corresponds with the skills of the individual.

The therapist can glean from history and initial contact with the person. The therapist should have a clear understanding of the person's language skills through the efforts it has taken to establish rapport and trust.

Slide 37

Adaptations of Therapy

2) Frequency of Sessions

- In the beginning stage of therapy, it may be useful to have sessions held more frequently than one would with a neurotypical person.
- It takes more time to establish a therapeutic relationship as compared to a neurotypical person.
- For some people, it may be recommended to have therapy two times per week for a relatively brief period of time, and then weekly.

Fletcher et al. (Eds.), 2015

Slide 38

Adaptations of Therapy

3) Shorter Sessions

- There may be a challenge to maintain the person's attention and focus on therapeutic issues that last the usual 45-60 minutes.
- Allow for a degree of flexibility with regard to the length of any given therapy session.
- For some people, a 30-minute session is the time period for which their cognitive reserve will allow them the maximum benefit.

Fletcher et al. (Eds), 2015

Keep in mind that each session length might change from week to week. The therapist must recognize the behavior that will indicate that the person has reached the end of their attention span relative to topic of the therapeutic discussion.

Slide 39

Adaptations of Therapy

4) Duration of Therapy

- Increase length of treatment to allow for needed repetition.
- Increase length of treatment to allow for newly acquired skill sets to be generalized.
- Increase length of treatment to build upon therapeutic relationship and needed time to work on goals and objectives.
- Effective termination process may take longer.

Fletcher et al. (Eds.), 2015

Slide 40

Adaptations of Therapy

5) Utilize a More Structured and Directive Approach

- Structure is often needed in therapy to help bring and maintain focus on the therapeutic material being addressed.
- A more directive approach can be useful to facilitate meaningful interaction between the therapist and the person.
- Silence can be perceived as rejection.

Fletcher et al. (Eds.), 2015

The therapist can provide structure by taking the lead in drawing the person out. The therapist can ask the person to describe a situation or event that is under discussion. After a discussion about an event, the therapist can then bring up feeling states associated with the event.

Slide 41

Adaptations of Therapy

6) **Communication with Other Care Providers**

- With appropriate permission, therapist should communicate with others (care providers, parents, psychiatrist, residential staff, etc.).
- Therapist should not work in isolation, but be part of the holistic treatment/habilitation/care planning team.
- If individual is living with natural family, employing a family systems approach can be incorporated as an adjunct to individual therapy.
- Other caregivers can provide important collateral information.

Fletcher et al. (Eds.), 2015

It is not uncommon for the person who lives with the natural family to express conflicts concerning the family system. In this situation, it may be useful to invite one or more family members into a session, with the person's permission. Another example is an individual in a group home setting and the issues brought in therapy are directly related to a problem the individual is having with a particular staff person. In this situation, the therapist might consider having contact with the staff, with the client's permission.

It is because of the nature of the level of dependence on others, as compared to a neurotypical person, that it is important to include those others in the therapist's approach.

Slide 42

Adaptations of Therapy

7) Modify complexity of interventions to be in sync with the person's developmental framework

- Repetition is important in order for the person to internalize the material discussed in therapy.
- Discuss one therapeutic issue at a time with attention to beginning, middle and end stages of the material discussed.
- Break down interventions into smaller pieces to ensure understanding before moving on to the next topic of discussion.
- Use reflection to ensure understanding the materials discussed.

Fletcher et al. (Eds.), 2015

Basically, keep it simple. Repetition is important. Go slow. Make sure the person understands.

Slide 43

Adaptations of Therapy

8) The therapist needs to be supportive

- Provide a lot of support.
- Give recognition to even small improvements.
- Provide a sense of hope.

Fletcher et al. (Eds.), 2015

Many of our clients come in with a pervasive feeling of defeat, inadequacy and failure. Their self- perception of lifelong failures is greater than their perception of lifelong successes. It is therefore important for the therapist to provide positive communication at any opportunity. Furthermore, instilling a sense of hope can be transformative.

Slide 44

Adaptations of Therapy

9) The therapist needs to be flexible

- For neurotypical people, when progress is not made, the therapist might assume resistance. With people who have IDD, the therapist needs to adjust and consider an alternative approach.
- An elective approach or at least the knowledge and skills of using more than one model is suggested.
- A supportive approach can be beneficial.

Fletcher et al. (Eds.), 2015

We know we work with people who have intellectual or developmental disabilities, and as such, when we look to support a person properly, we have to take into account the differences in how they learn. Even when a particular therapeutic model is being used, it might help for the therapist to consider adding elements from an alternate model of therapy.

Slide 45

Adaptations of Therapy

10) Use of visual supports

Employing visual supports, such as graphics and pictures, can help a person increase their understanding of the therapeutic process:

- Flip charts
- Games
- Social stories
- Handouts
- Multisensory approach

Fletcher et al. (Eds.), 2015

In addition, homework assignments with visual supports can support the individual to practice at home. A pictorial method can be used to help identify feeling states. In this way, clients can monitor their daily feeling state.

For some people with disabilities who learn best visually, adding supports such as graphics and pictures might be very helpful.

Slide 46

Theoretical Orientation

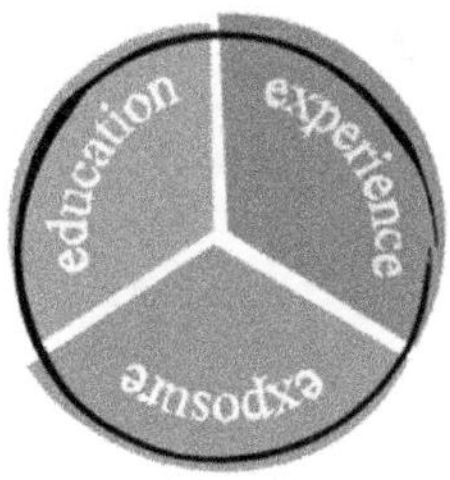

Just as with the general population, people with intellectual disability and co-occurring mental illness respond to a variety of therapeutic approaches.

A clinician's approach should be informed based on the need of the identified person, rooted in sound, evidence-based theory and supported by education, experience and exposure, relative to providing the treatment.

Fletcher et al. (Eds.), 2015

Along with traditional psychotherapy, approaches such as art therapy, music therapy and even pet therapy address the emotional needs of people who are less able to participate in talk therapy.

Slide 47

Therapy Techniques Can Be Adapted

- Cognitive Behavior Therapy (CBT)
- Dialectical Behavior Therapy (DBT)
- Trauma Focused (TF-CBT)
- Group Therapy (GT)
- Support Therapy (SP)
- Other approaches that can be modified
  - Interactive Behavioral Treatment (IBT)
  - Eye Movement Desensitization and Reprocessing (EMDR)
  - Positive psychology

Fletcher et al., 2011

Models of therapy that are used with the neurotypical population can be adapted for persons with IDD.

Slide 48

Cognitive Behavior Therapy (CBT)

- CBT is evidenced-based practice
- Based on theory that faulty thinking patterns and beliefs cause both maladaptive behavior and negative emotions
  Targets:
  - Faulty thinking patterns
  - Maladaptive behaviors

- CBT is designed to help client identify and change:
  - Dysfunctional thinking
  - Behavior
  - Emotional responses

Jackson & Gentile, 2011

Albert Ellis, Ph.D., and Aaron Beck, MD, are early originators of CBT.

Slide 49

Characteristics of CBT

1. Thoughts cause feelings and behaviors
2. Time limited to between 16-30 sessions, approximately
3. Emphasis placed on current behavior
4. Teaches the benefits of remaining calm or neutral when faced with difficult situations:

   If you are upset by a problem, then you have two problems:

   - The problem
   - Your upsetness

Jackson & Gentile, 2011

Slide 50

Characteristics of CBT (cont.)

5. Based on relational thought
6. It is structured and directive, based on the notion that maladaptive behaviors are the result of skill deficits.
7. Based on the assumption that most emotional and behavioral reactions are learned; need to unlearn and find new ways of reacting.

Jackson & Gentile, 2011

Slide 51

Cognitive Behavior Therapy

CBT is effective in helping clients improve functioning and in identifying the beliefs, feelings and behaviors associated with the trauma responses.

Overall functioning is improved through skills development and more adaptive cognitive appraisals of events that trigger intense responses.

CBT teaches people to monitor thoughts and change thought patterns that lead to problems. There is a strong evidence base showing utility for persons with IDD if proper adaptation is made (Gaus, 2007).

Jackson & Gentile, 2011

Slide 4

CBT is "problem-focused" (undertaken for specific problems) and "action-oriented" (therapist tries to assist the client in selecting specific strategies to help address those problems). Strategies may be presented in a variety of concrete media. For example, a client who is working on impulsive behavior may carry a picture of traffic lights representing "Stop. Think. Go." to prompt them to process emotions and thoughts before taking action.

Adaptations in CBT need to include consideration to:

- Meaningfully include past knowledge in current discussions
- Ability to evaluate ideas and reflect on actions taken
- Have insight into and ability to express thoughts and feelings
- Delays in processing verbal information and forming a response — receptive and expressive language deficits

Slide 52

Trauma-Focused Cognitive Behavioral Therapy

- People are provided knowledge and skills related to processing the trauma; managing distressing thoughts, feelings and behaviors; and enhancing safety.
- TFCBT combines trauma and sensitive interventions with DBT.

Slide 53

Adaptations of CBT for persons with IDD

- Increase the number of sessions to help the person understand abstract concepts.
- Use repetition to help the person with internalization of the material under discussion.
- Involve care providers to assist the person in identifying cognitive distortions.
- Enlist care providers to assist with homework assignments.

Jackson & Gentile, 2011

Slide 54

Dialectical Behavior Therapy (DBT)

- Established by Marsha Linehan (1993).
- DBT is an evidenced-based practice.
- DBT is a structured, skill-based approached.
- The efficacy of DBT is improved when the focus is on building replacement skills rather than merely attempting to eliminate problematic behaviors.

Linehan, 2993

Slide 55

Dialectical Behavior Therapy

DBT is a type of CBT and focuses on helping people:

- Learn to regulate their emotions
- Improve ability to cope with stress

DBT comprises two main components:

1. Weekly individual sessions
2. Weekly group sessions

Linehan, 1993

Slide 56

Dialectical Behavior Therapy

DBT is a comprehensive treatment program addressing deficits in emotion regulation, distress tolerance and interpersonal relationships accomplished through:

- individual psychotherapy
- skills training groups
- supervision/case consultation groups

Linehan, 1993

DBT was originally developed by Marsha Linehan (1993a; 1993b) for the treatment of individuals diagnosed with borderline personality disorder.

It is now best described as being designed for the severe and chronic, multidiagnostic, difficult-to-treat client. DBT has been adapted to persons with IDD by Charlton and colleagues (Charlton, 2006; Charlton & Dykstra, 2011).

Slide 57

Adaptations of DBT for Persons with IDD

- Principles of treatment remain the same, but the presentation and language are modified
- Concepts are pared down or simplified
- Handouts are rewritten to increase attention and aid in understanding
- Much individual feedback is provided
- Repetition is used to assist with learning, retention and generalization
- Shorter time for individual and group treatment

Charlton & Dykstra, 2011

Slide 58

Group Therapy

- Group Therapy (GT) affords the opportunity to address problems with the support of others who may have common issues and goals.
- The result is a sense of universality as clients realize that others share similar struggles.
- GT can be process-oriented, and there is benefit in witnessing the resourcefulness of the group members who are in a similar situation.

Fletcher & Duffy, 1993

Slide 59

Group Therapy

- Group members can gain a sense of reassurance and hope in their own recovery
- GT provides a safe environment to experience validation and normalcy
- GT benefits include
  - Improved interpersonal relationships
  - Improved problem-solving skills
  - Improved acceptance of self, leading to improved self-esteem and acceptance

Fletcher & Duffy 1993

Slide 60

Interactive Behavioral Treatment (IBT)

A group therapy treatment for trauma that uses person-to-person interaction, psychodrama and therapeutic interventions as an interactive method to address trauma and related conditions.

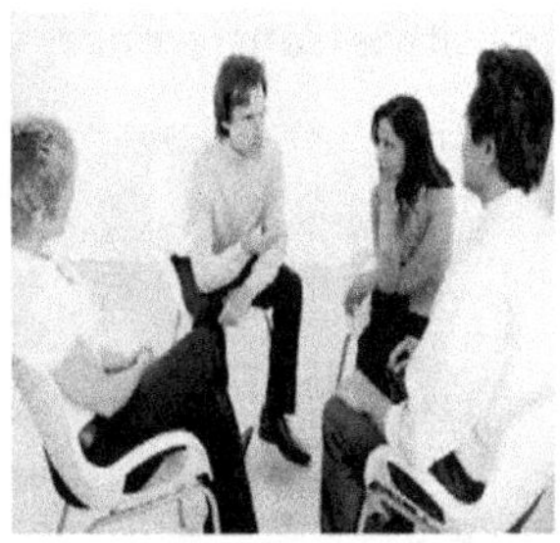

Razza & Tomasulo (2005).

Interactive behavior therapy modifies the typical psychodrama session, which has three stages: (1) warm-up, (2) enactment and (3) sharing (Tomasulo, 2013).

Normally, the first stage would prepare group members for interactive role-playing. The second stage would see the enactment happen, and the third stage would be used for reflection on the role play.

The cognitive limitations of people with intellectual disability made this format unworkable, so positive interactive behavior therapy developed a four-stage model, with stage 4 being affirmation that identifies the strengths and positive aspects of each interaction or "enactment" (Tomasulo, 2013).

Slide 61

Supportive Psychotherapy (SP)

- Supportive therapy (SP) incorporates a variety of therapy theories.
- It is interactive between therapist and client.
- SP is based on the belief that a supportive relationship can serve to help the client make a positive change.
- Therapist assumes a strong empathetic stance and nurturing positive transference, which strengthens the relationship.

Jackson & Gentile, 2012

Slide 62

Supportive Psychotherapy (SP)

- SP primarily focuses on "here and now" issues.
- Therapist facilitates improved affect regulation, improved healthy emotional response to stress and improved interpersonal relationships.
- Modification with people who have IDD
  - Reduce complexity by shrinking down time into smaller units
  - Augment with games, drawings, role play, etc.
  - Therapy may involve family and/or others who have significant impact on the client.

Jackson & Gentile, 2012

Slide 63

Eye Movement Desensitization and Reprocessing (EMDR)

- First developed by Francine Shapiro upon noticing that certain eye movements reduced the intensity of disturbing thought.
- EMDR uses a person's own rapid, rhythmic eye movements.
- Treatment consists of eight phases with precise intentions.

Shapiro, 2012

EMDR is now recommended as an effective treatment for trauma in the Practice Guidelines of the American Psychiatric Association.

EMDR integrates elements from both psychological theories (e.g., affect, attachment, behavior, bioinformational processing, cognitive, humanistic, family systems, psychodynamic and somatic) and psychotherapies (e.g., body-based, cognitive-behavioral, interpersonal, person-centered and psychodynamic) into a standardized set of procedures and clinical protocols.

Slide 64

Positive Psychology for People with ID/MI

There has been a recent shift in the conceptualization of intellectual disability, with increased attention directed toward the importance of identifying and enhancing the strengths and capabilities of people with intellectual disabilities as a means to promote meaningful participation, community inclusion and quality-of-life outcomes.

Positive psychological approach seeks to increase human flourishing and optimal functioning. For people with ID and MI, their strengths and virtues are recognized and developed to enable them to thrive.

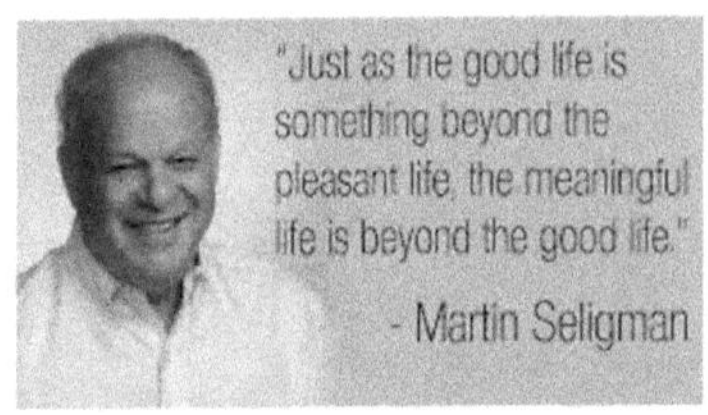

Shogren, Wehmeyer & Singh (Eds.), 2017

Slide 65

Summary

By adapting empirically validated psychotherapy techniques and treatments, a clinician can provide effective therapy for people with IDD/MI.

With some consideration to cognitive abilities, including expressive and receptive language, psychotherapy techniques can be effectively adapted to meet the needs of people who have IDD/MI.

References: Module IX

Adler-Tapia, R. L., & Settle, C. S. (2009, March). EMDR with children: The full works. *Counseling Children and Young People* [a divisional journal of the British Association for Counselling and Psychotherapy], 12-15.

American Psychiatric Association (2013). Recovering emotionally from disaster. Retrieved February 2015 from http://www.apa.org/topics/trauma/index.aspx.

Anderson, G., & Kazantzis, N. (2008). Social problem solving skills training for adults with mild intellectual disability: A multiple case study. In *Behaviour Change,* 25 (2), 97-108.

Brown, J. (2011). *The skills system instructor's guide: An emotion-regulation skills curriculum for all learning abilities.* Bloomington, IN: iUniverse.

Charlton, M. (2006). Dialectical behavior therapy for children with developmental disabilities. *NADD Bulletin,* 9(5): 90-97.

Charlton, M., & Dykstra, E. J. (2011). Dialectical behaviour therapy for special populations: treatment with adolescents and their caregivers. *Advances in Mental Health and Intellectual Disabilities.* 5 (5), 6–14.

Charlton, M., & Tallant, B. (2003). Trauma treatment with clients who have dual diagnoses: Developmental disabilities and mental illness. *National Association for the Dually Diagnosed Annual Conference Proceedings.* Kingston, NY: NADD Press.

Fletcher, R. (Ed.). (2011). *Psychotherapy for Individuals with Intellectual Disability.* Kingston, NY: NADD Press.

Fletcher, R., Barnhill, J., & Cooper, S-A. (2016). *Diagnostic Manual – Intellectual Disability (DM-ID-2): A Textbook of Diagnosis of Mental Disorder in Persons with Intellectual Disability* (2nd ed.). Kingston, NY: NADD Press.

Fletcher, R., & Duffy T., Group therapy for persons with mental retardation. In Fletcher, R., Dosent, A. (Eds.), (1993), *Mental Health Aspects of Mental Retardation*. New York, NY: Lexington Books.

Gaus, V. L. (2007). *Cognitive Behavioral Therapy for Adult Asperger Syndrome.* New York: Guilford Press.

Harvey, K. (2009). *Positive Identity Development: An Alternative Treatment Approach for Individuals with Mild and Moderate Intellectual Disabilities.* Kingston, NY: NADD Press.

Herman, J. (1992). *Trauma and Recovery.* New York: Basic Books.

Hollins, S., & Sinason, V. (2000). Psychotherapy, learning disabilities and trauma: new perspectives. *The British Journal of Psychiatry*, 176, 32-36.

Jackson, C. & Gentile, J. (2012) Psychotherapy. In Gentile, J. P., & Gillig, P. M. (Eds.), *Psychiatry of Intellectual Disability: A Practical Manual.* Oxford, UK: John Wiley & Sons, Ltd.

Linehan, M. (1993a). *Cognitive-behavioral treatment of borderline personality disorder.* New York: Guilford Press.

Linehan, M. (1993b). *Skills training manual for treating borderline personality disorder.* New York: Guilford Press.

Linehan, M. (2000). Commentary on innovations in Dialectical Behavior Therapy. *Cognitive and Behavioral Practice*, 7, 478-481.

Morasky, R. (2007). Making counseling/therapy intellectually attainable. *NADD Bulletin*, 10(3), 58-62.

National Association for the Dually Diagnosed (2018). Psychotherapy and other therapies for people with ID/MI. [Training in NADD Clinical Certification Competencies, St. Louis, MO, January 31–February 2, 2018.]

Palay, L. (2012). *Autism and trauma: Calming anxious brains.* Columbus, OH: Centre for Systems Change: Disability Policy and Social Welfare.

Prout, H. T., & Browning, B. (2011), The Effectiveness of Psychotherapy with Persons with Intellectual Disabilities. In Fletcher, R. (Ed.) *Psychotherapy for Individuals with Intellectual Disability*, Kingston, NY: NADD Press.

Razza, N., & Tomasulo, D. (2005). *Healing trauma: The power of group treatment for people with intellectual disabilities.* Washington, DC: American Psychological Association.

Razza, N., Tomasulo, D., & Sobsey, D. (2011). Group psychotherapy for trauma-related disorders in people with intellectual disabilities. *Advances in Mental Health and Intellectual Disabilities*, 5 (5), 40-45.

Sequeira, H., Howlin, P., & Hollins, S. (2003). Psychological disturbance associated with sexual abuse in people with learning disabilities: Case-control study. *The British Journal of Psychiatry*, 183, 451-456.

Shapiro, F. (2012). EMDR therapy: An overview of current and future research. *European Review of Applied Psychology*, 62, 193-195.

Shogren, K., Wehmeyer, M., & Singh, N. (Eds.), (2017). *Handbook of Positive Psychology in Intellectual and Developmental Disabilities.* New York: Springer Series on Child and Family Studies.

Sobsey, D. (1994). *Violence and abuse in the lives of people with disabilities: The end of silent acceptance?* Baltimore, MD: Paul H. Brookes Publishing Co.

Sumners, J., Fletcher, R., & Bradley, W. (2017). People with Intellectual and Developmental Disabilities and Mental Health Needs. In Wehmeyer et al. (Eds.), *A Comprehensive Guide to Intellectual and Developmental Disabilities.* Baltimore, MD: Paul H. Brookes Publishing Co.

YAI National Institute for People with Disabilities. (n.d.). Coping: Helping people with DD better cope with their daily problems [DVD/CD-ROM].

Wittman, J. P., Strohmer, D. C., & Prout, H. T. (1989). Problems presented by persons of mentally retarded and borderline intelligence in counseling: An exploratory investigation. *Journal of Applied Rehabilitation Counseling*, 20, 8-13.

Module X

Trauma-Informed Supports

Slide 2

Learning Objectives

Participants will

- Identify risks of individuals with IDD for developing trauma-related disorders.
- Recognize how trauma history can present as challenging behavior.
- Identify methods for adapting trauma treatment and supports for individuals with IDD.

Slide 3

Trauma

- Trauma is the emotional response to a terrible event like an accident, rape or natural disaster.
- Immediately after the event, shock and denial are typical.
- Longer-term reactions include unpredictable emotions, flashbacks, strained relationships and even physical symptoms, such as headaches or nausea (APA, 2013).

Slide 4

A major trauma could be:

- Sexual assault/physical assault
- Natural or manmade disasters
- Catastrophic illness
- Loss of a loved one
- Humiliation
- Bullying
- Deprivation and powerlessness to act on one's own behalf

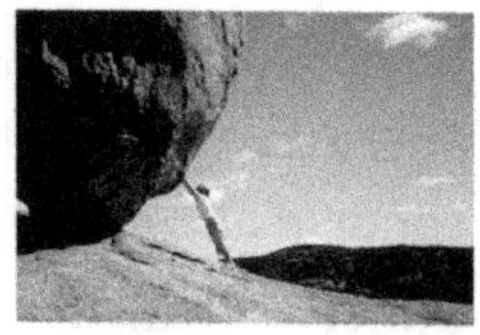

Palay, 2012

Not all trauma results in lasting problems for a person. Whether or not the trauma leads to longer-term issues and lasting stress depends on:

- Duration
- Intensity of stressor
- Time of day
- Warning/no warning
- Intentionality/preventability
- Scope/numbers affected
- Support system during and after traumatic event(s).
- Difficult relationships/poor attachment to others. This is especially true if the trauma has been caused by another person or people.
- Previous history of traumas/stressors/abuse
- History or family history of mental illness
- Inherent resilience/vulnerability
- Substance abuse

Slide 5

Types of Trauma

- **Single or event** — occurs one time (car accident, one instance of abuse, witnessing a death).
- **Complex** (in contrast to single) — over time, prolonged (repeated abuse, target of bullying, moving frequently, living in a situation of continuous conflict).
- **Direct** — death of a loved one, car accident, illness.
- **Vicarious** (in contrast to direct) — through experience of others (hearing about abuse from a friend, being a therapist listening to others' experiences, child or abused parent).

Those who experience single trauma may have a better prognosis (more likely to build resilience) vs. complex trauma, which does not have a definitive endpoint after which recovery can commence. For example, ongoing bullying or repeated abuse can result in multiple triggers and timelines for potential disorders to develop.

These types of trauma are not mutually exclusive. People who experience trauma may experience one, two, three or all four different types.

Slide 6

Simple and Complex PTSD

"Big T" Traumas

Simple post-traumatic stress **results from a one-time incident, such as a rape, violent assault or injury.**

"Little t" Traumas

Complex post-traumatic stress **is a complex set of responses that follows chronic, multiple and/or ongoing traumatic events such as taunting, teasing, tormenting or prolonged abuse.**

Harvey, 2009

Complex PTSD is a result of prolonged and repeated trauma and occurs in situations where a person is captive, unable to flee or is under the control of the perpetrator (Herman, 1992).

Cognitive behavioral therapy (CBT) has yielded positive results amongst individuals with learning disability and PTSD just as it has in the general population. An adapted CBT therapy developed a modified self-report scale from 0 to 10 rather than 0 to 100; allowing the victim to use the past tense when relating the traumatic event (rather than using the present tense to explain the story as if it were occurring presently); and allowing a therapist to attend with the victim at the site of the original traumatic event because the person may not be sufficiently independent to do so on his/her own.

Francine Shapiro (2012), the founder of EMDR, asserts that small but traumatic events can accumulate to have a similar traumatic effect on an individual.

Slide 7

Possible Trauma Events for Individuals with IDD

- Abuse: verbal, physical, sexual
- Bullying
- Identified as being different
- Being restrained or forced seclusion (re-traumatizing)
- The "R" word, other disparaging language
- Constant threats (perceived or actual)
- Moving away from family, loss, grief
- Uncertainty of safety and basic needs being met
- Witnessing violence
- Loss of home or job or support services
- Add medical and dental problems, costly prescriptions

These are the events that people with IDD are most likely to encounter in their lives and also that, due to lack of protective factors, can lead to lasting trauma.

Discussion: Consider if these are single, complex, direct or vicarious. They can be more than one. A vicarious trauma can be complex, such as witnessing violence repeatedly over a long period of time or repeated loss (frequent change in staff or housing).

Slide 8

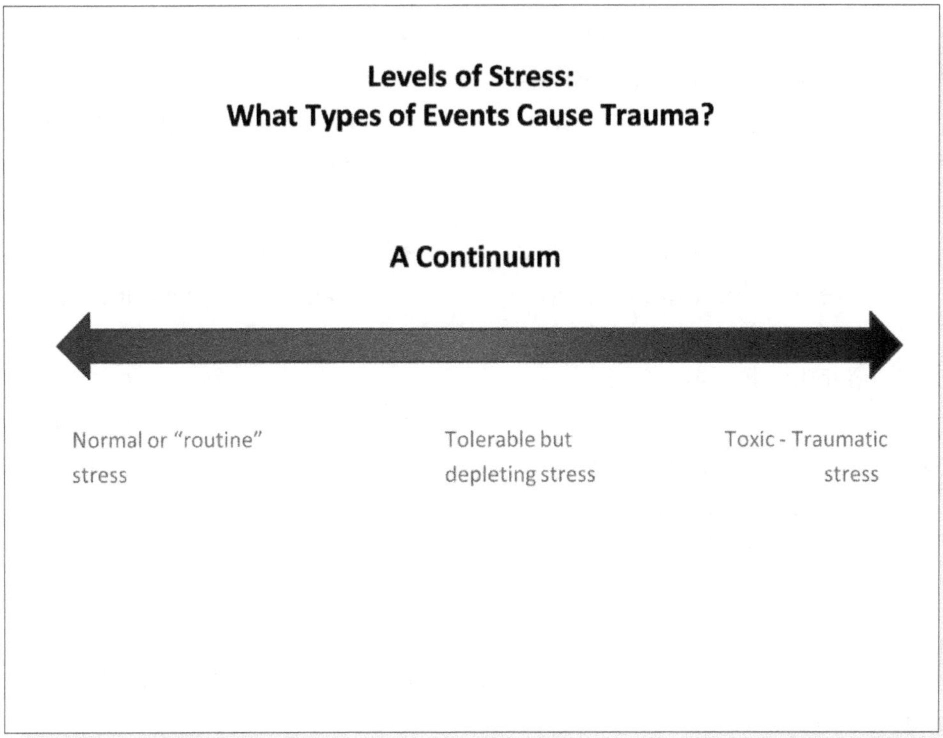

Activity: Depending on class size and facility space, there are two modifications with this exercise. Either with a partner at your seat or by getting up and standing, identify which part of the continuum they place themselves on at designated places in the training room. Modify these examples based on their relatability to the cultural and geographic experiences of the group.

- A severe thunderstorm or snowstorm and subsequent power outage (no heat, no access to communication devices, food is spoiled).
- Health insurance denial.
- Internet disconnected for three days and no access to Wi-Fi or email.
- Your family moves and you have nowhere to live.
- You have to start taking a new prescription, but you don't know what it is for, the dosage or the expected side effects.
- Your best friend leaves one day and never returns.

- You come down to your kitchen in the morning to make coffee and there is a stranger in your home.
- Traveling to an unfamiliar place where you don't understand the language and nobody understands you.
- Losing your home suddenly (due to fire, economics, change in caregivers, other circumstances).
- Seeing your peers date, go to the prom, drive, leave home and go to college while you don't do any of those things.
- Having your symptoms or ailments questioned or dismissed.
- Not seeing your parents or friends for weeks or months.

Discussion: Variables determine why one may place themselves at different points on the scale:

- Perception of the event (ongoing event)
- Available supports (technology, resources)
- Coping strategies
- Meaning that the person attributes to the event
- History of being exposed to those stressors in the past (experience)
- Lasting impact

After participants have connected the situation to their place on the continuum, add more information about the event to increase stress level, e.g., a repeated occurrence of insurance denial, your second or third friend leaves, you face the above scenarios without language, a cell phone or access to other resources.

Slide 9

Trauma

People with intellectual/developmental disabilities are at greater risk for being victimized or abused.

Some experts believe as many as 90 percent of people with intellectual disabilities have some level of traumatic stress. Sobsey (1994) reports that people with disabilities are twice as likely to experience abuse.

Sobsey, 1994

People with intellectual/developmental disabilities are also at great risk of experiencing longer-term trauma due to the build-up of everyday stresses and losses, which can be unique to their experiences.

- Feeling different
- Not being accepted
- Not being able to do what others do
- Moving to a new home or significant change at home
- Being misunderstood
- Knowing that one has a disability and is "different" than others
- Having symptoms or ailments questioned or not believed
- Failing at a task
- Getting confused and overwhelmed

(Adler-Tapia & Settle, 2009)

Slide 10

People with Disabilities Are at Greater Risk of Being Victimized

- More than one in five people from ages 12-19 report sexual violence.
- Three times more likely to experience violent victimization as adolescents and adults.
- Three times more likely to experience rape, sexual assault, aggravated assault and robbery.
- Three times more likely to be sexually abused as children.
- 1.6 times more likely to experience abuse or neglect as children.
- 1.5 times more likely to experience repeated abuse or neglect as children.
- This includes women with disabilities, people with cognitive or developmental disabilities, people with psychiatric illness and people with multiple disabilities.

People with disabilities are devalued.

In general, throughout our society, people with disabilities are viewed as "less than" someone who doesn't have a disability — less smart, less capable, less able and even less deserving.

People with disabilities are not seen as credible.

People with disabilities are seen as unreliable, less credible and more prone to fantasizing. Because of this myth, people with disabilities who report abuse often aren't believed or they are viewed as less credible. The victims are silenced. Abusers know this myth exists and they use it to their advantage: "No one will believe you, even if you do tell."

People with disabilities are isolated.

People with disabilities are often segregated and isolated in communities. While there have been policy and practice shifts away from putting people with disabilities in institutions and toward community-based care, many people with disabilities still live in institutions or nursing homes, which can be just as isolating. Even people with disabilities living in the community experience isolation, as social segregation between people with disabilities and those without persists.

Compliance is expected.
Many people with disabilities, especially people who have an intellectual or cognitive disability, are taught and expected to follow the directions of those "in charge" and comply with someone else's wants, needs or demands. There's a belief that if a person with a disability just does what he's told, he'll be safe and get along OK in life. This is a dangerous belief and practice, because anyone who's taught and expected to automatically do what she's told is more vulnerable and at risk of abuse. Abusers of people with disabilities rely on compliance.

People with disabilities are seen as "easy targets."
Sexual assault and physical abuse are motivated by wanting to exert power and control over another person. Someone who is devalued, taught to be compliant and seen as less credible by others is easier to have power over and easier to control.

The problem is hidden.
Few people in general want to talk about or report when they have been raped or physically abused. The stigma that surrounds these types of interpersonal violence breeds silence. Add to that silence the myths, expectations of compliance and devalued views held about people with disabilities. The result? People with disabilities who are abused are doubly silenced — who they are and the hurt and harm they experience is not widely known, understood or taken seriously.

Slide 11

Risk Factors

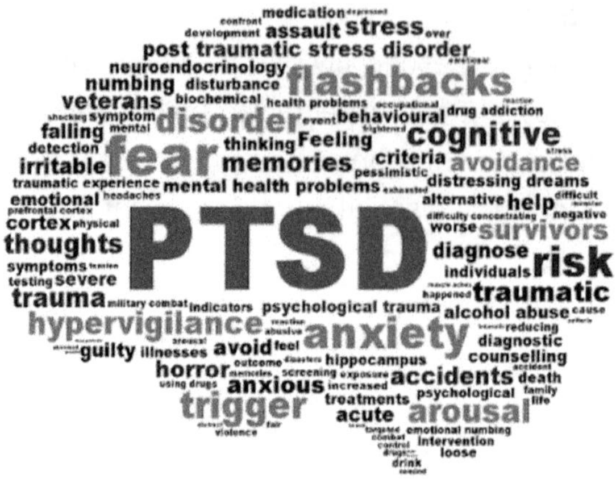

Everyone is at risk. Everyone will be exposed to events that could be sufficient to result in PTSD. However, we don't all have PTSD in this room.

Some are more at risk than others. For individuals with IDD, the range of potentially traumatizing events is greater.

Slide 12

Risk Factors for Developing Trauma Disorders

Risk Factors	Protective Factors
Multiple traumas	Timely and appropriate care
Acquiescence/passivity	Social supports
Lack of control	Safety awareness
Underdeveloped/ineffective coping skills	Previous experience
Communication difficulties	Good communication skills
Mood or anxiety disorder	Wellness supports
Age at time of event	Coping skills
Likely to have less inductive and deductive reasoning	Experiences cognitive dissonance
Isolation and exclusion	Stable housing and work

Type of trauma ties back to the single/direct/vicarious/complex chart earlier. The type of trauma that someone encounters is going to play a role in determining whether a person develops a disorder or shows resilience.

Slide 13

DSM-5: Trauma- and Stressor-Related Disorders

Include: Reactive Attachment Disorder, Post-traumatic Stress Disorder, Acute Stress Disorder.

PTSD is the most common.

- History of exposure to traumatic events (stressors)
- Presence of intrusion symptoms: reliving trauma, flashbacks
- Avoidance behaviors in effort to escape distress
- Alterations in arousal and reactivity following the trauma (e.g., irritable aggressive behavior or self-destructive behavior)
- Symptoms persist longer than one month after trauma

Trauma brings the past into the present.

In the DSM-IV-TR, Anxiety Disorders is one large chapter. Now in the DSM-5, Anxiety Disorders continues to be a chapter with two subsequent chapters (one of which is Trauma- and Stressor-Related Disorders). Their proximity shows both their interconnectedness and individuality. Even though anxiety is part of these disorders, the DSM-5 puts it in its own category.

Slide 14

People with IDD often manifest PTSD differently than what is typically recognized as PTSD in the DSM–5.

Some individuals may have flashbacks but are not able to communicate that experience. What they do communicate, rather, may be misunderstood as a psychotic disorder.

It can be a challenge to identify that a traumatic event has even happened for an individual with a disability, especially when the individual lacks well-developed communication skills and when the event happened long in the past. Some of the events most likely to cause PTSD, such as sexual abuse, occur without witnesses.

The general underdiagnosis of PTSD among people who have IDD leads to a large portion of those with PTSD never receiving treatment. One study of people who have IDD and PTSD as a result of sexual abuse found that only 39 percent of victims received treatment from a therapist (Sequeira, Howlin, & Hollins, 2003).

Slide 15

DM-ID-2 PTSD

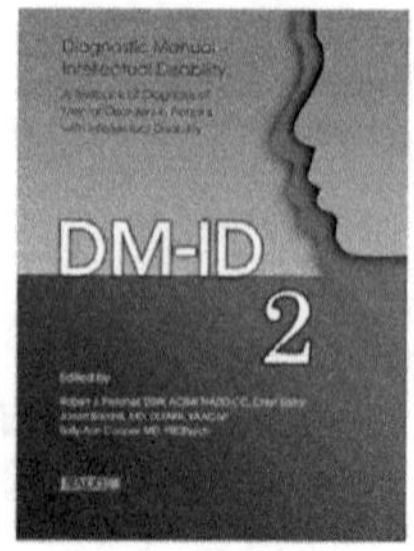

Behaviors

A. Agitation/property destruction
B. Obsessive behavior
C. Paranoia
D. Noncompliance
E. Aggression
F. "Shutdown"
G. Escape behavior

Symptoms

A. Arousal (hyperarousal)
B. Avoidance (hypervigilance)
C. Mistrust based on abuse experiences
D. Dissociation
E. Fight response based on triggering of amygdala and sympathetic nervous system
F. Freeze response
G. Flight response

The DM-ID provides information to help recognize signs and symptoms of mental illness. It lists behavior changes that may indicate certain mental health problems that are noticeable.

Slide 16

Trauma and ASD: Symptoms and Diagnosis

Pathology	Trauma symptomology	Autism traits
Impaired stress response	• Sensitivity to traumatic reminders • Alternation in neuroendocrine stress response system	• Sensitivity to traumatic reminders • Alternation in neuroendocrine stress response system
Disturbance in sense of self and identity	• Suicidality • Self-mutilation • Low self-esteem • Risk-taking • Depersonalization	• Self-mutilation • Low self-esteem • Depersonalization
Interpersonal and relationship problems	• Attachment disorders • Social withdrawal • Promiscuity • Antisocial behavior	• Attachment disorders • Social withdrawal • Antisocial behavior
Affect dysregulation	• Use and abuse of substances to regulate mood, sense of self and behavior • Attention problems • ADHD symptoms • Impulsivity • Hypervigilance	• Attention problems • ADHD symptoms • Impulsivity • Hypervigilance

http://www.traumainformedcareproject.org/

There can be overlap between symptoms of PTSD and behaviors characteristic of autism, even when there isn't PTSD. This can complicate diagnosis of trauma when present in autism. When considering a mental health disorder, consider change in baseline, rapid increase in frequency or severity of behavior and the underlying cause of the pathology.

Slide 17

Trauma and the Mind

When a trigger/stressor is introduced:

- **Amygdala** activated by stressors, activates release hormones
- **Cortex** processes information
- **Limbic system** activated: fight, flight or freeze
- **Hippocampus** is working memory
  - stores experiences and cause
  - breaks down when there is too much stress
  - interrupts learning and remembering behavioral tasks when overworked

Prolonged stress causes permanent damage due to increased levels of cortisol and adrenaline.

When the fight-or-flight response is activated in people with a trauma history, they do whatever is necessary to feel safe (from real or perceived threats). If this happens over and over, there is a quick and conditioned path worn in the brain that easily stimulates the "fear reaction."

During repeated stress (complex trauma), the amygdala communicates to the cortex much more strongly than the cortex can communicate with the amygdala, and the path from the cortex to the amygdala is weakened, so new ways of thinking and behaving develop a new connection from cortex to amygdala.

The hippocampus shrinks, but the amygdala gets larger, therefore less stress in needed to be activated and cause a fear reaction in brain and body.

Slide 18

Trauma and the Body

The body stores trauma. The physiological response to threats (real or perceived) takes its toll over time and can manifest as somatic symptoms:

- Gastrointestinal issues
- Exaggerated pain response
- Migraines
- Muscle tension and soreness

Our bodies were not designed for repeated (chronic) stress. Fight or flight is the biological response to acute stress. Over time, the body adjusts to repeated stress by adapting — instead of incidental fight or flight for long-term survival, the person may adapt with hypervigilance (cannot rest, always feeling threatened) or collapse (depression, constant freeze).

Be aware that these can be healthy adaptations to unhealthy experiences to help a person cope and adjust.

Slide 19

Trauma and Emotions

Emotional states of trauma include anxiety, anger, horror, helplessness and sadness. An individual's experience can fluctuate and include:

- Avoidant behavior, overreaction
- Increased arousal
- Exaggerated startle response, hypervigilance
- Difficulty concentrating
- Outbursts of rage and fear

Slide 20

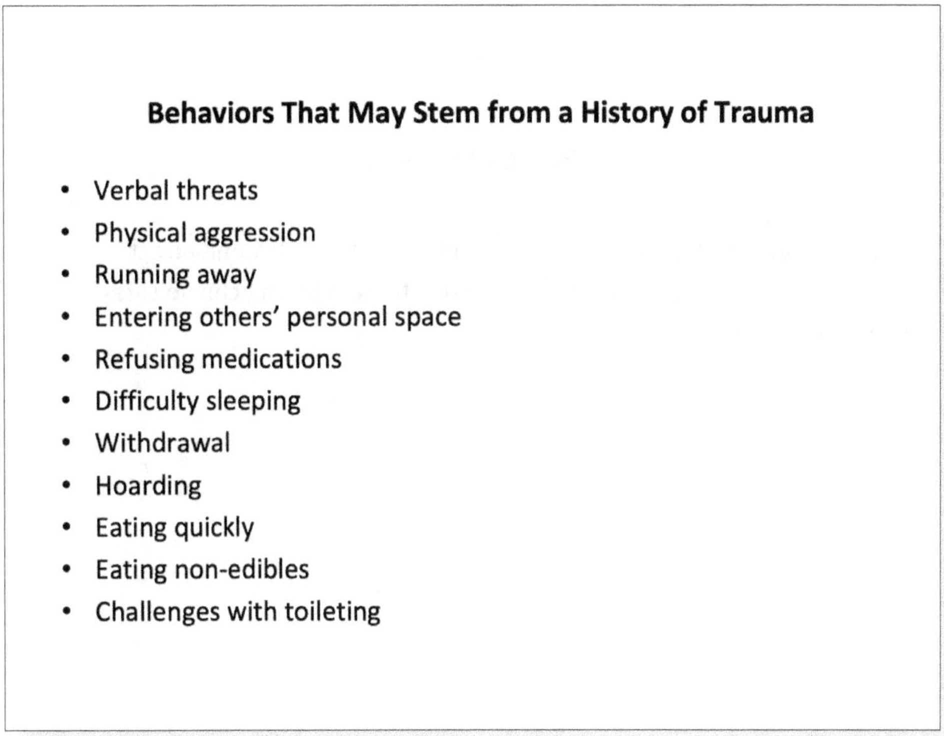

Trauma sets people up for challenging behavior. A trigger or reminder of past trauma may arouse fear or panic response in a non-threatening situation and appear as behaviors.

Slide 21

Trauma-Informed

Being trauma-informed means understanding how trauma affects a person and knowing effective strategies to help them achieve safety and wellness.

Slide 22

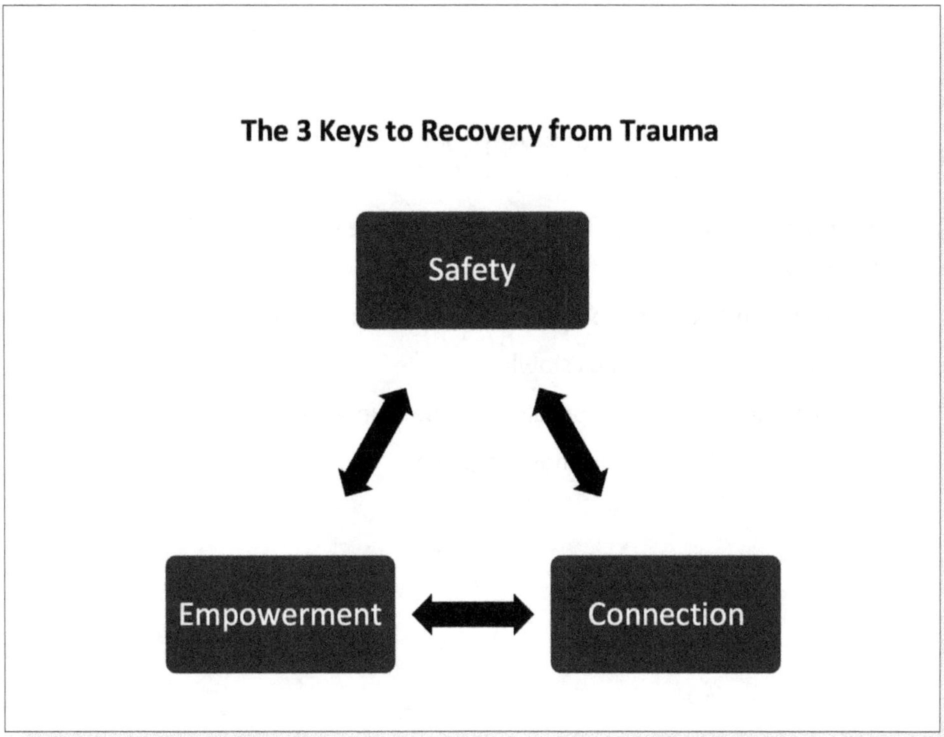

This model was introduced by Karyn Harvey, 2012.

Safety includes ensuring basic needs such as housing, emergency response, health needs, identification and possible reconnection to support systems.

Connection includes processing the traumatic experience at the person's safe and manageable pace with someone he/she trusts. This may include building rapport with new support persons and development of healthy and supportive relationships (friendships, therapy, intimate, family, professional).

Empowerment includes development or rediscovering a positive sense of self and self-identity. A person takes a more active role in his/her recovery by making healthy choices, engaging in self-care and helping others.

Slide 23

Trauma Approach: Safety

People need to feel safe from threats that are real or perceived. This includes:

- Be mindful of behavior that can stem from trauma history
- Introduce relationships slowly
- Creating a structured, predictable, flexible environment
- Be aware of your own body language

When the fight-or-flight response is activated in people with a trauma history, they do whatever is necessary to feel safe (from real or perceived threats). If this happens over and over, there is a quick and conditioned path worn in the brain that easily stimulates the "fear reaction."

Slide 24

Techniques to Help People Feel Safe

- Redirection/Refocusing
- Reframing
  - Change the topic or setting or activity to avoid triggers
- Awareness of your own body language
- Find more supportive and comfortable staff, home, job, neighborhood
- Teach coping skills: breathing, humor, prayer, music

Establish a safety option to provide the person coping or control if the trigger is encountered or anxiety begins to escalate.

Slide 25

Safety: Proactive Supports

Recovery is in not linear. Be mindful and attentive to threats to healing.

- Avoid any kind of re-traumatization from our support strategies (seclusion, isolation, punitive consequences).
- Create a psychiatric advance care directive: Help the person make a plan with steps for support strategies for any setbacks or triggers.

Provide warnings when one might be likely to encounter triggers or reminders of a past traumatic event.

Slide 26

Promote Safe Communication

- Be open to listening
- Show empathy, not judgment
- Be sensitive to the person's triggers
- Use kind words and a calm tone
- Engage in kind actions
- Validate emotions
- Define expectations and roles
- Use visual cues
- Have a predictable staff and activity schedule

- Identify past traumatic events and triggers, evaluate when exposure to triggers is likely in the schedule.
- Provide warnings when one might be likely to encounter triggers or reminders of a past traumatic event.
- Establish a safety option to provide the person coping or control if the trigger is encountered or anxiety begins to escalate.
- Use humor (whenever appropriate).
- Allow the person to make activity choices within a consistent and predictable schedule. This helps the individual begin to establish a sense of security and control.
- Use active listening and validation. Express desire to listen and help. It's OK to say, "I'm sorry."
- Always be aware of your body language. Non-verbal aspects of communication speak louder than words.

Slide 27

Trauma Recovery: Connection

- Include individuals in hiring staff, choosing therapists, other team members.
- Build relationships with trusted people first; expand to new members once rapport is established.
- Create and develop valued roles in the community.
- Support meaningful activities.

- Personalize communication to build rapport.
- Label emotion, reflect content.
- Focus on the positive.
- Avoid "why" questions.
- Make comfortable eye contact.
- Refocus as needed.
- Be clear, concrete, concise.

Slide 28

Trauma Recovery: Empowerment

- Provide and honor real choices.
- Support informed decision-making.
- Encourage leadership and organization of others in need of healing support.
- Create and nurture opportunities for self-care, including healthy diet, exercise and sleep.
- Assist in the use of tools and resources.

http://pid.thenadd.org/

Resilience: Some variables associated with better mental health outcomes lead to being informed; getting involved in leisure activities such as physical activity; and practicing self-care (can include staying active, connecting with your loved ones, rest, pleasant activities, etc.).

Slide 29

Kristina

Kristina is a 24-year-old woman who lives in a group home with two other women. She has anxiety and mild intellectual disability. Kristina is generally a happy and social person. She has a job in a plant nursery watering flowers. When she has free time, she likes to go shopping, go to movies and go out to eat. She does best when her schedule and work are predictable. Kristina tends to stick to activities with which she feels successful.

Kristina has a history of being teased when she was at school, specifically being called names and being told she's *stupid* and *ugly* and excluded from activities. Sometimes at work when a customer asks her a question she can't answer, she will hear her old classmates' voices in her head and run to the breakroom to cry.

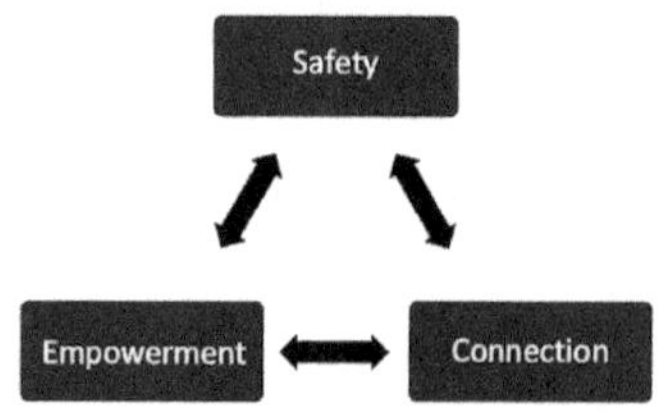

Using the recovery components of safety, connection and empowerment, how can we support Kristina in her trauma recovery?

Slide 30

Therapeutic Approaches

- DBT – Dialectical Behavior Therapy
  - Supportive counseling
  - Group therapy
- TF-CBT
- EMDR
- Individual psychotherapy
- Workbook, journaling, guided imagery
- Positive identity development

There are a wide variety of different intervention packages for trauma treatment for persons with IDD that have an evidence base to support effectiveness. Module IX of this training manual, *Adapting Therapy Practices*, expands on the approaches listed on this slide in greater detail.

DBT (Dialectical Behavior Therapy) for trauma focuses on mindfulness, emotional regulation, distress tolerance and interpersonal effectiveness. It helps people learn to ways to cope with stress and trauma memories.

Trauma-focused CBT is effective to help manage the intrusive anxiety and fear that can accompany trauma memories.

Eye Movement Desensitization and Reprocessing (EMDR) Therapy is a structured therapy that encourages an individual to safely and briefly focus on a trauma memory while simultaneously experiencing bilateral stimulation (typically eye movements), which can result in a reduction in the vividness and emotion associated with the trauma memories.

Tools such as workbooks, journaling and imagery can be used to support skill development and reinforce progress in between formal therapy sessions.

Art therapy, dance, music, pet and play therapy are also creative and healthy ways to refocus attention and expression.

Slide 31

For people who experienced trauma as a child, they may experience memories that are out of sequence or incomplete. As a way to avoid painful or distressing events, they may not have a complete picture of themselves in their youth or developing stages. A lack of foundation or protective factors can disrupt or distort identity. People with negative developmental experiences may also isolate themselves or avoid relationships or activities that foster connection or the social support necessary to recover.

Slide 32

Positive Identity Development

The presence of an intellectual/developmental disability impacts exposure to new experiences and the person's understanding and integration of those experiences.

This requires the organization and delivery of identity-related supports and counseling for persons with IDD across the life span.

Harvey, 2009

Identity forms through the accumulation of experience and the integration of experiences and interpretations of experience.

These experiences begin in infancy when children begin to recognize themselves. It is likely that persons with IDD will move through stages of identity development at a slower or different rate from persons in the general population.

A critical role for care providers and families exists in the need to support persons with IDD in the development of a healthy, accurate self-identity.

Slide 33

Many people with IDD have a largely negative sense of identity, which is constituted of all the good things the person is not. Specific therapeutic approaches can help to create a more positive sense of identity.

Harvey, 2009

"The therapist facilitates the discovery of self and then helps to strengthen and reinforce that sense of self from session to session."
– Harvey, 2009.

Slide 34

How Is Identity Developed?

- Accumulation of experience
- Learning from experience
- Inductive and deductive reasoning
- Timing
- Attribution of meaning

Steve Dahl, 2019

These five factors all contribute to identity. People have experiences that help them learn about themselves, and then they start to generate rules about themselves from those experiences. If I am friendly in a number of different experiences, and I understand that I am friendly in them, then I learn I am a friendly person. If I have a number of experiences where I do well with tasks, and I understand that, then I will learn I am industrious. Ask the participants if they remember where "industrious" fits into identity theory. Simply getting older may help generate a sense of identity, such as puberty. Finally, being able to find meaning in events shapes identity.

Positive effects on identity

- Completion of tasks
- Achievements

- Roles in relationships
- Making meaningful choices
- Risk-taking

Negative effects on identity

- Limited experiences
- Trauma and abuse
- Stereotypes
- Stigma
- Marginalization
- Learned helplessness

Slide 35

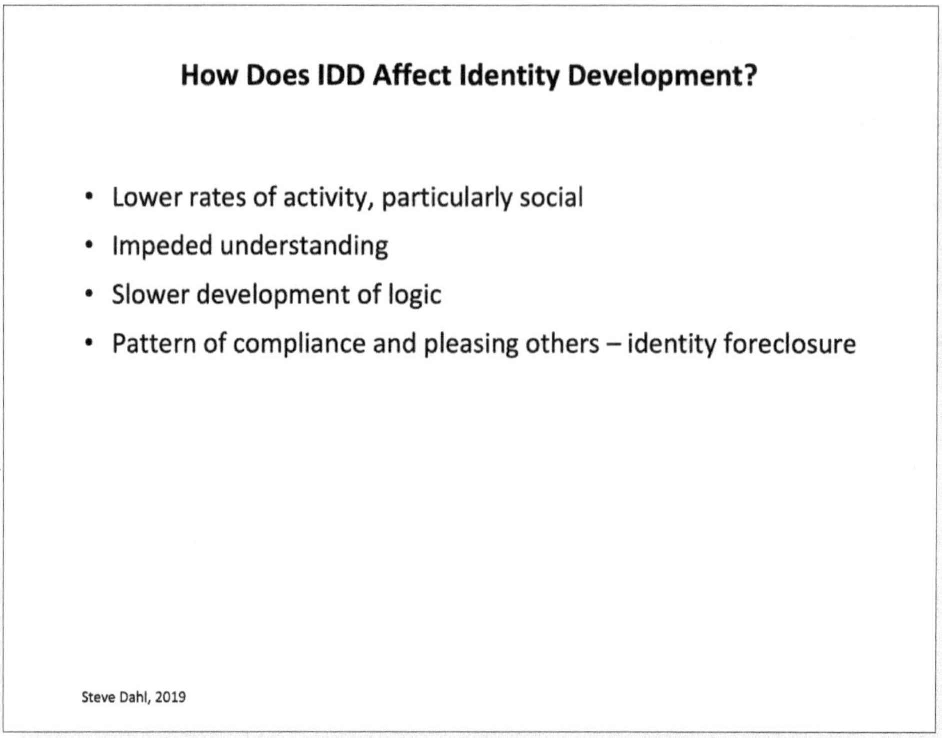

These four elements all change the development of identity for people with intellectual or developmental disabilities. Review each of these for the participants and ask if the people they support have had or show any of these factors. The pattern of compliance is sometimes seen as a personality trait among people who have Down syndrome.

Slide 36

Small Group Activity

- Review the factors that contribute to identity development
- How would each be different as a result of having IDD?
- How can this increase trauma risk and impede trauma recovery? (safety, empowerment, connection)

Have participants work in groups of two, three or four, and pick one person they support. Have the groups discuss how the intellectual or developmental disability may affect their sense of identity.

Slide 37

Resources

Trauma-Informed Project-resources and publications
http://www.traumainformedcareproject.org/resources.php

My Book About Recovery by Karen Harvey (2007)—available free at: *https://aaidd.org/docs/default-source/events/harvey-my-book-about-recovery.pdf?sfvrsn=2*

http://pid.thenadd.org/

Trauma and Recovery: The Aftermath of Violence—from Domestic Abuse to Political Terror by Judith Herman, MD (1992)

Behind Closed Doors: The Story of Four Women Struggling to Reconcile Violence within the Psychiatric System (brief documentary): https://vimeo.com/2709542

Healing Neen (brief documentary): https://vimeo.com/15851924

References: Module X

American Psychiatric Association, (2013). *Diagnostic and Statistical Manual of Mental Disorders. (5th ed.).* Arlington, PA.

Dahl, Steven. (2015). *Introduction to trauma-informed care.* St. Paul, MN: Minnesota Department of Human Services.

Fletcher, R., Loschen, E., Stavrakaki, C., & First, M. (Eds.). (2007). *Diagnostic Manual – Intellectual Disability (DM-ID): A Clinical Guide for Diagnosis of Mental Disorders in Persons with Intellectual Disability.* Kingston, NY: NADD Press.

Ford, G. R., Improving Lives: EMDR Psychotherapy for People with I/DD Experiencing Trauma and Distress. Presentation. NASDDDS, November, 2010.

Harvey, K. (2009). *Positive Identity Development.* Kingston, NY: NADD Press.

Harvey, K. (2012). *Trauma-Informed Behavioral Interventions.* Silver Spring, MD: American Association of Intellectual and Developmental Disabilities.

Harvey, K. (2012). *Trauma-Informed Behavioral Interventions: What Works and What Doesn't.* Silver Spring, MD: American Association of Intellectual and Developmental Disabilities.

Herman, J. L. (1992). *Trauma and Recovery.* Riverhead, NY: Basic Books.

Palay, L. Trauma and Neural Integration: Everyday Strategies. Presentation. (2012).

Razza, N. & Tomasulo, D. (2005). *Healing Trauma: The Power of Group Treatment for People with Intellectual Disabilities.* Washington, DC: American Psychological Association.

SAMHSA's Concept of Trauma and Guidance for a Trauma-Informed Approach. SAMHSA's Trauma and Justice Strategic Initiative. July 2014.

MODULE 10

Sobsey, R. (1994). *Violence and abuse in the lives of people with disabilities: The end of silent acceptance?* Baltimore, MD: Paul H. Brookes Publishing.

Sequeira, H., Howlin, P. and Hollins, S. (2003). Psychological disturbance associated with sexual abuse in people with learning disabilities: Case-control study. *British Journal of Psychiatry*, 183, 451-456.

Trauma Informed Care Project. www.traumainformedcareproject.org.

Vera Institute of Justice, Center on Victimization and Safety. 2019

Van der Kolk, B. A. (2005). Developmental trauma disorder. *Psychiatric Annals*, 35 (5), 401-408.

Van der Kolk, B. A. (2012). Trauma, Attachment and Neuroscience: New Therapeutic Treatments.

Module XI

Childhood and Adolescence

Slide 2

Childhood and Adolescence

Portions of this module were developed originally by Phil Smith, Ph.D.
Boggs Center on Developmental Disabilities
Rutgers Robert Wood Johnson Medical School

Mental wellness for youth with IDD and MI has been less fully explored than the phenomenon in adults.

There have been many books and materials written for adults, but Baker and Blumberg's book for NADD is the first book entirely dedicated to these questions in youth, and it was not published until 2013. The fact that youth are in schools adds a level of complexity, as there is a dedicated service element for them, but in-home and after-school supports differ in each state and province, and the constellation of services may differ from one community to the next.

One of the significant complexities is that development for typical children is likely to look very different than it does for children with IDD.

Slide 3

This module describes issues of typical childhood and adolescence development and details how they are relevant to youth with IDD.

Slide 4

Learning Objectives

- Describe the stages of typical development for younger children and adolescents
- Describe how disability affects self-image/self-esteem
- Describe the issue around development and support for various challenges of maturation

Slide 5

Issues of Development

- There is a typical pathway or sequence of development in which certain cognitive, social and emotional things are seen in each stage for typical people.
- Functioning and behavior are influenced by stages of development.
- Intellectual/developmental disabilities often change development due to difficulties in learning, different patterns of interaction and lack of typical experiences, but most stages still occur (American Academy of Pediatrics, 2013).

"Child development" refers to a child's process of learning to do more complex skills as the child gets older. Milestones usually refer to the sets of age-specific skills that children typically acquire by certain ages, such as gross motor skills, fine motor skills, language, cognitive thinking skills (learning, understanding, problem-solving, reasoning and remembering) and social skills (interacting, developing relationships, cooperation and responding to others' feelings).

Skills such as taking a first step, smiling for the first time and waving goodbye are called "developmental milestones." Children reach milestones in how they play, learn, speak, behave and move (crawling, walking, etc.).

All children develop at their own pace. However, the developmental milestones give a general idea of the changes to expect as a child gets older. The presence of an intellectual/developmental disability can impact the timeline in which these milestones occur. The delay in reaching milestones, or reaching them much later than the general population, is often the first indication that the child may have an intellectual or developmental disability.

Things that are common in smaller children, such as tantrums, generally fade as development occurs. However, in a child who develops at a slower pace, those changes occur at later ages, which makes it very important to understand the manner in which intellectual/developmental disabilities affect maturation. Is it a tantrum due to delayed emotional maturation, is it a learned behavior, or is it impulse control disorder?

Slide 6

It's All About Family

- Support for youth and adolescents with IDD must always consider the family.
- Support for the child must fit within the family system.
- Cultural perspectives of family must always be taken into account.

Baker, 2013, Baker & BLumberg,2013

There are many resources around working with families in:
Baker, D. J., & Blumberg, E. R. (2013). *Mental Health and Wellness Supports for Youth with IDD.* Kingston, NY: NADD Press.

Husband, K. (2019). Medical family therapy for parents of children with intellectual or developmental disabilities. *NADD Bulletin*, 22, 21-25.

Slide 7

Typical Stages

Approximate ages

- Newborn, ages 0-1 month
- Infant, ages 1 month-1 year
- Toddler, ages 1-3 years
- Preschooler, ages 4-6 years
- School-aged child, ages 6-13 years
- Adolescent, ages 13-20

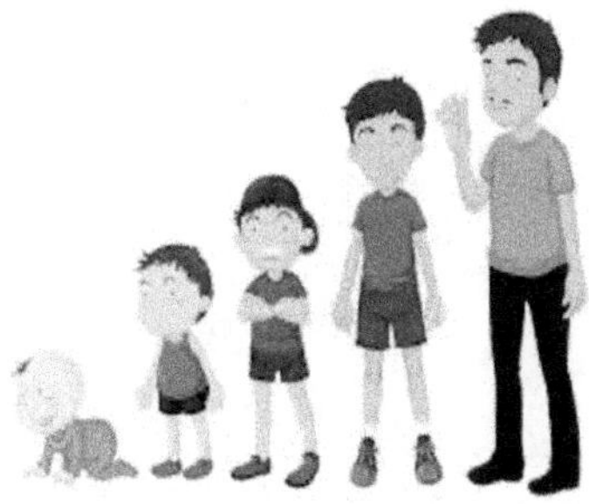

The American Academy of Pediatrics indicates some of the following as some of the first indicators that a newborn has signs of developmental delay:

Newborn/infant — feeding difficulties, blinking response absent in presence of bright light, poor eye focus or tracking, excessively stiff or loose movements of extremities, does not grasp or hold objects, lower jaw abnormalities, lack of response to loud sounds, does not babble, no smile response (American Academy of Pediatrics, 2013a).

Maturation and movement through stages depends on a wide variety of things, including cognitive changes due to development, physical changes, the presence of enriching environments and learning through inductive and deductive reasoning. Development also includes the development of a sense of self and identity, which also is impacted by IDD (Black & Baker, 2013). Proper maturation and development of identity are critical for mental wellness.

Slide 8

Characteristics of Typical Younger Children

- Often significant issues with attachment and attachment disorders
- Typical developmental tasks related to delaying gratification, task completion and development of a sense of identify
- Many problems related to impulsiveness and lack of empathy

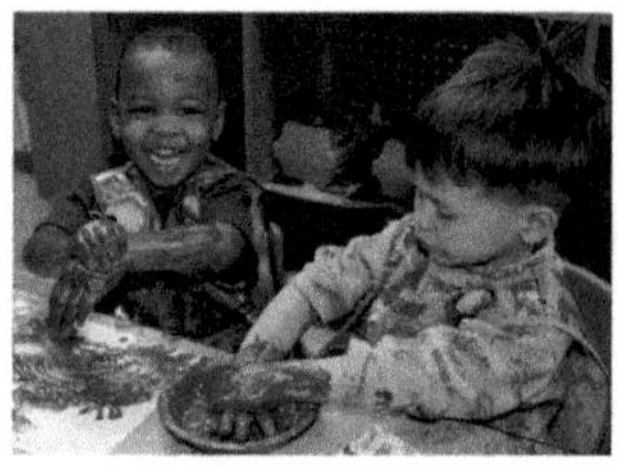

Attachment is a normal stage of child development and describes the reciprocal, enduring relationship that develops between infant and caregiver/parent. Later development can be influenced by the quality and timing of attachment (Papalia, Olds & Feldman, 1999).

It is critical for IDD providers to understand what typical children and youth are like. Many things that might be completely typical for a young person can be seen as problem behaviors by an IDD provider who works only with adults. All children need guidance and instructions on these things. What people don't realize is that young people are not just small adults. Working with youth presents an all new type of differential diagnosis: Is this pattern of actions occurring because this person is only 12?

Slide 9

Characteristics of Adolescence

Teen life is complex for all young people, as they ...

- Physically mature
- Sexually mature
- Emotionally mature
    - Desire independence
    - Sense of identity is built
    - Heightened focus on peers
    - Sexual awareness

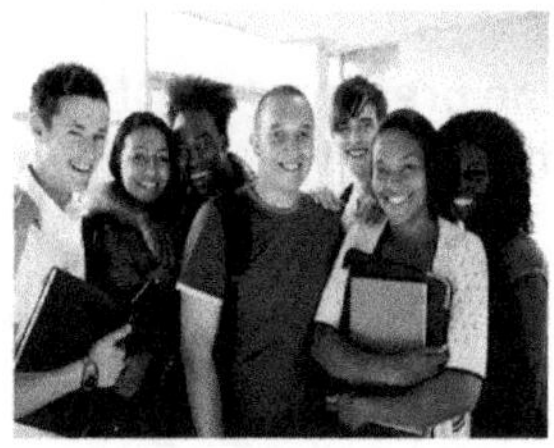

Shelov Remer Altmann, 2009

As with younger children, typical adolescents present an all new type of challenge. Teen years are difficult for all people. It is really interesting that this stage of life is difficult for all people, and conflict and strife are endemic. Efforts to become more adult presents stressors to relationships with care providers. Recall that until very recent times, adolescents were essentially seen as adults. Adoption of adult roles generally occurred in early teen years. The lengthening of childhood through adolescence is a modern occurrence.

During adolescence, in a typical teen the person turns from a child into more of an adult. Maturation occurs physically, emotionally and sexually, and the young person must learn to successfully navigate all of these changes. Parenting and support are critical, and typical forms of parenting and support must be adapted to fit the learning style of the youngster with IDD.

Slide 10

Adolescence and Disability

An adolescent with an IDD experiences the same life complexities as other adolescents.

The presence of IDD or a physical disability can make learning and making sense of the world more complex.

These maturational changes may be delayed by physical disability or intellectual/developmental disability that makes learning much harder. Impaired intellectual ability often results in difficulties with inductive and deductive reasoning, which makes it much harder to figure out how the world works.

Parent, V., Birtwell, K., Lambright, N., & DuBard, M. (2016). Combining CBT and behavior-analytic approaches to target severe emotion dysregulation in verbal youth with ASD and ID. *Journal of Mental Health Research in Intellectual Disabilities*, 10, 60-82.

Slide 11

Who am I? What am I to do in life? These are two of the central questions in the development of a unique identity. Identity development is among the most important developmental tasks of life, beginning in infancy but often being resolved during adolescent years. It must be noted that adults also experience a continually forming sense of self. Identity development is never complete. Erikson identified the goal of adolescence as achieving a coherent identity without confusion regarding identity (Erikson, 1959).

Identity often is accepted to include physical and sexual identity, occupational goals, religious and cultural beliefs and ethnic background. The presence of intellectual disability is a relevant aspect as well.

Identity forms through the accumulation of experience and the integration of experiences and interpretations of experience. These experiences begin in infancy when children begin to recognize themselves. Bullock and Lutkenhaus (1990) noted that 2-year-olds who see themselves in a mirror with a dot on their nose will then touch their noses. They recognize the image in the mirror as being them, early evidence of the understanding of self. Language use at this age similarly reflects the development of the sense of self, as does representational play (Bullock & Lutkenhaus, 1990). During later childhood, the sense of identity further develops and often is described in terms of qualities, skills and characteristics. While this pattern continues into adulthood, where it often includes a focus on various social roles, in younger children the terms are simple, concrete and unitary; in older children, they become more abstract (Berg, 1999).

Slide 12

Problems with Self-Esteem

Often include:

- Body image
- Weight problems
- Shyness
- Embarrassment

And for someone with IDD, awareness of disability.

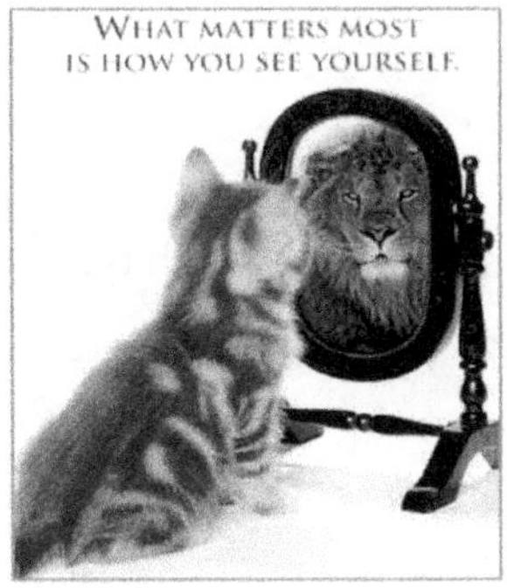

The top four issues are often true for all people. If I were to ask you what you dislike about yourself, you would have no trouble coming up with a million things. If I asked what you loved about yourself, it would not be nearly as easy, and you might have to stop to think. Our society is very good at helping us know what things are wrong with us and not nearly as good at teaching us to appreciate ourselves for who we are. As adults, we can often keep these things in perspective. We know that advertising is trying to make us feel we need things to be better or more accepted and loved. We know movies show people who don't look like most people, being impossibly attractive. Young people haven't yet figured that out in many cases.

This problem is magnified for teens with IDD.

Slide 13

Exercise

Please come up with ten words that describe you, ten things that make you who you are.

Slide 14

Risk-Taking Behavior

- All teenagers take risks as a normal part of growing up.
- Changes in the teen brain make risk-taking more likely.
  - Time of great opportunity
  - Risks and problems as well
- Taking risks is a tool teens use to define and develop their identity.
- Adolescents need to take risks.
  - Healthy risk-taking can help prevent unhealthy risk-taking
  - Help create opportunities for healthy risks

Romer, 2010

Risk-taking is a common part of adolescence for most people. Taking risks can be a way for youth to figure out how the world works and what life is like. The problem lies in youth who take risks that are foolish. We have to teach the distinction between healthy and unhealthy risk-taking. That is challenging enough for typical youth, but for youth with IDD it is a greater task. We also have to recognize that for adolescents with IDD, what we might see as a problem behavior may be a manifestation of completely typical teen behavior.

Slide 15

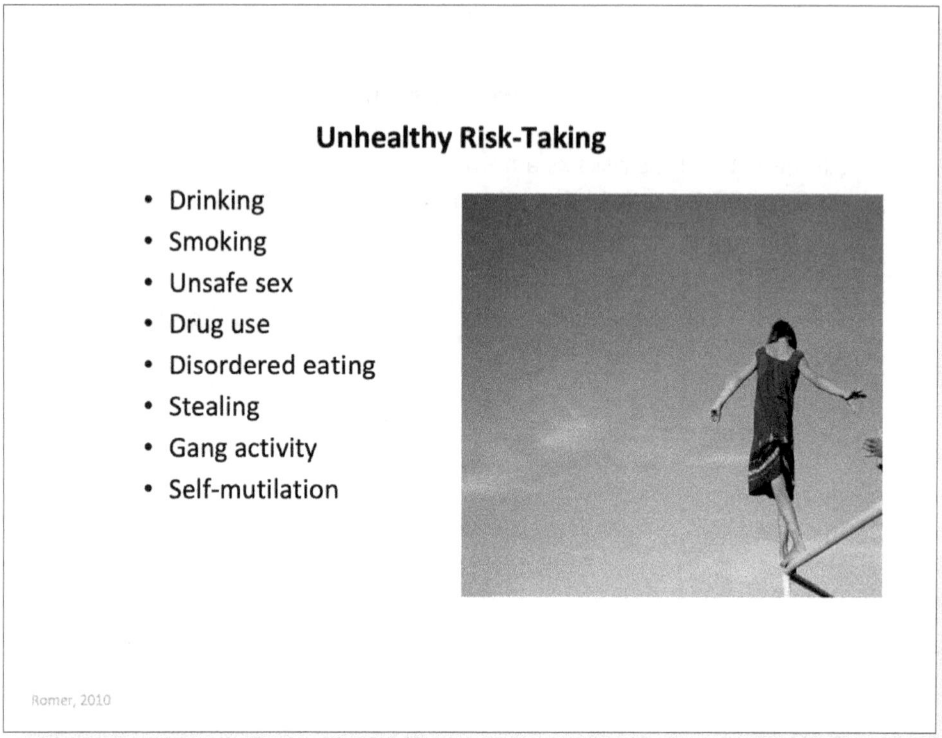

These are the unhealthy kinds of risks. The danger in all of these is evident. In each of these, there is a fine line between unhealthy and healthy. We can teach that, but we know that despite the well-known and publicized dangers of tobacco, many, many people still love their cigarettes, chew and cigars. When does a low-fat diet become anorexia? What is the difference between fudging on taxes and stealing a cell phone? Some of these are exactly the kinds of social judgment calls that people with IDD are notoriously bad at.

Slide 16

Healthy Risk-Taking

- Sports
- Developing artistic abilities
- Volunteer activities
- Travel
- Making new friends
- Hobbies
- Exploring community

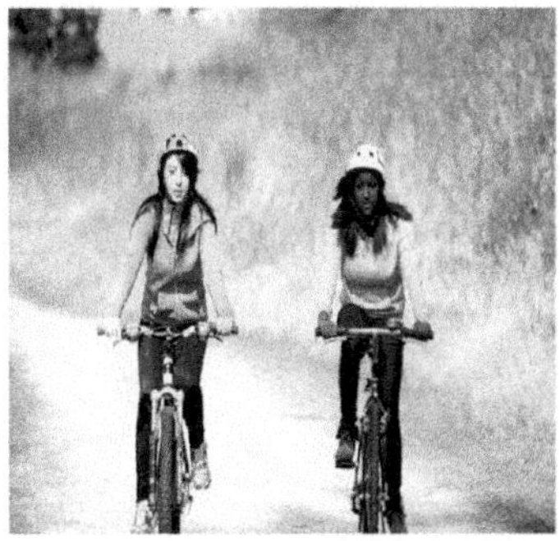

Romer, 2010

These kinds of risks are the activities that can lead to a sense of mental wellness, the preventative buffers that can protect us from some kinds of mental health disorders. They reduce stress and improve optimism and well-being (Cannon, 1932).

Slide 17

Exercise

- Identify two things you do that are examples of healthy risk-taking.
- Then think of one negative risk-taking thing you do, but don't write it down or share it.

Slide 18

Supporting Risk-Taking

All such activities contain the possibility of failure.

- How can we help provide supports that include realistic goals?
- What skills do young people need to make good choices about taking risks?
- What are some challenges unique to younger individuals?

Failure is a normal part of growing up and a logical outcome of trying anything new. We have to teach youth with IDD to expect failure at times. We also have to teach the reasonable progression of goals from simpler things to more complex things. Nobody learns to hit a baseball on a pitch from a major-league pitcher. We learn to swing a bat in Tee-ball. We learn to hit a slow Wiffle ball. Trying new things often requires a kind of shaping process.

Slide 19

Sexuality

- Key milestones of adolescent development
  - Attaining an adult body
  - Capable of reproducing
  - Intimate relationships
  - Complex emotions
- Individuals with disabilities may be hindered in this area of development
  - Functional limitations
  - Social isolation
    - Fewer social activities
    - Less likely to have intimate relationships
  - Lack of information on parenthood, birth control and STDs

Watson, Griffiths, Richards & Dykstra, 2002

Historically, the sexual behaviors of people with IDD and/or mental illness (MI) have been ignored, prevented and/or punished by those in charge of their care (Owen & Griffiths, 2009). To explain where we are today, we must examine where we have been.

In the United States and Canada, public perception and professional response to natural sexual behavior in youth and adults with intellectual disabilities and/or mental health disorders have changed over the years. In the early 1900s, sexual behavior of individuals with IDD or MI was seen as immoral and criminal, a scourge on society that needed to be eradicated through segregation and sterilization.

By the middle of the twentieth century, sexual behavior was no longer seen as harmful to society, but harmful to individuals with IDD/MI. During this time, parents and professionals engaged in close monitoring to prevent sexual behavior; education focused on prevention of abuse and exploitation.

The last part of the 1900s focused more on individual rights as an adult sexual being. Because sexuality is such a value-laden and emotionally charged area, there are still wide variations in how youth and adults with IDD/MI are educated about sexuality; however, service provision today primarily focuses on enabling and nurturing healthy intimate relationships.

Societal attitudes toward sexuality in youth in general present additional challenges for this population. While sexuality has always been a large part of society, instruction on sexuality for youth has been largely a family responsibility in modern western society until very recent times. Sex education and sexuality education for youth depended largely on individual family preferences and mores and varied widely. In more recent time, such education has been provided by schools and other community institutions and resources, with considerable controversy (Black & Baker, 2013).

Slide 20

Development of Sexuality

- Children and adolescents with IDD, like all individuals, are sexual persons.
- Most of their behaviors are "typical."
- The problem is they are often unable to distinguish between behaviors that are publicly and privately appropriate.
- Attention to medical, functional and behavioral issues may shift focus away from addressing sexuality.

Watson, Griffiths, Richards, & Dykstra, 2002

The World Health Organization (1976) defined sexual health as "the integration of the physical, emotional, intellectual and social aspects of sexual being in ways that are positively enriching, and that enhance personality, communication, and love ... every person has a right to receive sexual information and to consider sexual relationships for pleasure as well as for procreation."

Sexuality develops in persons with IDD in the same manner as persons without IDD. Social judgment in areas of sexuality is a critical concern. Society is often very intolerant of sexual misbehavior, unless one is a politician.

Slide 21

Supports

- Avoid judgment and projection of personal values or discomfort
- Ensure the privacy of each child and adolescent
- Promote self-care and social independence among persons with disabilities
- Advocate for appropriate sexuality education
- Help provide knowledge and/or identify a source of information
- Lack of attention to issues of sexuality can lead to misinformation and problem behavior

What to Teach

1. Teach age-appropriate information.
2. Teach appropriate behavior/what TO DO.
3. Teach sexuality as personal identity formation and self-awareness.
4. Teach the right to choose and the right to refuse.
5. Teach healthy boundaries.

Slide 22

Sex Education

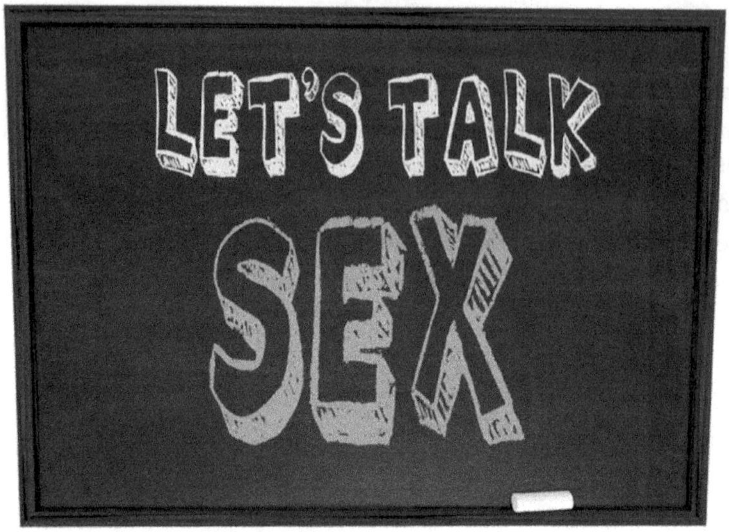

We need to directly teach appropriate ways of telling someone you are interested in getting to know them better. We need to teach how to ask for a date or how to let someone know you'd like the relationship to progress to a deeper level.

Slide 23

Sex Education

- Provided by someone with special expertise
- Children with disabilities have the right to the same education about sexuality as their peers
- May need modifications
  - Simplifying information
  - Using special teaching materials as needed
    - Anatomically correct dolls
    - Role-playing
    - Frequently reviewing and reinforcing the material
    - IEPs/IHPs should include provision of sexuality education

Black & Baker, 2013

In the area of sexuality, professionals often focus on what behavior is inappropriate and what NOT TO DO. The individual with IDD/MI is then filled with ideas about what is wrong but doesn't understand what behaviors are acceptable and desirable. Instead, we need to teach what TO DO.

Slide 24

Sex Education

- Remember this is developmental and questions are completely normal.
  - Sexual thoughts or actions are not negative risk behaviors.
- Parents/youth workers can help adolescents make safe and healthy choices regarding sexual behavior by:
  - Maintaining open lines of communication
  - Ensuring access to appropriate information and resources
  - Providing complete and accurate sex education so adolescents with IDD can make informed decisions
- A team process
  - Planned and coordinated by support team
  - Parent input
  - Not just DSP

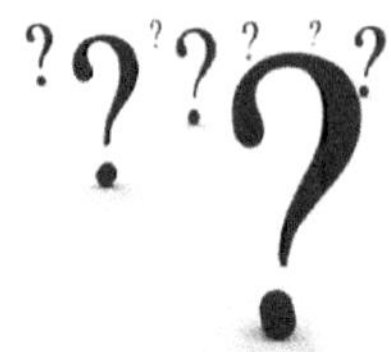

Black & Baker, 2013

Sex and sexuality education often occurs within schools. It is often wholly inadequate to the needs of students in the general population. For students with typical learning profiles, sex and sexuality education need to be more comprehensive and thorough.

The needs of students with IDD are even greater. Education in this complex and challenging area must involve all interested stakeholders. Sex education and sexuality education belongs in schools, families, medical or clinical professional visits and other logical points of contact for youth with disabilities. The question remains, though, does this overly impede the development of a sense of privacy about sexuality? If it is discussed with too many people, overgeneralization may occur and the bus driver may be seen as an appropriate source of sexuality education. Those experiences must be established through careful team involvement and participation (Black & Baker, 2013).

It is imperative that the experiences youth have not be "informed" by the media. The media often presents inappropriate examples of sexual behavior, and youth with IDD/MI are vulnerable to seeing those examples as "positive examples" to be emulated. Young people in general have this vulnerability, which has been known since Bandura's Bobo doll research in 1977, and the added complexities of IDD/MI make this far more likely to occur. Understanding that popular media is simply entertainment, even when couched as "reality TV," requires abstract thinking that may be difficult for many youth in this target population. Unfortunately, good examples in popular media are few. As such, exposure to media may need to be filtered carefully (Bandura, Ross & Ross, 1961).

Slide 25

Privacy

- Teach which behaviors are acceptable to do only when they are alone
  - Provide guidelines about when
  - Review expectations
  - Provide guidelines about where
  - Ensure the guidelines are followed
- Identify and recognize cues in the environment (a closed door)
- Social cues for public settings
- Create cues for alone time (a sign on the door)

Richards, et al, 2012

Privacy in sexual behavior is very important. Most typical youth very quickly figure out what is and what is not appropriate to do in front of others. Youth with disabilities are likely to need extra instruction. Especially when one needs assistance in hygiene, personal care does not seem very personal anymore, and privacy can become public. Persons with disabilities can often be treated in dehumanizing ways by well-intentioned educators and care providers. This can easily become a problematic pattern. Cues may need to be taught and communication requesting privacy needs to be honored (Black & Baker, 2013).

Slide 26

Working Together

- Empower young people to set limits.
- Assist lower-functioning individuals with achieving and maintaining privacy.
- When supervising or assisting with personal care:
  - Be considerate
  - Ask permission
  - Remember they still need privacy
  - Seek to minimize discomfort

Slide 27

Intimate Relationships

- Another important consideration is developing and maintaining intimate relationships.
  - Emotional intimacy
  - Physical intimacy

- Developmentally appropriate information about sexuality can help individuals with IDD attain a life with more personal fulfillment.

Walsh, Margaret

Many human rights statements call for the full range of choice regarding sexuality being available to individuals with IDD. This has been a complex issue and is often one of the most difficult areas to address in disability supports. It is relevant to all persons, and as society often struggles with expression of sexuality, the struggle gets played out in disability supports as well (Black & Baker, 2013).

Creating environments where youth with IDD feel safe to openly discuss their sexuality can be challenging for care providers. Caregivers and family members may feel uncomfortable or lack the knowledge to discuss these issues in an informed manner.

The Massachusetts Department of Health and the Massachusetts Department of Developmental Services produced the following resource guide to assist parents and caregivers in discussing sex and sexuality: https://www.mass.gov/files/documents/2016/07/xe/hrhs-sexuality-and-disability-resource-guide.pdf

Slide 28

Sexual Orientation

- In addition to physical development of sexual characteristics, exploration of sexual orientation is a normal part of sexual development.

- Sexual orientation is the pattern of to whom one is physically and emotionally attracted. There is a growing list of terms used to describe one's sexual orientation, but the majority fall into one of the three following categories:
  - Heterosexuality (Straight)
  - Homosexuality (Gay/Lesbian)
  - Bisexuality

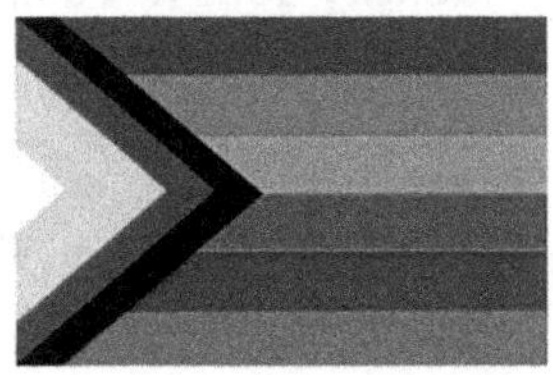

APA, 2008

Sexual orientation refers to an enduring pattern of emotional, romantic and/or sexual attraction. Sexual orientation also refers to a person's sense of identity based on those attractions, related behaviors and membership in a community of others who share those attractions. Research over several decades has demonstrated that sexual orientation ranges along a continuum, from exclusive attraction to the other sex to exclusive attraction to the same sex. There are an increasing number of terms used to describe one's identity along this continuum. However, most fall into one of three categories: heterosexual or straight (having emotional, romantic or sexual attractions to members of the other sex), homosexual — gay/lesbian (having emotional, romantic or sexual attractions to members of one's own sex) and bisexual (having emotional, romantic or sexual attractions to both men and women) (American Psychological Association, 2008).

LGBTQ+ is a term meant to be inclusive of lesbian, gay, bisexual, and transgender persons, as well as those who identify as queer, questioning, intersex, asexual, etc.

Slide 29

Gender Identity

- Gender Identity – an individual's inherent sense of being male, female, a blend of male and female or an alternative gender.
- Transgender – when an individual's gender identity does not correspond with their biological sex.
  - Often beginning in youth
  - May or may not be presented outwardly for others to see
- Genderqueer/Gender-fluid/Non-Binary – those whose gender identity does not align with a binary understanding of gender

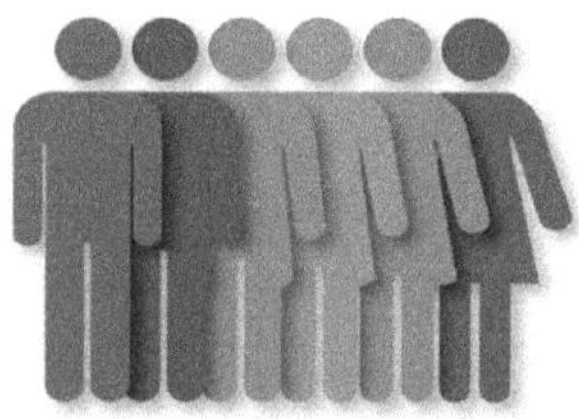

APA, 2015

Gender Identity is the deeply felt, inherent sense of being a boy (or man), a girl (or woman) or an alternative (e.g., genderqueer, gender-nonconforming, gender-neutral) that may or may not correspond to a person's sex assigned at birth. Since gender identity is internal, a person's gender identity is not necessarily visible to others.

The American Academy of Pediatrics in collaboration with the Human Rights Campaign produced a thorough review and set of recommendations regarding support for transgender children in 2016. The resource is available at: https://hrc-prod-requests.s3-us-west-2.amazonaws.com/files/documents/SupportingCaringforTransChildren.pdf?mtime=20200713125239&focal=none

Slide 30

Sexual Orientation and Gender Identity

- IDD + LGBTQ = greater risk of bullying and harassment
- Competent, compassionate care providers should be sought
- Access to the LGBTQ+ community
- Support from caregivers is vital

Walsh, Maragaret

As we know, individuals with intellectual disabilities (IDD) are often victims of harassment and discrimination simply because they have a disability. People with IDD who also identify as LGBTQ+ face even further risk of bullying and harassment because of their sexuality or how they express their identity.

Providing access to the LGBTQ+ community will help them develop positive sexual identities and a sense of belonging. Without encouragement and support from those who care for and about them, their ability to fully embrace and express their sexuality will be inhibited.

Slide 31

Peer Pressure

- Peer pressure is one thing all teens have in common.
  - Need for acceptance, approval and belonging is vital during the teen years.
  - Teens who feel isolated or rejected are more likely to engage in risky behaviors to fit in with a group.
- During adolescence, people begin to spend a lot more time with their friends and less time with their family.
  - More susceptible to the influences of their peers.

Peer acceptance is incredibly important to all people, but during the teen years, as one tries to forge an identity beyond just being a member of a family, peer acceptance and involvement becomes a greater issue. This has positive sides, but in the case of peer pressure to do things that are wrong or foolishly risky, peer pressure can become a significant concern. The creation of a healthy sense of identity beyond family and peer group has a buffering effect.

Slide 32

Peer Pressure

- Pressure isn't always negative.
  - Pressure into negative behaviors
  - Away from positive behaviors
  - Positive influences, such as doing well in school, having respect for others and avoiding taking negative risks
- Handling peer pressure depends largely on how adolescents feel about themselves.

Learning to handle peer pressure is a part of maturing. Positive role models can provide positive peer pressure. This can be specifically nurtured in young people with IDD.

Slide 33

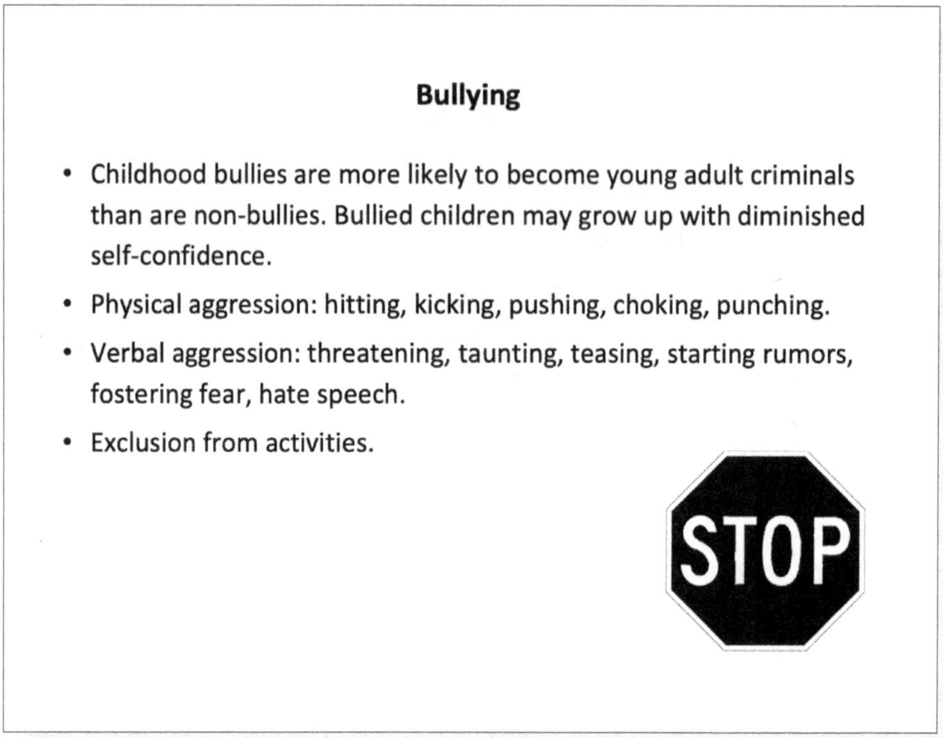

Bullying is a growing concern worldwide, amplified largely by horrific events. Some countries, such as Norway, have efforts on a national basis to address bullying; in most of the world it is a local effort, often managed by schools.

Slide 34

Bullying

- Done by someone with more power or social support to someone with less power or social support.
- Often includes the abuser blaming the target for the abuse.
- Often leads to the target blaming him or herself for the abuse.
- In most bullying situations, the target cannot stop the bullying by his or her own actions.

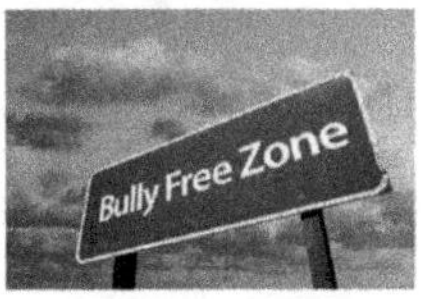

Many adults who have been bullied remember it as a terrible period in their lives. Youth with IDD are often particularly targeted for bullying due to obvious differences in appearance, skills or actions and are often seen as being vulnerable by bullies.

(https://www.stopbullying.gov/resources/facts)

Slide 35

Exercise

- **How do you think the way bullying is portrayed in popular TV shows/movies can affect a young person with IDD?**
- **What happened and how did the bullying resolve?**

Higher rates of bullying experienced by people with IDD can be, at least partially, attributed to societal factors. "Negative attitudes toward people with disabilities go unchallenged as efforts to promote equality through policy are deemed to be insufficiently implemented" (Mepham, 2010).

"[There is still a] prevalent belief that people with intellectual disabilities are not affected by bullying and they do not understand what is happening to them" (Roberts & Hamilton, 2010).

"Early studies on independent living and community-based arrangements for people with intellectual disabilities indicated that quality of life is significantly impaired for victims" (Flynn, 1989; Halpern, Close, & Nelson, 1986).

People with intellectual disability themselves rate bullying as a leading stressor (Bramston, Fogarty & Cummins, 1999).

Slide 36

Stopping Bullying: What Doesn't Work

- **Denial:** ("She would never do that;" "I'm sure he didn't mean to hurt you;" "Boys are just like that;" "Sticks and stones may break bones, but words will never harm").
- **Telling the victim to solve the problem:** ("Just make sure you're never alone with that kid;" "Say no;" "Stand up for yourself and hit back;" "Wear less revealing clothes;" "Pretend it doesn't bother you").
- **Broad-brush educational efforts alone:** ("Soft is the heart of a child;" Sensitivity training; "Hands are for helping, not hurting").

None of these strategies works as a general intervention despite what Hollywood movies have shown about punching the bully back. If the efforts the child makes alone were effective, the need for intervention would not have been raised to this level.

Slide 37

Stopping Bullying: What Works

- Consistent enforcement of effective consequences that are predictable, inevitable, immediate and escalating.
- Monitoring to make sure consequences and education are effective.
- Effective counseling for youth who bully after enforcement of consequences has generated some anxiety.

These strategies do work and generally require effort beyond what the bullied youngster alone can do. In schools, these interventions are often implemented on a school-wide basis, starting with a national anti-bullying campaign in Norway designed by Dan Olweus. Below are a number of resources and supporting documents regarding bullying prevention:

- https://www.stopbullying.gov/resources/laws/federal.
- https://www.stopbullying.gov/sites/default/files/2017-10/school-climate-infographic.pdf.
- U.S. Department of Education, National Center for Education Statistics, 2017–18 School Survey on Crime and Safety (SSOCS), 2018.

Slide 38

Stopping Bullying: What Works

- Effective support for targets, including protection from repeat victimization.
- Empowering bystanders to tell adults, support targets and discourage unacceptable behavior.

Effective support for victims of bullying is important. A culture of non-bullying should be created. This often involves specific instruction about bullying and responses to it.

Slide 39

Cyberbullying

Cyberbullying is bullying that takes place using electronic technology. Examples of cyberbullying include:

- Mean text messages or emails
- Rumors sent by email or posted on social networking sites
- Embarrassing pictures, videos, websites or fake profiles posted online

Baker, 2013

More information is available at stopbullying.gov

Slide 40

Why Cyberbullying is Different

- Cyberbullying can happen 24 hours a day, seven days a week, and reach a young person even when he or she is alone.
- Cyberbullying messages and images can be posted anonymously and distributed quickly to a very wide audience. It can be difficult and sometimes impossible to trace the source.
- Deleting inappropriate or harassing messages, texts and pictures is extremely difficult after they have been posted or sent.

Baker, 2013

More information is available at stopbullying.gov

Slide 41

How Much Does It Happen?

- The 2020 Indicators of School Crime and Safety (National Center for Education Statistics and Bureau of Justice Statistics) indicates that, nationwide, about 24 percent of students were in schools where bullying occurred at least monthly.
- The 2020 Indicators of School Crime and Safety (National Center for Education Statistics and Bureau of Justice Statistics) indicates that 15 percent of students experienced cyberbullying at least once a week. The cyberbullying summary shows 36.5 percent lifetime victimization rates.

Baker, 2013

Cyberbullying is a significant problem for many people, notably young people. As more and more of our lives go online, cyberbullying can become more significant than bullying in real life.

(https://nces.ed.gov/pubs2020/2020063.pdf, https://cyberbullying.org/statistics)

Slide 42

How to Prevent Cyberbullying

- Be aware of online activity
- Monitor online activity
- Talk about online activity
- Teaching online safety
- Set rules

Baker, 2013

Slide 43

If Cyberbullying Occurs

- Keep evidence of the activity
- Don't respond
- Use blocking technology
- Report to service providers
- Report to law enforcement if appropriate
- Involve schools

Baker, 2013

More information is available at stopbullying.gov

(https://nces.ed.gov/pubs2020/2020063.pdf)

Slide 44

Gangs

- Gang violence has spread to communities throughout the world. In the U.S., these are the statistics:
  - More than 24,500 different youth gangs around the country
  - More than 772,500 teens and young adult members
- Teens join gangs for a variety of reasons:
  - Seeking excitement
  - Looking for prestige
  - Protection
  - Make money
  - A sense of belonging
- Few teens are forced to join gangs; most can refuse to join without fear of retaliation.

Gang involvement is a particularly risky form of peer involvement, with peer pressure to commit criminal acts being a huge problem. Gang involvement leads to any number of terrible outcomes. Youth with IDD often join gangs as a route to having friends. Gangs can be organized around location, ethnicity or loyalty. In the United States, gang activity has diminished somewhat from its height but remains a plague on many communities.

Slide 45

Steps to Conflict Resolution

- **Set the stage.** Agree to try to work together to find a solution peacefully and establish ground rules (e.g., no name-calling, yelling, or interrupting).
- **Gather perspectives.** Each person describes his/her perspective. Listeners pay attention to what the others say they want and why.
- **Find common interests.** Establish points everyone agrees on. Identify common interests; can be as simple as a shared need to save face.
- **Create options.** Brainstorm possible solutions in which both people gain something. Think win-win!
- **Evaluate options.** Each teen discusses feelings about solutions. Negotiate to reach a conclusion acceptable to both.
- **Create an agreement.** The teens explicitly state their agreement and may even want to write it down.

Conflict resolution is of critical importance. Conflict between peers can lead to acts of bullying and violence. These six steps are an excellent introduction to conflict resolution. Once again, this framework can and should be taught.

Slide 46

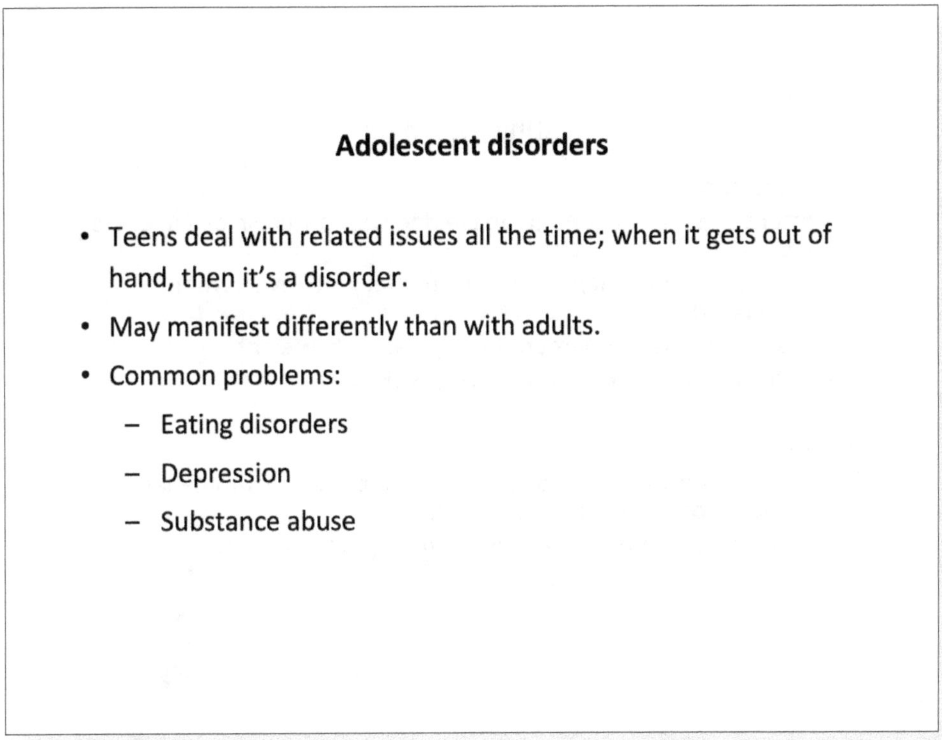

As discussed earlier, in modern times, adolescents are not just young adults. There are maturational differences, and some mental health disorders presents differently. We will review three of the most common problems.

Slide 47

Eating Disorders

- Anorexia nervosa
  - Intense fear of becoming obese does not diminish as weight is lost.
  - Disturbed body image — claims to "feel fat" even when emaciated.
  - Loss of at least 25 percent of original body weight.
  - Refusal to maintain normal body weight.
- Bulimia
  - Recurrent episodes of binge-eating (rapidly consuming large amounts of food in a short time).
  - Often followed by purging via vomiting or laxatives.

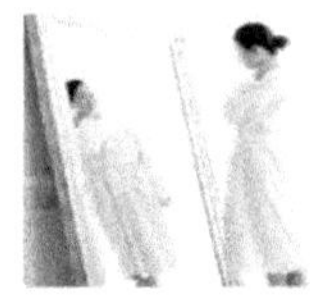

Eating disorders are dangerous and present significant health risks. Most people want to look attractive. Media presents impossible images of what beauty looks like, and young people are at tremendous risk for trying to emulate these ideals. Eating disorders were previously seen as the province of only young women, but young men have begun to evidence increasing rates of eating disorders as well. Eating disorders are often seen as control issues.

Slide 48

Eating Disorders: Causes and Solutions

- Causes
  - Adolescent focus on body image
  - Cultural emphasis on appearances
  - Other unmet emotional needs
- Response
  - Requires formal treatment
  - May include: lectures, group therapy, assertiveness training, drug therapy and nutritional counseling
- Cautions
  - Avoid arguing; you're not going to talk them out of it.
  - Be careful to avoid criticism.

Eating disorders must be diagnosed and treated by competent professionals and may require inpatient treatment if the weight loss becomes severe to the point of risking health. Most communities have skilled professionals who are knowledgeable about this. Be careful to not mistake a person who is thin as having an eating disorder. Eating disorders are driven by intense irrational fear, not by a desire to be healthy.

Slide 49

Early Onset of Mental Illness

- Environmental stress does not cause mental illness but can trigger onset.
- Biological events, chemical imbalance or disturbance requires psychiatric treatment.
- Untreatable mental illness places children at the risk of developing severe forms as adults, more reluctant to seek proper treatment.
- Poor functioning in school, development, social relationships, family life.
- Therapy can support but is insufficient to treat many severe illness driven symptoms and behaviors.
- Observation is key to diagnosis: intensity, frequency, impact.

Early detection of mental illness is very important. Mental health disorders can start in childhood. Effective treatment can follow the diagnosis. Competent mental health professionals can assist in providing the proper supports.

Slide 50

Triggers for Emotional Crises

- Onset of illness (medical or mental)
- Birth of sibling
- Onset of puberty/adolescence
- Start or end of school
- Out of home placement
- Sex and dating issues
- Changes in staff and teacher relationships
- Surpassed by younger siblings or peers
- Inappropriate expectations of others
- Physical, sexual or emotional abuse
- Illness/aging of parents
- Death of parent, caretaker or family member
- Loss of peer or roommate

Any of these triggers should result in observation of a young person to see how the young person manages the stress. Additional support can be placed as a preventative in any of these circumstances. A show of hands regarding each of these that attendees have faced can be illuminating about the number of stressors that typical people face.

Slide 51

Exercise

Consider wellness strategies you can use to support a young person with IDD who might experience one of the emotional crises listed on the previous slide. Discuss with the group.

Slide 52

Child Adolescent Depression

- Not just bad moods and occasional sadness
- Serious problem that impacts every aspect of a teen's life
- Requires treatment and can lead to:
  - Problems at home and school
  - Drug abuse
  - Poor adjustment and self-image
  - Negative identity
  - Homicide, violence or suicide

Depression may manifest very differently in youth as opposed to adults. Depression was not accepted as occurring in youth until fairly recent times. This needs to be considered separately from moodiness that is very common in youth (and adults) and also not confused with labile moods (rapid mood changes). Youth with IDD probably experience depression at a similar rate as typical youth.

This is a particular concern for youth with ASD (Wigham, S., Barton, S., Parr, J. & Rodgers, J. [2017]. A systematic review of the rates of depression in children and adults with high-functioning autism spectrum disorder. *Journal of Mental Health Research in Intellectual Disabilities*, 11, 1-21).

Slide 53

Depression Signs and Symptoms

- Sadness or hopelessness
- Irritability, anger or hostility
- Tearfulness or frequent crying
- Withdrawal from friends and family
- Loss of interest in activities
- Changes in eating and sleeping habits
- Restlessness and agitation
- Feelings of worthlessness and guilt

Slide 54

Depression Signs and Symptoms

- Lack of enthusiasm and motivation
- Fatigue or lack of energy
- Difficulty concentrating
- Thoughts of death or suicide
- Physical complaints (far more likely in youth than adults)

Which of these are different from adults? The biggest difference is in the physical complaints, such as stomachaches. This symptom is far more common in youth with depression. The technical term "somatic complaint" is often used for this.

Slide 55

Warning Signs of Teen Suicide

- Talking or joking about suicide.
- Saying things like "I'd be better off dead" or "I wish I could disappear forever."
- Speaking positively about death or romanticizing dying ("If I died, people might love me more").
- Writing stories and poems about death or dying.

Suicide is an impulsive act, and youth are more impulsive than adults. This is a significant concern, and any specific worry that a teen might be suicidal or thinking about suicide (suicidal ideation) should be evaluated by a trained professional who will interview the young person and ask a specific set of questions.

Slide 56

Warning Signs of Teen Suicide

- Engaging in reckless behavior or having a lot of accidents resulting in injury.
- Giving away prized possessions.
- Saying goodbye to friends and family in dramatic ways.
- Seeking out weapons, pills or other ways to kill themselves.

These additional warning signs are of increased concern, of course with the last one being the greatest danger.

Slide 57

Talking Tips for Depressed Teens

- Offer support
  - Let them know you're there for them. Avoid asking lots of questions (teens don't like to feel patronized).
  - Make it clear you're ready and willing to provide whatever support they need.
- Be gentle but persistent
  - Don't give up if they shut you out.
  - Talking about depression can be very tough for teens.
  - Be respectful; show you are concerned and willing to listen.

These strategies are all important and represent the things a non-licensed professional can do. We shouldn't always put all of the responsibility on therapists and doctors. All of us can play a very important role in support.

Slide 58

Talking Tips for Depressed Teens

- Listen without lecturing
  - Resist criticizing or passing judgment; when they talk, at least they are communicating.
  - Avoid offering unsolicited advice.
- Validate feelings
  - Don't try to talk them out of depression.
  - Acknowledge the pain and sadness they are feeling.
  - Make them feel like you take their emotions seriously.

Listening without lecturing is critical but can be very difficult for adults in helping professions. We want to offer advice and guidance, but sometimes the best thing to do is listen and then validate what the young person says. Validation is important for any person, but particularly a young person with IDD.

Slide 59

Substance Abuse

- Experimenting
  - Teens may try alcohol, cigarettes, inhalants or other drugs one or more times but not go any further.
  - Usually do not have any problems as a result of substance use.
- Substance abuse
  - Experimenting leads to regular or frequent use.
  - Substance abuse results in problems at home (more arguments), at school (such as failing grades) or with the law.
- Substance dependence (addiction)
  - Physical and/or psychological dependence.
  - Use takes up a significant portion of the teen's activities.
  - Continues despite causing harm and is difficult to stop.
  - An ongoing, and possibly fatal, disease.

Substance abuse is a critical concern for all of humanity. We have become increasingly aware of the damage caused by substance abuse, from car accidents to overdose. Experimenting with substances can be a typical part of adolescence, but that does not mean we simply accept it. Young people with IDD are vulnerable to making significant mistakes.

Slide 60

Health Care

- Adolescents — facilitate a transition to more active role in healthy behavior, medication management, appointments.
- Help young people to understand their disability or diagnosis and health concerns.
- Identify reliable resources for further information
- Teach healthy lifestyle skills, promote wellness.
- Empower them to be more involved in asking questions and making decisions.
- Provide guidance in knowing how and when to acquire or decline further help and support.

One of the tasks of childhood and adolescence is learning to take care of one's health. As a youngster moves into teen years, a more and more active role should be played in this, with the hope of becoming as independent as possible in adulthood. Young people should be specifically taught these items.

Slide 61

Community Safety

- Who/what is dangerous?
  - Help identify potential danger and make decisions beforehand about safety and trust.
  - Build awareness by reviewing everyday dangers often: fire safety, traffic, crime, internet threats, risk-taking behavior.
  - Build confidence to act safely "in the moment."
    - Discuss potentially threatening situations.
    - Practice or role-play appropriate response.
    - Review who/how to ask for help.

The world can be risky. Even in low-crime areas, there are significant risks. In high-crime areas, the risks become greater and more pronounced. Instruction on community safety is needed. Everything from crossing the streets to answering a phone can have some element of risk. We need to teach our young people how to safely navigate life so they don't have to live in a bubble.

Slide 62

Safety Tips

- Teach the person to always let someone know where he/she is going and for how long.
- Routines
  - Many children with IDD depend on routines.
  - Avoid routines that others can predict to victimize children.
- Talk about safety often.

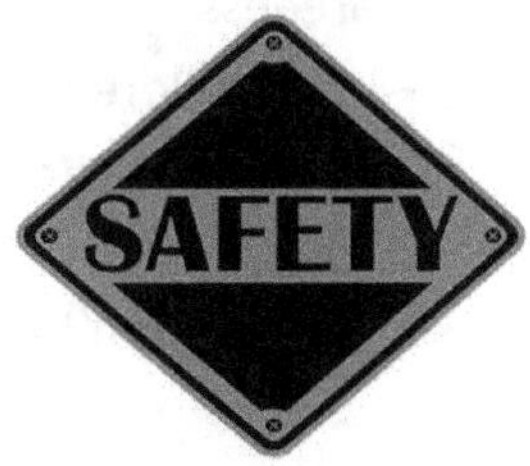

These are some general tips regarding safety.

Slide 63

Potential Victimization

- Appearance of safety doesn't mean there is no threat.
- Grooming — The establishment of trust through repeated interaction to increase access to a potential victim and decrease likelihood of discovery.
- Awareness
  - Can children recognize they are being "set up"?
  - Are parents/care providers able to tell when children don't see it?
  - What "Don't talk to strangers" means.

Victimization is a serious problem for youth with IDD and adults as well. Recognition of threats and grooming is necessary. Creating an awareness of these kinds of concerns can help, even if they might lead to uncomfortable discussions.

Slide 64

Internet Safety

- Keep the computer in a high-traffic area.
- Monitor use of other digital devices.
- Establish limits for which online sites children may visit and for how long.
- Remember that Internet technology can be mobile, so make sure to monitor cell phones, gaming devices and laptops.
- Surf the Internet with children and let them show you what they like to do online.
- Ask questions about their interests and have them show you what they are searching.
- Bookmark/shortcuts to apps and safe websites for immediate access.
- Continually dialogue with children about online safety.

Young people require a level of supervision with computer and Internet resources to ensure maximum benefit while maintaining safety and security.

These are some tips that can be used in a family, classroom, workspace or residential setting to promote safe habits.

Slide 65

Technology Safety

- Know who young people are communicating with online.
- Note numbers of outgoing/incoming calls with no contact information.
- Open a family/group/house email account to share with younger children.
- Brainstorm screen names and email addresses that do not contain information about gender, identity or location and avoid being suggestive.

Some of these tips and strategies are things we can do for young people and other are approaches we cooperate on together. Rather than control or isolate teenagers, it's helpful to be involved: Validate their activities and relationships and empower them to take a role in making sure they are safe.

Slide 66

More Technology Safety

- Teach children never to open emails/messages from unknown senders and to use settings to block messages from people they do not know.
- Be aware of other ways children may be going online — with cell phones, laptops, tablets, games or from friends' homes or the library.
- Remind children that anything they send from their phones can be easily forwarded and shared.
- Familiarize yourself with popular acronyms at sites like netlingo.com and noslang.com.

Tech safety should be taught. Online activity can lead to less problematic issues, such as computer viruses, and more problematic issues, such as victimization. Online bullying has become more of a concern as well.

Slide 67

Social Networking: Benefits

Gain social confidence and become more secure in new situations, such as going to college, joining a sports team and meeting new friends.

Learn about his or her diagnosis and health needs.

Find support in online communities — especially true for kids who have unique interests or feel isolated.

Make friends who are interested in the same things or may be dealing with similar issues.

The concerns previously mentioned bear notice, but there are positive things about social networking online as well. Youth from the community of people with Asperger's syndrome in particular have seen great benefit (please note that Asperger's is no longer in the DSM-5 but is still a widely recognized and used term, and we use it here as the community of people with Asperger's syndrome continue to use it).

Slide 68

Social Networking: More Benefits

Keep in touch with family members who live far away by sharing updates, photos, videos and messages.

Be creative sharing ideas or through poetry, blogging or journaling.

Increasing media literacy and expand vocabulary and communication skills.

Generate topics for discussion in "live" conversations and with peers in school and other offline settings.

These are all significant benefits that can lead to wellness.

Slide 69

Supporting Young People to Develop Goals

Set realistic expectations by considering:

- Strengths, abilities and interests.
- Opportunities, resources and feasibility.

Be careful not to devalue someone's ambitions.

Break larger goals into mini-goals or objectives.

- See progress quickly.
- Even on a daily basis if needed.

Establish incentives that are meaningful to the person.

Be flexible. Use setbacks as building blocks to modify goals or create new dreams (turn disappointment into opportunity).

All people need goals. Young people, in particular, need to have goals. They are often frustrated with not being adults yet, and setting future goals can be of great benefit. Having positive goals also leads to mental wellness. Both small and big goals are beneficial. Sometimes people have goals that others see as being silly or foolish dreams. Telling somebody their dreams are foolish never helps in the long run.

References: Module XI

American Academy of Pediatrics. (2013a). Age & stages, http://www.healthychildren.org/English/ages-stages/Pages/default.aspx. Retrieved February 2015.

American Academy of Pediatrics. (2013b). Outlook for children with intellectual disabilities, http://www.healthychildren.org/English/health-issues/conditions/developmental-disabilities/Pages/Outlook-for-Children-with-Intellectual-Disabilities.aspx. Retrieved February, 2015.

American Academy of Pediatrics (2016). Supporting and caring for transgender children. Retrieved September, 2020, from https://www.aap.org/en-us/Documents/solgbt_resource_transgenderchildren.pdf.

Baker, D. J., & Blumberg, E. R. (2013). *Mental Health and Wellness Supports for Youth with IDD*. Kingston, NY: NADD Press.

Husband, K. (2019). Medical family therapy for Parents of Children with Intellectual or Developmental Disabilities. *NADD Bulletin*, 22, 21-25.

Bandura, A., Ross, D., & Ross, S.A. (1961) Transmission of aggression through the imitation of aggressive models. *Journal of Abnormal and Social Psychology*, 63 (3), 575-582.

Berg, L. (1999). Developmental play stages in child identity construction: An interactionist theoretical contribution. *International Journal of Early Childhood*, 31 (1), 11-24.

Black, R. S., & Baker, D. J. (2013). Sexuality and youth with the dual diagnosis of ID/MI. In Baker, D., & Blumberg, R. (Eds.), *Mental Health and Wellness Supports for Youth with IDD* (pp. 83-120). Kingston, NY: NADD Press.

Bramston, P., Fogarty, G., & Cummins, R. A. (1999). The nature of stressors reported by people with intellectual disabilities. *Journal of Applied Social Research in Intellectual Disabilities*, 12, 1-10.

MODULE 11

Bullock, M., & Lutkenhaus, P. (1990). Who am I? Self-understanding in toddlers. *Merrill Palmer Quarterly*, 36 (2), 217–238.

Cannon, W. B. (1932). *The Wisdom of the Body*. New York: Norton.

Cyberbullying research center. (2019). Summary of our cyberbullying research (2007-2019). https://cyberbullying.org/summary-of-our-cyberbullying-research. Retrieved September 2020.

Erikson, E. H. (1959). Identity and the life cycle: selected papers, *Psychological Issues*, 1, 1-171.

Flynn, M., (1989). *Independent Living for Adults with Mental Handicap: "A Place of My Own."* London: Cassell.

Halpern, A., Close, W., & Nelson, D., (1986). *On My Own: The Impact of Semi-Independent Living Programs for Adults with Mental Retardation*. Baltimore, MD: Paul H. Brookes Publishing Co.

Mepham, S. (2010). Disabled children: the right to feel safe. *Child Care in Practice*, 16 (1), 19-34.

National Center for Education Statistics. (2018). School Survey on Crime and Safety. U.S. Department of Education.

Owen, F. A., & Griffiths, D. M., (2009). *Challenges to Human Rights of People with Intellectual Disabilities* (pp. 119-288). London: Jessica Kingsley.

Papalia, D. E., Olds, S. W., & Feldman, R. D., (1999). *A Child's World: Infancy through Adolescence*. New York, NY: McGraw Hill.

Parent, V., Birtwell, K., Lambright, N., & DuBard, M. (2016). Combining CBT and behavior-analytic approaches to target severe emotion dysregulation in verbal youth with ASD and ID. *Journal of Mental Health Research in Intellectual Disabilities*, 10, 60-82.

Richards, D.A., Watson, S.L., Monger, S., & Rogers, C. (2012). The right to sexuality and relationships (pp. 103-128). In Griffiths, D., Owen, F., & Watson, S. L., (Eds.), *The Human Rights Agenda for Persons with Intellectual Disabilities.* Kingston, NY: NADD Press.

Roberts, B. & Hamilton, C. (2010). "Out of the darkness into the light." A life story from Ireland. *British Journal of Learning Disabilities*, 38, 127-132.

Romer, D. (2010). Adolescent risk taking, and impulsivity: implications for brain development. *Developmental Psychobiology*, 52 (3), 263-276.

Shelov, S., & Remer Altmann, T. (Eds.). (2009). *Caring for Your Baby and Young Child: Birth to Age 5.* New York: American Academy of Pediatrics.

Stop Bullying. Facts. https://www.stopbullying.gov/resources/facts. Retrieved September 2020.

Stop Bullying. Improving school climate to help prevent bullying. https://www.stopbullying.gov/sites/default/files/2017-10/school-climate-infographic.pdf. Retrieved September 2020.

Stop Bullying. Laws about bullying. https://www.stopbullying.gov/sites/default/files/2017-10/school-climate-infographic.pdf. Retrieved September 2020.

Watson, S., Griffiths, D. Richards, D. & Dykstra, L. (2002). Sex education. In Griffiths, D. M., Richards, D., Fedoroff, P., & Watson, S. L., (Eds.), *Ethical dilemmas: Sexuality and developmental disability.* Kingston, NY: NADD Press.

Wigham, S., Barton, S., Parr, J., & Rodgers, J. (2017). A systematic review of the rates of depression in children and adults with high-functioning autism spectrum disorder. *Journal of Mental Health Research in Intellectual Disabilities, 11,* 1-21.

World Health Organization. (1976). Document A29/INFDOCI/1. Geneva, Switzerland.

Module XII

Wellness and Aging

Slide 2

The purpose of this module is to discuss mental wellness among persons with IDD who are aging, considering the experiences of typical persons as well and how best to address their changing support needs.

Slide 3

Learning Objectives

- Describe the age-related health problems attributed to people with IDD, including dementia and the challenges in diagnosing.
- Describe the psycho-social aspects of aging with IDD and how to support a person to maintain healthy psycho-social contacts.
- Identify how to enhance supports in consideration of health and wellness factors affecting people with IDD as they age.

Slide 4

The WHO (World Health Organization) acknowledges that aging is a lifelong process of change and there is no generally accepted age that defines exactly when people become old.

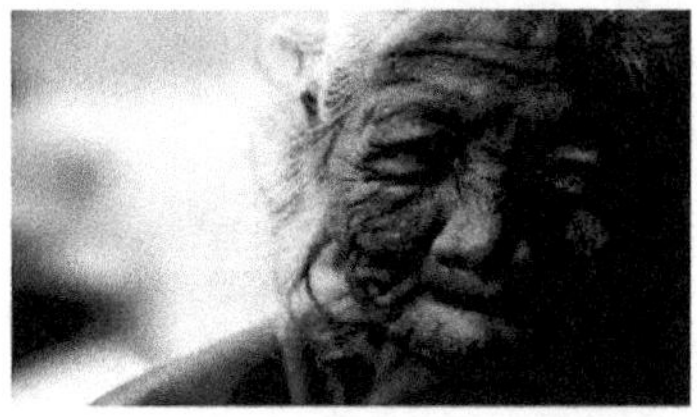

WHO, 2000

Aging has traditionally been seen as ongoing deterioration and viewed as an undesirable but inevitable end-of-life process. However, our thinking about the process of aging has changed in recent decades to acknowledge that it does not have to be an inescapable process of cumulative loss of health and function (Comfort, 1979).

The historical view on aging describes the process with a somewhat negative perspective, inferring that the general quality of health and life of an aging adult is low, and suffering is an expected component of aging for all people.

While this may have been and may continue to be true for some people, improvements in health care, economic and social conditions are changing the experiences of most people as they age. This is particularly true in developed and developing countries. Vulnerabilities still exist, but there is now a more concerted focus on disease and injury prevention and wellness in general. Supporting wellness opportunities during this stage in the life span, can enhance quality of life for individuals as they age.

Slide 5

Understanding Aging

For some people, the types of changes that occur toward the end of their lives may require more care and support.

As people who have a dual diagnosis age, understanding and supporting their mental wellness is crucial.

The process of aging applies to all people, intellectual/developmental disability or not. While many individuals in the general population tend to shift into a "caretaking setting" as they get older, many people with disabilities are already receiving supports under a model of care that can be adapted to changing abilities and needs.

An aging model of care focuses on a group. A disability model of care is person-centered and should maintain that individualized focus as one ages.

Slide 6

A New Perspective

Clinical definition: "Aging is a continuation of the developmental process and is influenced by genetic and other biological factors as well as personal and social circumstances."

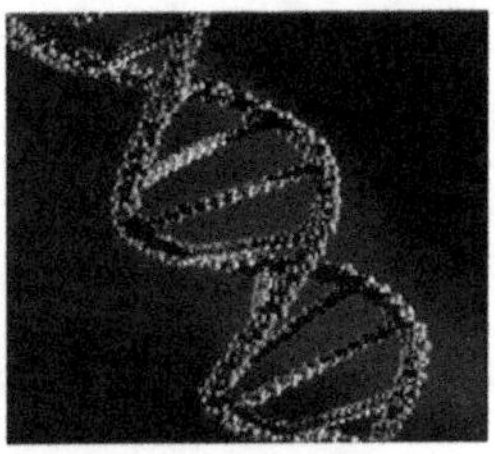

Holland, 2000

Viewed through this lens, aging is a natural biological process that may or may not involve some predisposed health and wellness vulnerabilities.

By assuming that aging will naturally lead to illness, we take on an illness-focused approach to disease management as opposed to a preventative approach that focuses on improving all components of health — physical, social, mental.

Ongoing research into prevention of age-related illnesses indicates that the most effective prevention strategy is to focus on improving one's own mental and physical well-being. By being attentive to healthy diet, an active lifestyle and mental wellness, one can help contribute to prevention of or reduction of severity of age-related illnesses.

Slide 7

A Diverse Process

The accumulation of changes over time occur at different rates depending on an individual's genetics, environment and lifestyle.

Physical and physiological changes make the body more susceptible to illness, but no certain pathology is predictable without consideration of lifestyle variables (Saxon et al., 2009).

All people age physically and cognitively in different manners and timeframes. There are actually more "differences in terms of changes and development among older people than among younger people" (Poindexter, 2002). There is great variation from person to person in the processes that occur.

While the prevalence of almost every long-term illness (chronic illness) and disability increases and health will naturally decline as people age, sickness is not a mandatory part of growing older whether or not a person has an intellectual/developmental disability (Talarico, 1998).

Slide 8

Exercise

What words come to your mind when you hear the word "aging"?

Slide 9

Aging and IDD

Due to factors associated with their disabilities and other health disparities, people with IDD generally have poorer health, greater need for support and experience greater health-related functional decline than do older people without IDD.

Bigby, 2004

Many people with IDD experience a combination of disability-related and age-related changes in health. In addition, they can have shortened life expectancy, increased numbers of medical problems and decreased rates of recommended preventative health interventions.

Slide 10

For some people who have IDD, aging can be complicated by the occurrence of what appears to be premature aging and shortened life expectancy, particularly for people with profound and multiple disabilities and frequently those with Down syndrome.

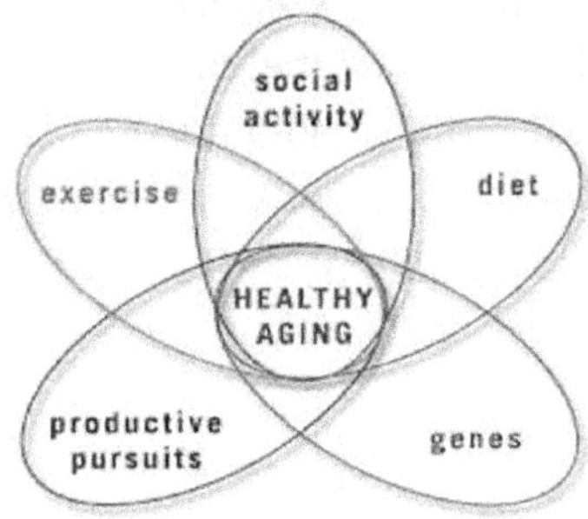

Life expectancy may also be compromised by previously poor health status and living conditions.

Slide 11

Aging in the General Population

Aging in the general population increases vulnerability to certain health issues:

- Memory and Alzheimer's disease
- Sensory problems: eye and ear conditions
- Digestive and metabolic disorders
- Urogenital conditions such as incontinence and prostate cancer
- Dental conditions such as periodontitis, gingivitis and tooth loss
- Skin conditions such as skin cancers, shingles, dry skin, pruritus, geriatric eczema

NIH, 2007

Aging is a genetically driven process Some of the information in our DNA is more likely to manifest toward the end of our lives after decades of environmental influences and lifestyle factors.

Other medical and health-related challenges in one's life can act as risk factors, but there is no blueprint or inevitable road map to determine the rate or severity of aging.

In addition to risk factors, there are protective factors that can support the aging process such as: balanced nutrition, activity, hobbies, injury prevention and social relationships.

Aging is not synonymous with disease. However, the body undergoes lessened reserve capacity during aging. In other words, organ systems are much more easily compromised and take longer to recover from injury or illness. Cell death increases and cell growth slows or stops. Body equilibrium is difficult to restore once it has been lost, causing changes in blood pressure and blood volume, dehydration and fluctuation of blood sugar.

Health issues identified on this slide are some examples of conditions related to biological aging.

Slide 12

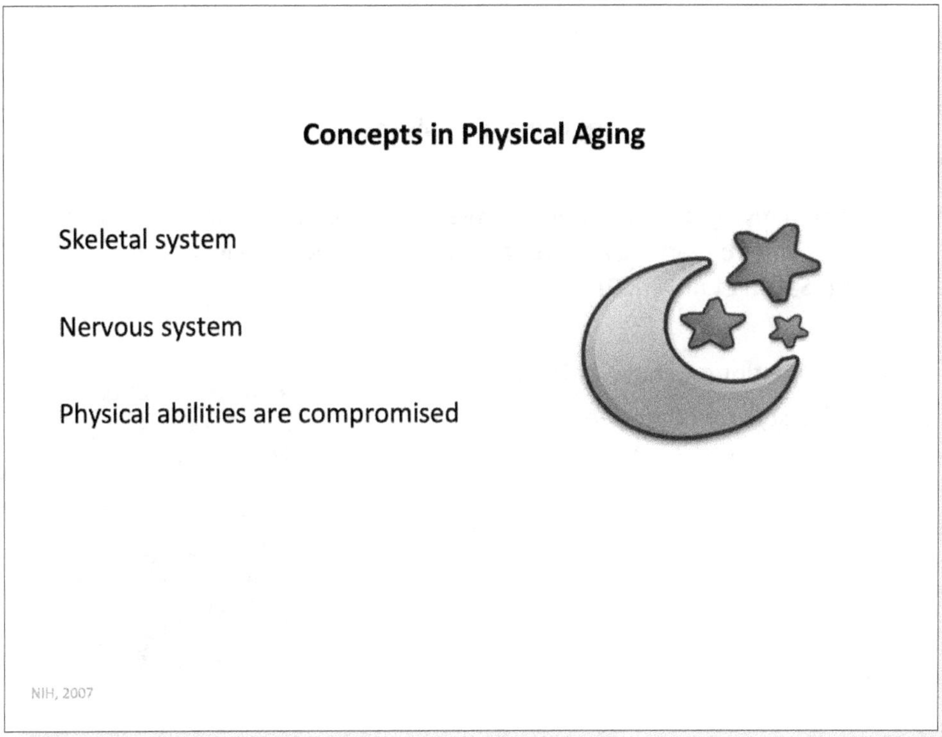

The skeletal system, including bones and joints, loses mass, which can cause osteoporosis, arthritis and bone breakage.

The nervous system slows down sensory integration; aging persons experience decreased functional neurons, reduced motor skills and less productive sleep.

Balance, coordination, muscle strength, sight and hearing are compromised.

Slide 13

Learning and Memory

Common myths and stereotypes have long implied that older adults are not able to learn new material or that poor memory is part of aging (Saxon et al., 2009).

People continue to have different learning styles as they age.

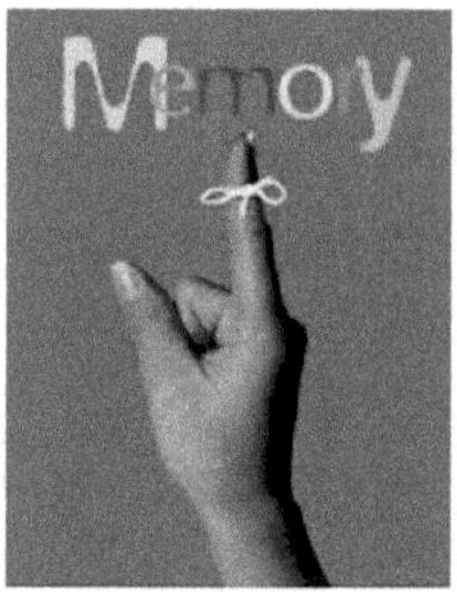

Older adults may be cautious about new information or have less opportunity to practice new skills.

Memory refers to ability to recall stored information. But memory also includes how often a person is required to recall specific information.

If one is not required to access certain information frequently or recently, they may have difficulty with retrieval.

Slide 14

Life Expectancy

As a result of advances in health care and community supports, life expectancy is increasing for people who have intellectual/developmental disabilities.

For example, life expectancy for people with Down syndrome has increased dramatically in recent decades, from 25 in 1983 to 60 today.

Bigby, 2004

Several hundred genetic causes of intellectual/developmental disability have been identified, and many are yet unknown. The commonality shared by this group is that, individually, each meets the criteria to be considered a person who has an intellectual/ developmental disability (based on limitations in cognitive functioning and adaptive functioning).

People with genetically caused IDD may not share commonalities in the way they age or the age-related issues they experience.

Genetic abnormalities frequently cause both cognitive delay and predisposition to specific health issues.

Lack of access to appropriate health services is also an impediment to maintaining good health for a person who has IDD.

While there have been significant advances in research and knowledge about IDD and medical care, many primary care physicians, the gateway to specialized health care, do not have the knowledge or experience to be able to identify the signs and symptoms of declining health in patients who have IDD.

Slide 15

The Differences in Aging with an IDD

- Genetics
- Environmental factors and lifestyle
- Access to specialized health and mental health services for people who have IDD or dual diagnosis
- Communication
- Accelerated aging

Baxter et al, 2006 and Ringaert and Waters, 2005

Genetic factors that result in both IDD and an increase in specific somatic health problems include a greater tendency to develop upper respiratory problems, early onset of hearing loss and genetic predispositions to Alzheimer's disease.

Institutional living and community living both may pose an increased risk of infection, lack of exercise choices, smoking, poor diet, alcohol and drug use and unsafe sex.

Lack of education about health promotion and prevention can affect diet and exercise. Poor nutrition and obesity are risk factors that can advance aging or lead to secondary chronic illnesses.

People with IDD often have health problems associated with their disability, of which a health care provider may not have knowledge.

People who have IDD may not have insight into what they are experiencing as they age. They also may not be able to describe what they are experiencing in a way that others understand. Symptoms can, therefore, go unnoticed until they are more pronounced.

Slide 16

Accelerated Physical Aging

There is evidence that people with IDD develop secondary conditions and diseases. As a result, they may age at a different rate than the general population.

Features of aging that can manifest as a gradual reduction in ability or capacity in an individual in the general population can occur more rapidly in someone with IDD.

Kailes, 2006

According to Isaacson Kailes (1998), typical aging does not involve a high rate of medical and functioning problems until between ages 70 and 75. But people with IDD can show these at higher rates up to 20 to 25 years earlier.

Sensory changes (hearing, smell, vision, balance, gait) can begin in the 40s and 50s, with significant limitations in the 70s and 80s. An individual with IDD may not have coping skills or the ability to make behavior modifications to adjust to reduction in acuity. Therefore the change is less gradual and appears at an earlier age.

Haverman et al. (2010) reports that people with IDD are at greater risk of health problems that can be prevented. Many of these lead to chronic disease, which greatly impacts physical health as they age.

Slide 17

Other age-related health issues are more frequent in people with particular genetically based syndromes.

- **Mitral valve prolapse and musculoskeletal disorders in people with Fragile X syndrome.**
- **Scoliosis in people with Prader-Willi syndrome.**
- **Recurrent upper respiratory and ear infections in people with Cri-du-Chat syndrome.**

Temkin, 2009

Fragile X syndrome is a genetically inherited syndrome that causes an error with the manufacture of a protein the brain requires for normal development and function. It is the most common inherited form of intellectual/ developmental disability. It results from a change or mutation in a single gene, which can be passed from one generation to the next.

Prader-Willi syndrome (PWS) is a genetic disorder that is complex in origin but results from an abnormality of the 15th chromosome.

Cri-du-Chat syndrome is a group of symptoms that result from missing a piece of chromosome No. 5 and is characterized by IDD. Infants with Cri-du-Chat syndrome have high-pitched cries similar to a cat, which is how the syndrome was named. Most cases of Cri-du-Chat syndrome are not inherited.

Slide 18

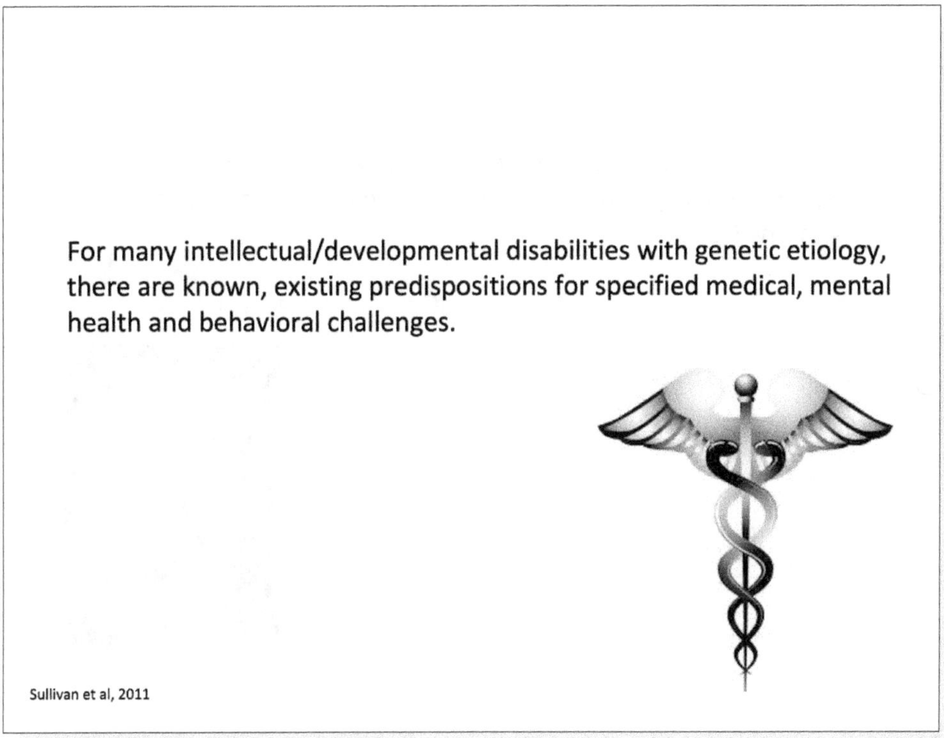

Mutations in genes that are related to brain activity can cause intellectual/developmental disability. Quite often, these mutations also cause physical abnormalities that lead to health vulnerabilities.

Slide 19

The most commonly known of these is the increased risk of precocious aging, dementia and increased sensory loss in people with Down syndrome.

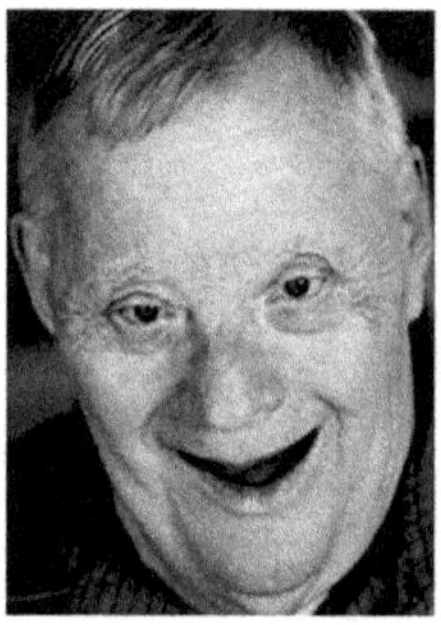

Wishart, 1996

People who have Down syndrome experience symptoms of aging at an earlier age than the general population. The additional chromosome on pair 21 is known to advance the chronological onset of aging and known to trigger the increase in amyloid precursor protein that is associated with Alzheimer's disease.

Slide 20

Sensory Changes and Aging

- Reduced acuity and alertness
- Increased masking and compensatory strategies
- Reduced potential for independence
- Increased social isolation
- Decreased attention span
- Increase in falls

As we age, our senses change and become less effective. People with IDD are already at risk of some sensory capabilities being compromised, so aging can be more limiting.

Sensory changes and limitations can manifest as problem behaviors or lead to misdiagnoses, such as mental health disorders, dementia or Alzheimer's.

Slide 21

Exercise

A **compensatory strategy** is a technique or modification to our behavior or environment that we use to compensate for a deficit, weakness, injury or perceived inadequacy in a specific area or skill.

Activity: Think of a compensatory strategy you use when you run into someone whose name you forgot or when you set a new security password to remember.

Discussion: In the same circumstances, would that compensatory strategy potentially be different for a person who has an IDD?

A compensatory strategy may be used by someone who experienced a traumatic brain injury or memory loss, but they are also things we all do in our everyday life. Examples include: calendars, appointment books, alarms, pill boxes, lists, creating acronyms, etc.

Slide 22

The prevalence of certain mental health issues increases with aging, including anxiety, depression, dementia and psychosis.

From the available research, it can be reasonably concluded that people who have IDD are more likely to develop a mental health issue as they age.

Patel, Goldberg & Moss, 1993

Although less common than behavioral disorders, major mental disorders still occur in older adults with intellectual/developmental disabilities with an overall prevalence of about 10 percent. Some disorders, such as dementia, increase with age. Dementia occurs at about the same rate as in the general population, except that it appears at a greater rate (and at a younger age) in adults with Down syndrome. As in the general elderly population, psychotic disorders may also increase with age (although psychoses which appeared in youth may stabilize). They are, however, less frequent than mood and anxiety disorders.

Slide 23

Prevalence of Mental Health Problems

The rate of psychiatric problems for people who have IDD is two to four times the rate of the general population as they age.

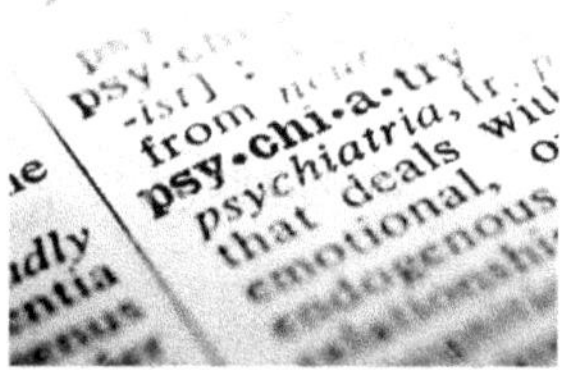

Torr & Davis, 2007

The overall prevalence of mental health problems in adults with IDD is higher than in the general population. Factors leading to this higher rate are associated with higher rates of exposure to traumatic events and/or development of PTSD, lack of coping skills, behavioral phenotypes (psychiatric issues of underlying genetic disorders), multiple prescribed medications and drug interactions, repeated pattern of broken relationships, limited choices and opportunities (Royal College of Psychiatrists, 2001).

Slide 24

Dementia

The DSM-5 defines dementia as Neurocognitive Disorder. It involves the "loss of memory plus impairment in at least one other cognitive function, such as aphasia, apraxia, agnosia; and disturbance in executive function, which is severe enough to interfere with activities of daily living and represents a decline."

APA, 2000, 2013

The diagnosis of dementia is made when symptoms have been present for a period (at a minimum six months), having ruled out treatable conditions or illnesses.

Dementia presentation may differ between people according to the severity of preexisting IDD.

Slide 25

Dementia Prevalence Rate

- 22 percent of adults 40+ who have Down syndrome develop dementia.
- The rate increases to 56 percent for adults 60+.
- For individuals with other types of IDD, the rate is comparable to that of the general population: 5 percent in adults 60+.

Janicki & Dalton, 2000 and Fletcher, et al., 2007

Research indicates that the increased prevalence of dementia in people who have Down syndrome is associated with the additional chromosome on pair 21, which can cause increased production of a protein believed to be responsible for the onset and progression of dementia. Nearly all adults who have Down syndrome over 40 years of age develop brain changes consistent with Alzheimer's, but not all develop significant symptoms (Fletcher et al., 2007).

Slide 26

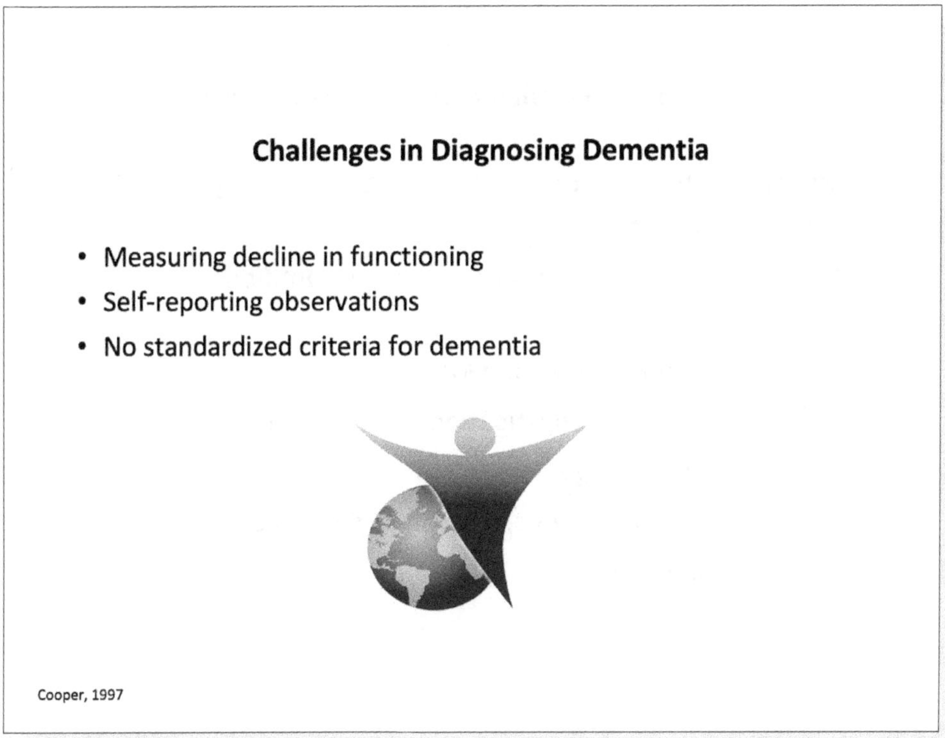

Baseline establishment for cognitive functioning and daily living tasks can be difficult for people who have IDD. This complicates measuring changes from baseline to determine if there is a decline in functioning and skills.

Many people who have IDD have difficulty answering questions about memory or higher cognitive functioning, which challenges the diagnostic process. As with other health and mental health conditions, limited communication skills and ability to articulate the experience of symptoms complicates diagnosis.

The lack of reliable and standardized diagnostic procedures for dementia complicates diagnosis in the early stages.

A careful assessment of baseline functioning should be obtained, utilizing knowledgeable informants and any written assessments from the past. A continuing data system should be implemented, and all observational criteria should be carefully followed and documented.

Slide 27

Diagnostic Overshadowing & Misdiagnosis

- Assumption that lack of cognition or sensory changes are due to IDD or MI
- Age-associated changes that may be misidentified as dementia:
    - Adjustment: grief and loss
    - Dehydration, constipation, nutritional imbalances
    - Sleep challenges
    - Visual impairments, cataracts, glaucoma
    - Urinary discomfort, UTIs

The conditions and symptoms listed above are more common as people age. They are also harder to identify and diagnose in people with IDD who cannot communicate symptoms and/or may be experiencing these challenges for the first time in their life. It is essential to address and rule out possible causes for decline when dementia is a suspected diagnosis.

Some symptoms may also be present as persistent behavioral problems, and because they are chronic, identifying a clear trigger/antecedent is challenging.

For some audiences, it may be useful to have a discussion about how symptoms manifest as behaviors when people primarily communicate through their actions.

Slide 28

Case illustration: Maria is a woman with Down syndrome. She is in her 40s and her health is failing. She suffers from digestive discomfort and sometimes has trouble hearing. She no longer has the energy to do the things she likes to do, and her favorite TV show, *The Office,* has gone off the air. Her life just seems to be slipping away. She gets crabby and takes her frustration out on staff, taking an occasional swing when she has energy and spitting at staff when she does not.

Exercise: Think about ways you could use these approaches to develop interventions to support Maria's wellness: positive behavior supports, mental health interventions and person-centered planning.

Encourage group participation. Correct answers are not limited to those below; they are listed as suggestions.

Consider the content reviewed in the previous slides and the implications of Maria's age and diagnosis. Evaluate her current health status and advocate for hearing screening and appropriate medical exams/appointments.

Rather than focusing on the TV program itself (reruns, DVDs, other shows etc.), identify what elements of the show Maria looked forward to seeing each week that we can possibly replicate for her by finding an "ensemble" community of her own in a part-time job, volunteer opportunity or similar setting.

Think about the role that hearing impairment can be playing in behavior challenges and what modifications we can make when addressing her or delivering instructions or information.

Slide 29

For people who have an intellectual/developmental disability, lifelong attention to preventable medical and mental health conditions is critical for healthy aging.

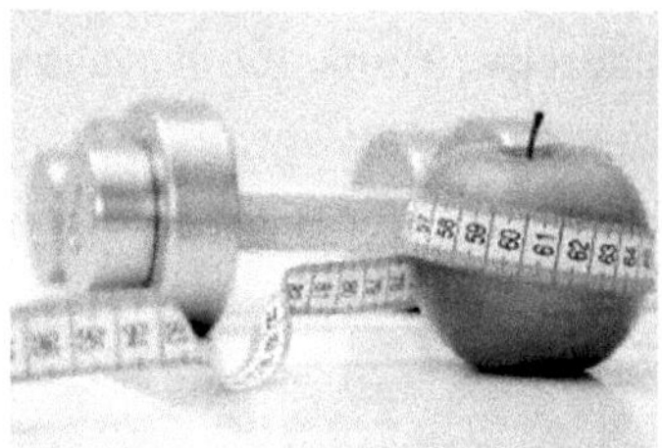

Health disorders in people with IDD frequently differ from those encountered in the general population in terms of prevalence, age of onset, rate of progression, degree of severity and presenting manifestations (Sullivan et al., 2011).

Implementation of best practice guidelines in preventative care throughout a person's life span increases the likelihood of healthy aging and the reduction of age-related health and mental health issues.

Evidence-based best practice guidelines for primary care physicians working with people who have an intellectual disability have been developed in Canada. These guidelines include an associated toolkit of information for general practitioners and direct support professionals on general issues in primary care, preventative care checklists, health watch tables and syndrome-specific charts, among other resources, etc. The tools have now been adapted for use in the U.S. health system.

Each of the health watch tables and syndrome-specific charts details conditions for which a person has a predisposition and tools for behavioral and mental health. The tools also include information on how to effectively communicate with a patient who has an IDD.

Slide 30

Best Practice Guidelines for Physicians

In 2011, Canadian Consensus Guidelines were developed for primary care physicians on evidence-based best practice in preventative health care for people with IDD.

In 2014, these tools were adapted by Vanderbilt Kennedy University Center for Excellence in Developmental Disabilities for use within the U.S. health care system.

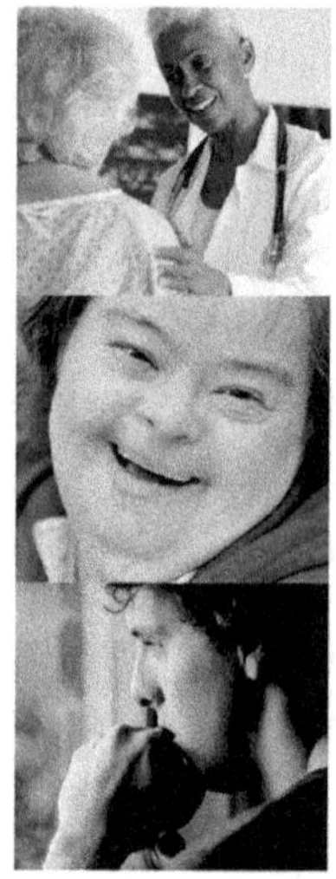

The Vanderbilt Kennedy University Center of Excellence in Developmental Disabilities has collaborated with the Utah Boling Center and the Tennessee Dept. of Intellectual and Developmental Disabilities, funded by Special Hope Foundation, adapting the Canadian Toolkit and guidelines for use within the U.S. health care system. This development provides primary care providers with the knowledge and tools needed to provide comprehensive, preventive health care to people with IDD.

Slide 31

Primary Care Toolkit

The Canadian Primary Care Guidelines and Toolkit are available at: https://www.cna-aiic.ca/en/nursing-practice/tools-for-practice/primary-care-toolkit

The primary care tools adapted for use in the US health care system are available at: https://iddtoolkit.vkcsites.org/

Slide 32

Creating a Supportive Setting

- Proper lighting
- Bold colors
- Reduce background noise
- Increase visual aids
- Non-slip surfaces
- Remove rugs
- Reduce clutter
- Check water and climate temperature
- Gentle soaps
- More seasoned food
- Visual aids
- Smoke detectors
- Clearly marked exits
- Rounded furniture

Adapted from Gilbride, M 2016

Slide 33

Creating a Supportive Setting

- Proper lighting
- Bold colors
- Reduce background noise
- Increase visual aids
- Non-slip surfaces
- Remove rugs
- Reduce clutter
- Check water and climate temperature
- Gentle soaps
- More seasoned food
- Visual aids
- Smoke detectors
- Clearly marked exits
- Rounded furniture

Adapted from Gilbride, M 2016

Support older people with clear, well-lit areas. Use bold colors to distinguish bedsheets from covers and tables from dishes and food.

Avoid caffeine and salt, but use natural seasoning to enhance taste as taste buds are lost to aging.

Use gentle soaps and increase moisturizers.

Temperature should be adjusted to climate and weather and not based on reporting by individuals whose sensory changes may compromise safety.

Slide 34

Activity: Help Tom

Tom has Down syndrome and has been experiencing early signs of dementia. He's been having trouble at mealtimes: He can eat finger foods, but he can't find food on the plate with his fork. And when he gets up to use the bathroom at night, he cannot find his way back to his room.

Help Tom using some ideas on the previous slide or your own.

Ideas to try:

- At mealtimes, reduce noise and watch Tom's body language. Try to serve food he likes. Distinguish plates from the table with a colorful placemat or bright dish. Leave nonperishable snacks around for Tom to be sure he eats enough and has access to food when he is hungry. Engage Tom in food prep so he recognizes food when it is served. Minimize patterns. Minimize new foods. Check false teeth or dental issues.

- Put a picture on Tom's door of himself — you may need a younger self he recognizes. Cover mirrors if they give the appearance of an intruder. Remove rugs in hallways. Restrict volume in shared spaces after certain hours. Color bedroom doors brightly. Consider automatic or sensor night lights.

Slide 35

The Social Aspects of Aging

As with all people, aging people with IDD deal with a variety of psycho-social changes and support as they age.

- Increasing social isolation
- Changing interests
- Declining energy
- Retirement

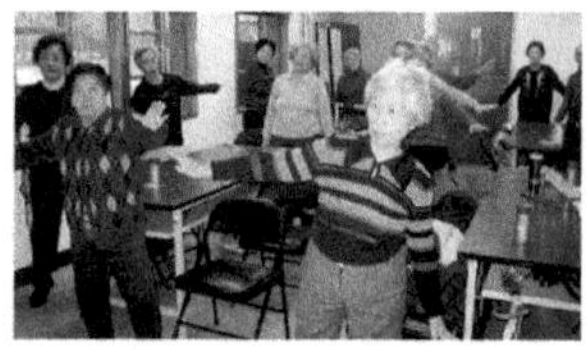

Temkin, 2009

Retirement from employment and/or supported leisure activities can have a profound impact on the well-being of all people. Transition planning for people with IDD is a critical element of supports to assist in reducing the potential social isolation, loss of income and boredom that can be experienced in this process.

Supports for people who have IDD should also acknowledge that interests change and energy declines as people age. Social and leisure activities, as well as expectations, should evolve in consideration of the changes a person goes through across their lifespan. Activities for which people have high enthusiasm and interest in their youth may not hold the same appeal later in life. Diverse and fluid support plans driven by the needs and wants of the person should be an accepted expectation of people as they age.

Slide 36

The Social Aspects of Aging

- Cognitive decline
- Financial and estate management
- Loss of family and friends
- Grief management
- Acceptance of mortality
- Lack of meaningful work or hobbies

Temkin, 2009

As previously noted, some cognitive decline is an expected outcome of aging. However, it can lead to frustration and declining overall wellness for the person if they lose previously achieved life skills.

Aging is associated not only with the increasing likelihood of the death of family members but also with the potential for the loss of knowledge about the past experiences of the person who has IDD.

As with the population generally, the experience of bereavement by people with IDD can be associated with considerable behavioral and emotional changes. When left unacknowledged and unresolved over time, the person will not receive the appropriate support. Loss and grief can also be expressed somatically as symptoms of declining health.

The acceptance of mortality is a healthy part of aging. People with IDD often have little opportunity to participate in the rituals of mortality like funerals and may not have the ability to understand the abstract concept of mortality without these experiences.

Slide 37

Social Value

Social value contributes to overall wellness for all people.

This includes people who have IDD who want to participate in and contribute to their communities in the same manner as all citizens.

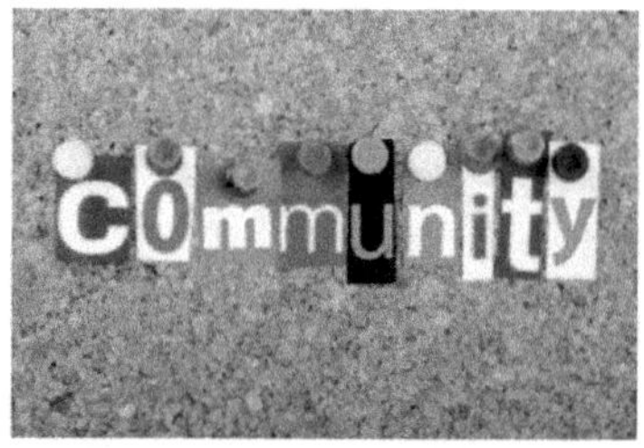

Activities and outcomes that enhance social value and contribute to mental and physical well-being can include:

- Practical, leisure or life-enhancing skills
- Improved or maintained dietary and general health status that prevents physical health factors from hindering typical activity
- A varied rhythm of life
- Recognition that challenge and productivity must continue throughout old age
- An increased and well-established social network
- Participation on a regular basis in the general life of the community with people who are meaningful to the person

Slide 38

Exercise

What social value did you experience from older people as you were growing up?

- Did you spend time around your grandparents?
- Were older people respected during your childhood?
- How can we ensure the people with IDD can continue to offer social value as they age?

Slide 39

Wellness

Wellness encompasses many components including:

- Promoting health and preventing illness, disease and injury.
- Optimizing mental and physical health.
- Managing chronic conditions.
- Engaging with life.

WHO, 2000

These four recommendations for healthy aging are identified as those that had the greatest potential for changing or improving the current situation in the area of healthy aging. Focus issues were identified as healthy eating, injury prevention, physical activity and tobacco cessation (Health Canada, 2002). Addressing these issues are shared components of wellness for the general and IDD population.

Health care providers serving adults and elders with intellectual/developmental disabilities must recognize that adult and older-age-onset medical conditions are common in this population and may require a high index of suspicion for clinical diagnosis throughout the person's life regardless of the person's ability to accurately self report.

Slide 40

Wellness

Key responsibilities for primary care and specialist health services:

1. **Maintenance of the physical and mental health of people with IDD**

2. **Early detection and treatment of both physical and mental health problems**

Poindexter, 2002

People in the U.S. and Canada are living longer than ever before. Many seniors live active and healthy lives. There are things all people can do to stay healthy and active as they age:

- Eat a balanced diet
- Activity for both body and mind
- Don't smoke
- Attend to regular preventative health care and get regular check-ups
- Practice safety habits

(NIH: National Institute on Aging, 2007)

Slide 41

Working Together

As people who have IDD age, there is ongoing need for collaborative supports and services to address the needs of the person in this stage of life to ensure that wellness is assured as an accepted part of aging for this population.

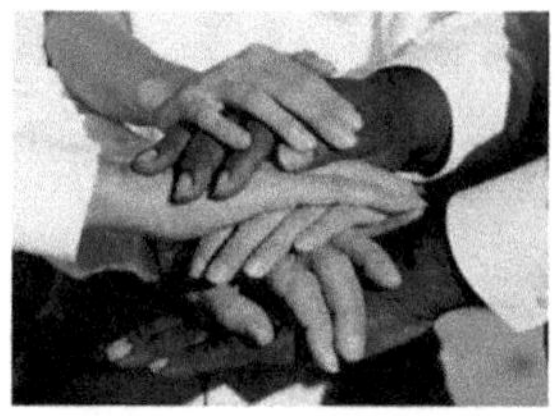

As noted in *Module VII: Positive Support Strategies and Wellness*, an interdisciplinary, collaborative system of services is needed for people who have a dual diagnosis across their life span, including as they age. There is great necessity for health services, senior services, mental health services and developmental services to make a coordinated effort to bridge service gaps for aging people.

Slide 42

End-of-Life Considerations

- Thinking ahead matters.
- Identify a person who will act in the best interest of the individual. Consider someone in his/her social or spiritual community.
- Help people understand there are options to plan for treatment, at a time when they might be unable to make informed decisions (advance directives, health care proxy, substitute decision-maker or power of attorney).

Support providers may be the first, and perhaps the most trusted, person that an individual and/or family looks to for guidance in serious decisions regarding wellness and health.

While not the legal, medical or psychiatric expert, the team should be familiar with resources and information that can help an individual guide their own treatment, or select a trusted person to see that their wishes are followed.

An advance directive is legally enforceable, completed at a time when the person is capable of making decisions, and is activated only when the individual is not capable of doing so (medically or psychiatrically).

Another document, a durable power of attorney (POA) for health care, can be prepared that appoints a person to make decisions on their behalf.

Share your knowledge of these options and encourage the family or the individual to further pursue these options if they feel it might be of benefit to them.

Medical issues that might arise at the end of life include:

- Do Not Resuscitate (DNR) orders
- Organ and tissue donation
- Physicians Orders for Life Sustaining Treatment (POLST) and Medical Orders for Life Sustaining Treatment (MOLST) forms in the United States. End of Life Planning and Advanced Care Directives in Canada.

Slide 43

For More Information about Healthcare Directives:

National Hospice and Palliative Care Organization
1-800-658-8898 (toll-free)
caringinfo@nhpco.org
www.caringinfo.org

Center for Practical Bioethics - US
1-800-344-3829 (toll-free)
center@centerforbioethics.org
www.practicalbioethics.org

OrganDonor.gov - US
Health Resources & Services Administration
www.organdonor.gov

National POLST Paradigm - US
1-202-780-8352
info@polst.org
www.polst.org

Put It In Writing - US
American Hospital Association
1-800-424-4301
www.putitinwriting.org

In Canada

Canadian Virtual Hospice
http://www.virtualhospice.ca

Canadian Hospice and Palliative Care Association
Toll Free: 1-800-668-2785
Email: info@chpca.net

Living Lessons® Hospice Palliative Care
Info Line: 1-877-203-4636
http://www.chpca.net

Organ Donation Canada
https://www.beadonor.ca

Wills and Estate Planning Canada
https://www.canada.ca/en/financial-consumer-agency/services/estate-planning/will-estate-planning

Advance Care planning and Directives – Canada Kit
https://www.dyingwithdignity.ca/download_your_advance_care_planning_kit

Slide 44

Advance Care Directive

- An advance healthcare directive, also known as a medical directive, is a legal document in which a person specifies what actions should be taken for their health if they are no longer able to make decisions for themselves because of illness or incapacity.
- In the United States, each state regulates the use of advance directives differently. A living will is one type of advance directive. It takes effect when the patient is terminally ill.

Slide 45

Power of Attorney

A "durable power of attorney for health care" is also called a "health care power of attorney." It's a legal document in which a person names a proxy (agent) to make all health care decisions if one becomes unable to do so.

A proxy or, substitute decision-maker, also known as a representative, surrogate or agent, should be familiar with the person's values and wishes. This means he or she will be able to decide when treatment decisions need to be made. A proxy can be chosen in addition to or instead of a living will.

Slide 46

- In Canada, a similar document is called a "power of attorney for personal care or for property." To be able to appoint a power of attorney, the person must be considered capable of making their own decisions around care and finances. This can be a challenge for people who have moderate to severe IDD. In these situations, decisions around care and finance may be made by an appropriate, identified substitute decision-maker. Separate acts govern substitute decision-making in each province and territory. For more information, search substitute decision-making for your province or territory.

- The Advance Care Planning in Canada: A National Framework and Implementation Project

Slide 47

Resources & Publications

Complex moral issues: End-of-life decisions for adults with significant intellectual disabilities.
ucedd.georgetown.edu/complex/

A caregiver's guide to the dying process.
hospicefoundation.org/HFA-Products/Caregiver-s-Guide-to-the-Dying-Process

The Center for Excellence in Aging & Community Wellness (CEACW)
A guide for supporting older people with intellectual disabilities and their families.
ceacw.org/

Slide 48

Resources & Publications

Options and Decision-Making at End of Life—Canada
canada.ca/en/health-canada/services/options-decision-making-end-life.html

Advance Care Planning—Canada
https://www.advancecareplanning.ca/resources-and-tools/

Powers of Attorney—Canada
canada.ca/en/employment-social-development/corporate/seniors/forum/power-attorney-financial.html

References: Module XII

National Institutes of Health (2007). 8 Areas of Age-Related Change. *NIMH Medline Plus*, 2 (1): *10-13.*

American Association of Geriatric Psychiatry (2008). *Geriatrics and mental health—the facts.* Available at: http://www.aagponline.org/prof/facts_mh.asp. Retrieved June 23, 2008.

American Psychiatric Association. (2000). *Diagnostic and statistical manual of mental disorders* (4th ed., text rev.). Washington, DC.

Baxter, H., Lowe, K., Houston, H., et al. (2006). Previously unidentified morbidity in patients with intellectual disability. *British Journal of General Practice*, 56, 93-98.

Bigby, C. (2004). *Aging with a Lifelong Disability: Policy, Program and Practice Issues for Professionals.* London: Jessica Kingsley.

Bigby, A. (2008). Beset by obstacles: A review of Australian policy development to support ageing in place for people with intellectual disability. *Journal of Intellectual & Developmental Disability*, 33 (1), 76–86.

Canadian Primary Care toolkit (2011). Implementation of Best Practice Guidelines.

Comfort A. (1979). *The Biology of Senescence* (3rd Ed). Edinburgh and London: Churchill Livingstone.

Cooper, S. A. (1997). Epidemiology of psychiatric disorders in elderly compared with younger adults with learning disabilities. *The British Journal of Psychiatry*, 170, 375-380.

Fletcher, R., Loschen, E., Stavrakaki, C., & First, M. (Eds.) (2007). *Diagnostic Manual – Intellectual Disability (DM-ID): A Clinical Guide for Diagnosis of Mental Disorders in Persons with Intellectual Disability.* Kingston, NY: NADD Press.

Gilbride, M. (2016). People with IDD and Growing Old: Understanding and Supporting Age-Related Changes.

Health Canada. Division of Aging and Seniors. (2002). Dare to Age Well: Workshop on Healthy Aging. Part1: Aging and Health Practices. Works and Government Services, Canada.

Holland, A. J. (2000). Ageing and learning disability. *The British Journal of Psychiatry*, 176, 26-31.

Isaacson Kailes, J. (1998). Dissemination Specialist, Rehabilitation Research and Training Center on Aging with Spinal Cord Injury, Downey, CA: Rancho Los Amigos National Rehabilitation Center, http://www.jik.com/awdrtcawd.html.

Janicki, M. P., & Dalton, A. J. (2000). Prevalence of dementia and impact on intellectual disability services. *Mental Retardation*, 38, 277-289.

Kailes, J. I. (2006). A user's perspective on midlife (ages 18 to 65) aging with disability. (pp. 194–204). In Field, M. J., Jette, A. M., & Martin, L. (Eds.), *Workshop on Disability in America: A New Look*. Washington, DC: The National Academies Press.

National Hospice and Palliative Care Organization (2019).

National Institute of Health. (2007). Global Health and Aging. Washington, DC.

Patel, P., Goldberg, D., & Moss, S. (1993). Psychiatric morbidity in older people with moderate and severe learning disability. II: The prevalence study. *The British Journal of Psychiatry*, 163, 481-491.

Poindexter, A. (2002). *Health Management of Aging Adults with Mental Retardation*. Kingston, NY: The NADD Press.

Ringaert, L., & Watters, C. (2005). The Canadian Centre on Disability Studies Discussion Paper on Seniors with Disabilities. Advancing the Inclusion of Seniors with Disabilities Report (third edition) for the Office of Disability Issues (ODI).

Royal College of Psychiatrists. (2001). *DC–LD: Diagnostic Criteria for Psychiatric Disorders for Use with Adults with Learning Disabilities/Mental Retardation.* London: Gaskell.

Saxon, S., Etten, M. J., & Perkins, E. A. (2009). *Physical Change and Aging: A Guide for the Helping Professions, Fifth Edition.* New York: Springer.

Sullivan, W. F., Berg, J. M., Bradley, E., Cheetham, T., Denton, R., Heng, J., Hennen, B., Joyce, D., Kelly, M., Korossy, M., Lunsky, Y., McMillan, S. (2011). Primary care of adults with developmental disabilities: Canadian consensus guidelines. *Canadian Family Physician*, 57, 541-53.

Talarico, L. D. (1998). Preventive gerontology: Strategies for optimal aging. *Patient Care*, 32 (9), 198-211.

Temkin, M. (2009). *Strategic Issues for Service Agencies.* Victoria, BC: Garth Homer Society.

Thorpe, L., Davidson, P., & Janicki, M. P. (2000). *Healthy Ageing - Adults with Intellectual Disabilities: Biobehavioural Issues.* Geneva, Switzerland: World Health Organization.

Torr, J., & Davis, R. (2007). Mental retardation and developmental disorders ageing and mental health problems in people with intellectual disability. *Current Opinion in Psychiatry*, 20 (5), 467-471.

The Vanderbilt Kennedy University Center of Excellence in Developmental Disabilities (2014). Health Care for Adults with Intellectual and Developmental Disabilities Toolkit for Primary Care Providers.

Wishart, J. G. (1996). Avoidant learning styles and cognitive development in young children. In Stratford, B., & Gunn, P. (Eds.), *New Approaches to Down Syndrome* (pp. 173-205). London: Cassell.

World Health Organization (2000). Ageing and Intellectual Disabilities - Improving Longevity and Promoting Healthy Ageing: Summative Report. Geneva, Switzerland: World Health Organization.

Module XIII

Justice System Considerations

Slide 2

This module contains information about the justice system as it relates to involvement with people who have an intellectual/ developmental disability.

The goal is to assist service providers and clinicians to become more familiar with the system as they advocate for people with IDD who may become involved with justice.

Slide 3

Learning Objectives

- Understand the historical perspective on IDD and criminal behavior.
- Be aware of the vulnerabilities that can lead to involvement with the justice system.
- Recognize support needs of persons with IDD involved with the justice system.

Slide 4

Through the early part of the twentieth century, it was accepted theory that people with intellectual/developmental disabilities were inherently criminal in their behavior and their nature.

In fact, there is evidence that the belief in the criminal nature of people with IDD was a primary contributor to the move to institutional living and mass sterilization.

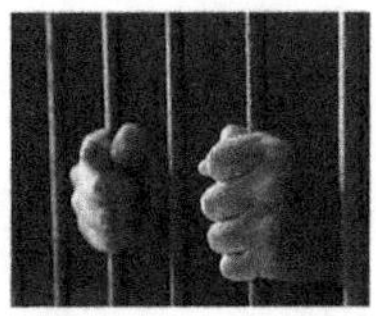

Luckasson (1988)

"In the early part of the twentieth century, several highly respected authorities not only believed that persons with intellectual disabilities were prone to engage in criminal behavior; they expounded the theory that such persons actually comprised virtually the entire offender population."

The president of what is now the American Association on Intellectual and Developmental Disabilities, Henry Goddard, in 1915 wrote that "a person with an IDD ... is a menace to society and civilization; ... he is responsible to a large degree for many, if not all, of our social problems" (quoted in Ellis & Luckasson, 1985, p. 418).

At the time, this was popular opinion in the psychiatric community.

Slide 5

The middle to latter part of the twentieth century brought different theories about IDD and behavior in general, leading to a more balanced understanding today.

There is no greater propensity to criminal behavior for a person with IDD than for a person without IDD.

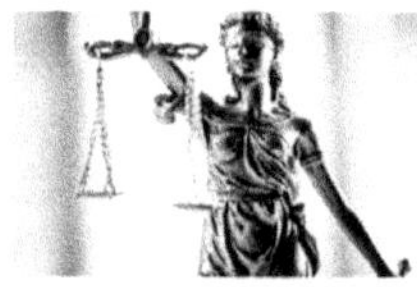

Bright (1989)

There has never been any reliable evidence to support the opinion that people with IDD are more inclined to commit criminal acts than those without (Endicott, 1991). The reasons people who have IDD engage in behavior that brings them into contact with the criminal justice system are varied and complex.

Slide 6

Prevalence Rates

Studies report a large range of estimates, from 2 percent to 40 percent, depending on methodology and diagnostic approach.

There is no strong evidence for different patterns of offending across types of abilities and disabilities.

Lindsay, Law & MacLeod (2002)

While definition, classification and diagnosis of IDD have become significantly less complicated in recent years, there are still challenges in capturing accurate prevalence rates of people with IDD who interact with the justice system. There are several potential reasons why this is the case.

- It is difficult to capture the actual numbers of individuals with IDD who commit crimes, due to underreporting to police.
- Criminal statistics traditionally do not represent true offending prevalence and incidence but rather actual arrest and conviction rates.
- Research focus has been placed on recidivism rates rather than on the path of criminal offending or the process of decision-making within the justice system for offenders with IDD (Jones, 2007).

Slide 7

Prevalence Rates

Establishing accurate or exact prevalence rates for specific conditions can be more effectively done depending on the visibility of the condition and the specific training provided to justice professionals around identification.

Lindsay, Law & MacLeod (2002)

Prevalence rates of people with IDD in the general population are between 2 and 3 percent. But studies in prisons indicate a prevalence rate among prison populations between 2 and 10 percent (Baroff, 1996, Denkowski, 1985; Smith, Algozzine, Schmid & Hennly, 1990). Statistics are higher for juveniles and jails (Griffiths et al., 2002).

Slide 8

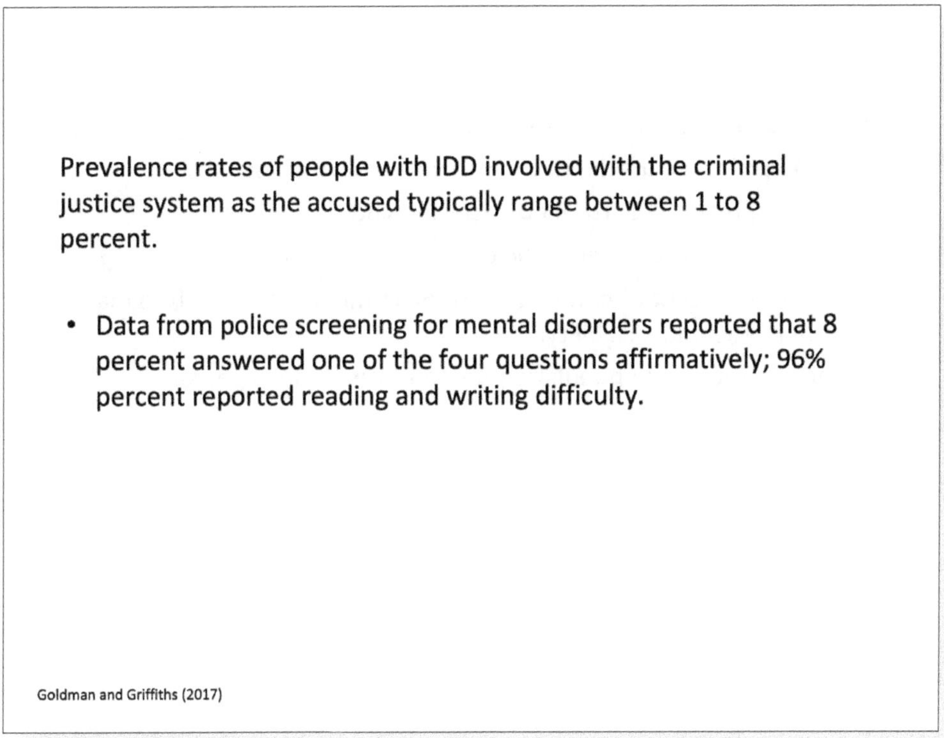
Prevalence rates of people with IDD involved with the criminal justice system as the accused typically range between 1 to 8 percent.
• Data from police screening for mental disorders reported that 8 percent answered one of the four questions affirmatively; 96% percent reported reading and writing difficulty.
Goldman and Griffiths (2017)

Slide 9

Of those screened by police services:

- 45 percent considered themselves to have a disability.
- 40 percent had attended a special school.
- 13 percent reported a coexisting mental health problem.

- Up to 24 percent of defendants in the criminal justice system may have intellectual disability.
- Rates in the prison population ranged from 0 to 9.5 percent.

Goldman and Griffiths (2017)

Slide 10

Counterfeit criminality refers to the concept in which criminal behavior is performed for reasons other than criminality or criminal gain.

Reasons include group membership or acceptance, the need to please peers, misunderstanding of the motives of others and the inability to see a setup.

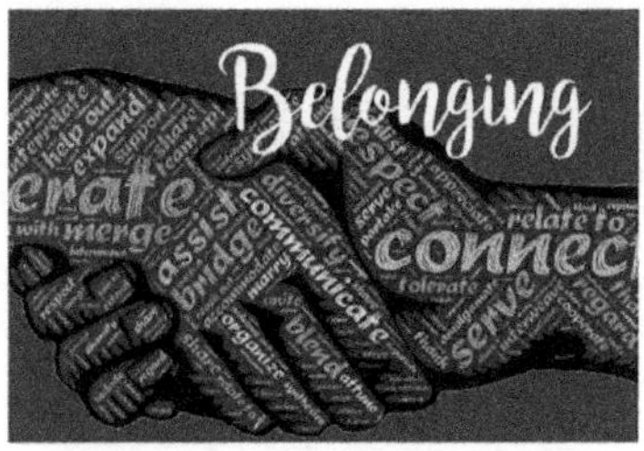

Hingsburger (2011)

The term "counterfeit criminalist" has previously been referred to as counterfeit deviance. David Hingsburger has popularized the term to refer to criminal behavior that is performed for reasons other than criminal gain. As prevention, he suggests "ensuring that people with disabilities both have safe places for socialization and the development of social networks and friendships as well as some tips for teaching and training to lessen the possibility that someone might engage in 'counterfeit criminality'" by:

- Assisting people with disabilities to learn about social interactions, including behavior to identify manipulation, using a person's disability against them and the different safety skills required to navigate in the community.
- Ensuring that there are options for self-advocacy and how people want to engage in self-advocacy.
- Providing the opportunity to practice social skills across different environments across situations.

- Helping people learn how to recognize when they are being taken advantage of and how to disengage from the situation.

- Assisting people to develop friendships and form social interactions.

- Training support people to be aware of the isolation potential for people with IDD and the signs this may be occurring (Hingsburger, 2011).

Slide 11

Vulnerabilities

- More susceptible to being "the fall guy" or doing something illegal to impress someone else or make friends.
- When questioned by police, may not understand questions asked or their rights.
- More likely to confess to crimes they did not commit.
- Past experience may lead them to believe that if they agree, people will usually leave them alone.

Luckasson (1992)

A person who has IDD frequently has specific vulnerabilities that can lead to initial involvement with the justice system. A person who has IDD faces challenges that can often make it difficult to end that involvement or avoid future involvement.

Slide 12

Vulnerabilities

- People with IDD are more often held in custody pre-trial due to the inability to follow recognizance orders.
- People with IDD are often on a fixed income and have few family ties or limited social support, which means they have difficulty securing funds for surety or bail.
- If a person is supported by a community-based organization, the organization cannot act as surety or secure bail on the person's behalf.

Luckasson (1992)

A person who has IDD frequently has specific vulnerabilities that can lead to involvement with the justice system and additional challenges once they are involved in the system.

Slide 13

Vulnerabilities

- People with IDD are more likely to be disciplined when in custody due to an inability to understand or follow institutional rules.
- People with IDD are more likely to have difficulty with others in custody due to an inability to understand institutional hierarchy or social rules.
- Frustration, fear or anxiety may manifest as challenging behavior that can lead to additional charges, the use of segregation and longer sentences.

Luckasson (1992)

Slide 14

When people who have IDD become involved with the justice system, they frequently experience prejudice, lack of understanding and fear. They often experience difficulties with:

- **Not being recognized as having a disability**
- **Being victimized at high rates**
- **Being denied opportunities for reparation**
- **Being denied due process**
- **Discrimination at sentencing, detention and release**

AAIDD and ARC (2014)

As is the case with all people, people who have IDD can become involved with the justice systems as victims, witnesses, suspects, defendants and people who are incarcerated or in detention.

People with IDD are often undiagnosed or misdiagnosed, as assessments are often completed by law enforcement personnel or those who are not specifically trained in assessments for IDD.

People with IDD are more vulnerable to victimization in many different forms, including sexual abuse, financial abuse, oppression, human trafficking, etc.

Victims of crime who have IDD and report the crime often have trouble having their cases investigated due to prejudicial beliefs and stereotypes about their competency to report and testify, their need for support or accommodation or their credibility.

People with IDD can have difficulty securing effective legal counsel. They frequently struggle with cost, credibility and accessing legal counsel familiar with the supports and accommodations the person will need.

People with IDD struggle with a multitude of challenges when sentenced, incarcerated and securing release. In detention centers, jails and prisons, people with IDD can have difficulty identifying, understanding and following prison rules, including those formalized by the institutions. They experience more violations than the general population, making release more difficult. They can be seen as noncompliant with one-size-fits-all treatment programs when they have challenges fitting in and following programs without support or modifications (Joint Position Statement, AAIDD and The Arc, 2014).

Slide 15

Common Characteristics

People who have IDD and commit crimes often share common characteristics:

- have mild IDD
- have no or minimal supports
- come from lower economic status backgrounds
- are isolated from their family and community
- are often homeless

Hayes (2012)

Slide 16

Common Characteristics (cont'd)

- lack productive activity during the day
- have substance abuse problems that affect their financial situation
- have high recidivism
- have high risk of mental illness

Hayes (2012)

Slide 17

Competence to Stand Trial

Competence or fitness to stand trial refers to the ability of the person accused to participate in their own defense. It is the most common forensic assessment in the United States.

It can also be referred to as "adjudicative competency."

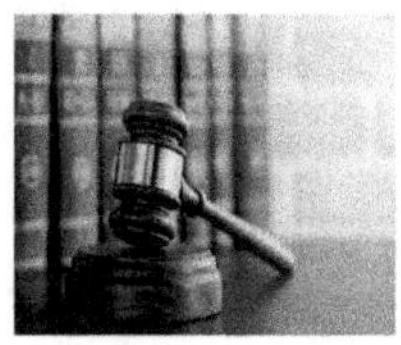

Hoge (2016)

A person with IDD may be found "unfit" to stand trial if they lack the capacity to understand the process of the trial; to understand the nature and importance of the evidence against them; and to give evidence to the court. However, neither the diagnosis of IDD nor of MI means a person will be found unfit to stand trial. A forensic assessment for competency will determine the nature of the specific cognitive impairments and if they affect the ability to participate meaningfully in the trial process (Freckleton, 2018).

A forensic assessment for fitness to stand trial is typically ordered by a judge. After the order for assessment is made, the proceedings are halted until there is a report issued by the psychiatrist completing the assessment. Court is then recalled to review the evidence and the psychiatrist's report. The judge will issue the final determination about fitness based on the assessment, evidence and lawyer's presentation.

There is a presumption of fitness to stand trial unless it is determined otherwise.

How long a determination of unfitness lasts depends largely on whether or not the person disagrees with the order.

Slide 18

Restoration of Competency

In Canada, having competency decisions appealed is done through a Review Board. Reviews of the incompetency decision must be made at regular and stipulated intervals after the initial order of incompetency to stand trial.

In the United States, a ruling of incompetency may be reversed and competency may be restored through educational interventions. Procedures in the United States vary by state.

Danzer, et al. (2020)

A review board is a specialized tribunal chaired by a judge or a person qualified by judicial appointment. It is made up of at least four other members, one of whom must be entitled, under the laws of the particular province, to practice psychiatry.

Slide 19

Forensic Psychiatry

Forensic psychiatry relates to the assessment, treatment and rehabilitation of people with serious mental illness who have come into contact with the law as a result of committing a crime.

After an order of unfit to stand trial has been made, the person is typically ordered to a hospital with forensic mental health treatment for mental health care.

Arboleda-Florez (2006)

Admission to a forensic mental health facility can be a necessary but challenging situation.

"The forensic pathway for persons with intellectual disability moves, often erratically, between the justice system and social services." Lunsky et al. indicate that a history of legal involvement and intellectual disability results in increased likelihood of police response to crises, but do not find an increase in the likelihood of crisis involving aggression (Hauser et al., 2014).

People with IDD are significantly less likely to successfully complete a competency restoration program, which can result in extended involvement with forensic psychiatry (Hauser et al., 2014).

Slide 20

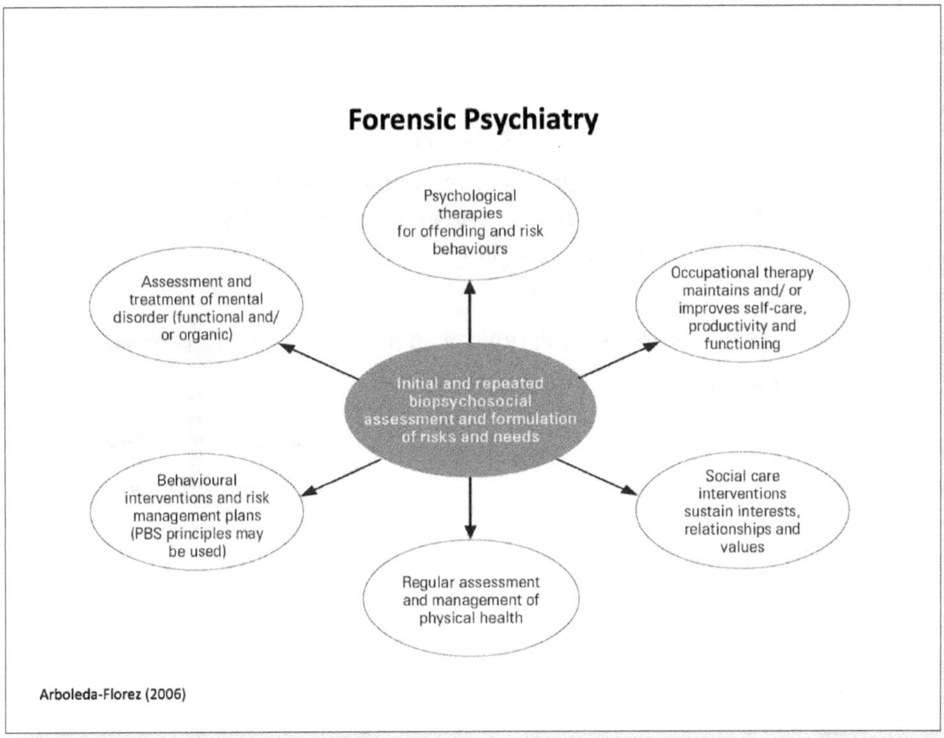
Forensic Psychiatry
Psychological therapies for offending and risk behaviours
Assessment and treatment of mental disorder (functional and/ or organic)
Occupational therapy maintains and/ or improves self-care, productivity and functioning
Initial and repeated biopsychosocial assessment and formulation of risks and needs
Behavioural interventions and risk management plans (PBS principles may be used)
Social care interventions sustain interests, relationships and values
Regular assessment and management of physical health
Arboleda-Florez (2006)

Slide 21

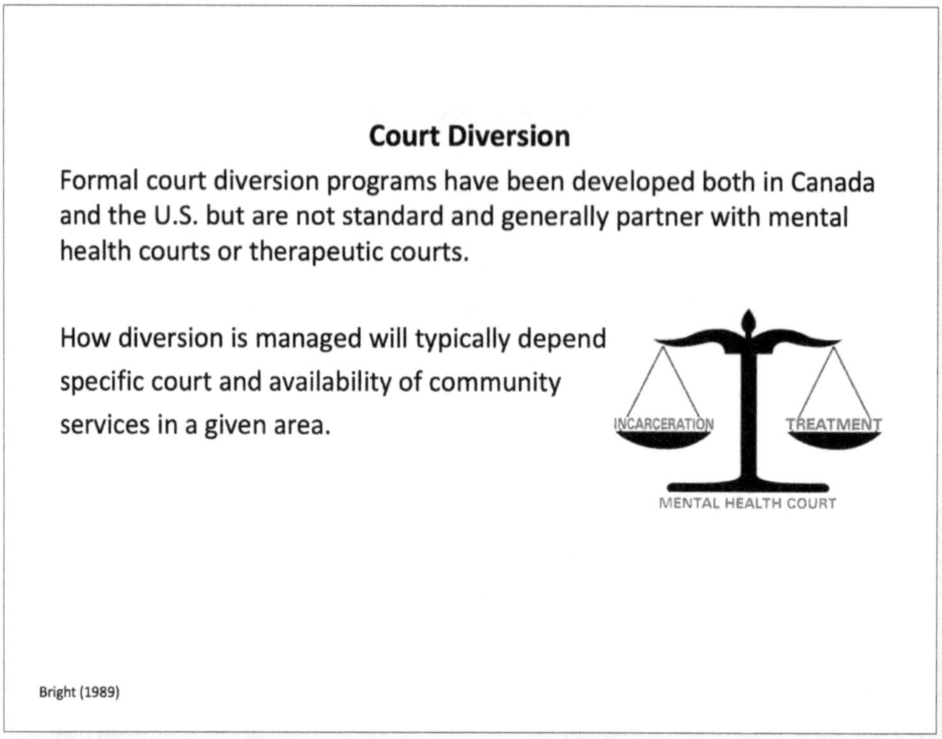

Diversion from the justice system for people with IDD was first proposed in the United States by Menolascino, 1974. He proposed a system of intervention that included prevention, advocacy and treatment options with residential, vocational and educational options.

Slide 22

Court Diversion

A diversion program in the criminal justice system is a form of sentence in which the criminal offender joins a rehabilitation program, which will help remedy the behavior leading to the original arrest, allow the offender to avoid conviction and, in some jurisdictions, hide a criminal record.

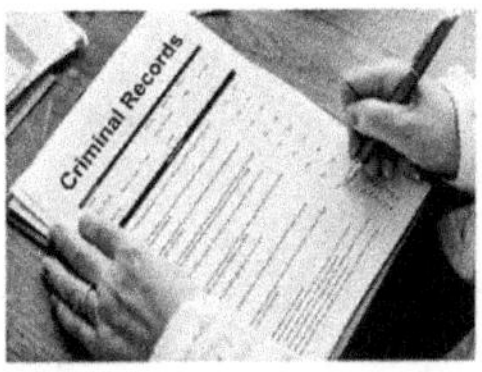

Diversion programs are offered at different points in criminal justice processing. There are pre-charge police diversion programs, post-charge programs and diversion from prison at the point of sentencing.

Diversion was described as a way of holding the accused accountable through means other than a trial. This approach can be used as long as society is still protected and when the accused accepts responsibility for their actions. Options for diversion could include community service, mediation, referrals to specialized programs for counseling, treatment or education (for example, life skills, drug or alcohol treatment, anger management), victim-offender reconciliation programs and similar measures aimed at restorative justice, or a letter of apology or essay.

(https://www.justice.gc.ca/eng/rp-pr/jr/rg-rco/2018/mar01.html)

Slide 23

Court Diversion

A diversion program in the criminal justice system is a form of sentence in which the criminal offender joins a rehabilitation program, which will help remedy the behavior leading to the original arrest, allow the offender to avoid conviction and, in some jurisdictions, hide a criminal record.

In the United States, the availability of diversion programs depends upon the jurisdiction, the nature of the crime (usually nonviolent offences) and in many cases the exercise of prosecutorial discretion. The programs are often run by a police department, court, a district attorney's office or outside agency.

Slide 24

Custody/Incarceration

Offenders who have IDD might find it difficult to follow rules for a variety of reasons.

- They may not have the ability to understand the implied social rules or recall and follow more concrete rules more often than others.
- Misconduct offenses must be documented, and frequent offenses can create an accumulation of misconduct reports.

Rickford & Kimmett (2005)

Inability to follow rules may be observed as disruptive behavior, aggressions or violence. In correctional facilities, inability or refusal to follow rules is often addressed with punitive measures such as removal of privileges, restraint or isolation.

For an offender who has difficulty understanding and following the rules, this can have a negative impact on success in seeking parole or early release.

Slide 25

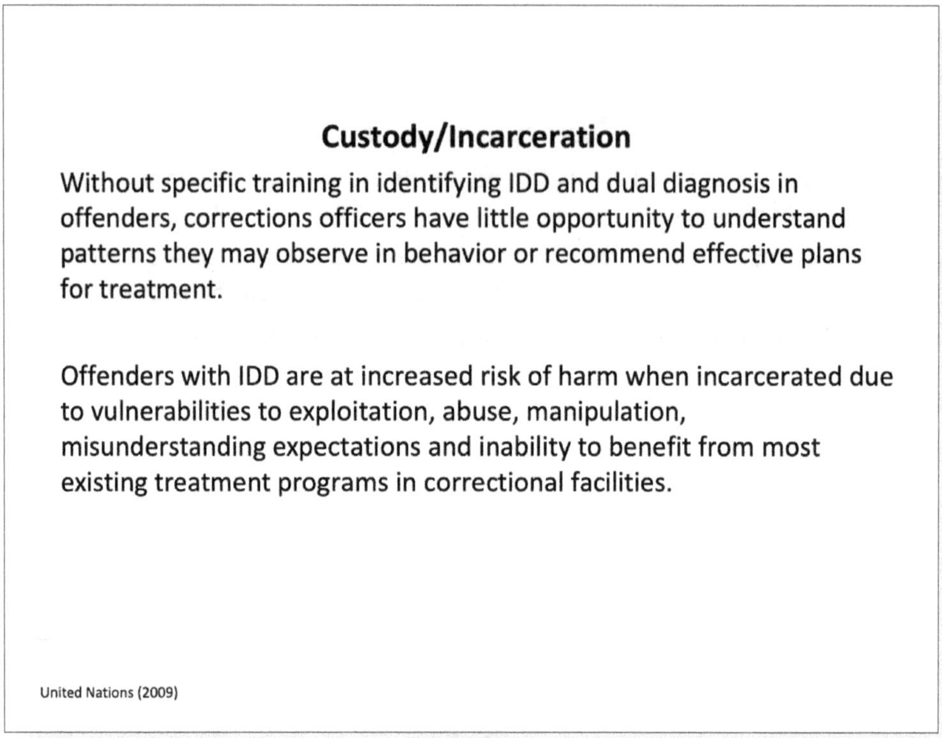

Existing treatment programs often rely on group work or strong receptive language skills. Programs in the criminal justice system are often not designed for offenders with IDD or for people who have cognitive challenges. People with these challenges experience greater difficulty understanding or benefitting from these types of programs.

Slide 26

Custody/Incarceration

The average length of stay in custody is frequently less than 35 days. This time period is often too short to provide effective treatment programming, particularly if the offender requires longer-than-average time to complete the program.

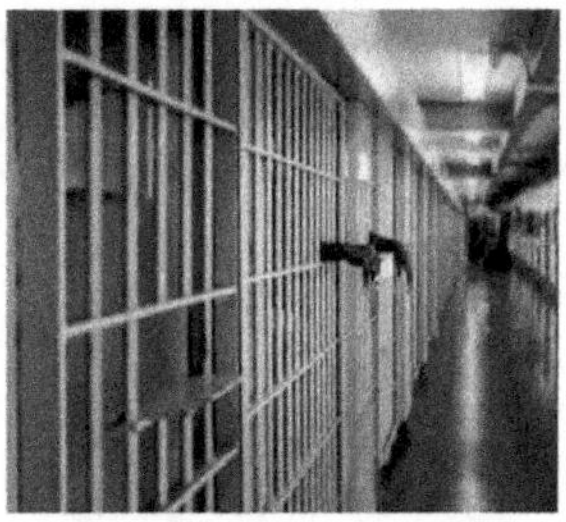

Endicott (1991)

Slide 27

Community residential settings more commonly call emergency services in response to behavioral crises. Organizationally, service providers should consider the following before developing crisis plans that include calling police:

- **Is law enforcement intended to assure safety?**
- **Should a person with disabilities be charged with a crime for aggression to care providers?**
- **Or aggression toward peers?**
- **Is it the responsibility of the provider to manage aggressive behavior?**

Ethical considerations are often involved in any decision to call emergency services, e.g., police services, to respond to a crisis incident involving aggressive/responsive behavior. Before considering this action as part of a crisis plan for a person, consideration must be given as to the goal of the intervention and all potential outcomes.

When police services are called to respond to incidents with people who have IDD/dual diagnosis, features of that response, such as sirens, lights, badges, uniforms, etc., could lead to potential trauma. For more information on crisis prevention and crisis planning, please refer to *Module VIII*.

Slide 28

Service providers, care providers and families typically involve police services for the following reasons:

- **Elopement, or the person with IDD is missing**
- **Generally unsafe behavior**
- **Failure to follow rules providers have in place**
- **Sexual misconduct**

Before building crisis plans that include calling police as an action step, service providers, caregivers and families may want to consider:

- What is the desired outcome of police involvement?
- Is the desired outcome a reasonable expectation of police services?
- Is calling police the most effective and safe response to the concern presented?

After careful consideration, the decision may truly be that police involvement is the most appropriate and effective response for the person. Please refer to *Module VIII: Crisis Prevention and Intervention: Reducing Risk* for more information on crisis prevention and crisis planning.

Slide 29

Special Needs Offenders:
Role of Special Needs Units

- Identification of vulnerable populations
- Provision of treatment while incarcerated
- Maintaining safety while incarcerated

Bright (1989)

Special needs offenders are identified as "those who are mentally ill and/or developmentally disabled person or persons with special needs who are in conflict with the law" (Howlett, 2005).

Special needs offenders are among the groups of people that are in a particularly vulnerable position in detention centers, jails and prisons and are in need of additional care and protection. It is often assumed that special needs offenders make up a small percentage of the general offender population. However, for a number of reasons, their proportions have been growing in recent years (Griffiths, Taillon-Wasmond & Smith, 2002).

Slide 30

Challenges within the Justice System

"Prisons are designed to provide secure containment of prisoners and to maintain order with a hope that punitive procedures will produce an inhibiting effect on criminal behavior."

However, as Gardner, et al., point out, the assumption of the system is that the offender has alternate prosocial behavior that they can choose. For people with IDD, this is often a false assumption.

Gardner, et al. (1998)

Prisoners with intellectual disabilities are likely to be in need of special health care services, such as behavioral therapy, speech therapy, occupational therapy and physiotherapy. Studies have shown that people with intellectual disabilities face a higher prevalence of psycho-social or psychiatric disabilities than the general population, and they will therefore need greater access to appropriate treatment (Rickford & Kimmett, 2005).

Slide 31

Treatment and Rehabilitation

- Treat co-occurring disorders
- Problem-solve common issues and stressors
- Identify what role the disability has and tailor treatment accordingly

Bright (1989)

Treatment programs within correctional facilities are often designed for group work or for people who have strong receptive language skills. For a better understanding of adapting treatment approaches and therapies, refer to *Module IX: Adapting Therapy Practices.*

Recommended among these are positive identity development, skill development, vocational training and employment readiness.

Slide 32

Treatment and Rehabilitation:
Preventing Recidivism

- Support with understanding social skills and problem-solving
- Education about following laws
- Work with impulse control, emotional regulation and problem-solving skills

D'Zurilla and Nezu (2001)

D'Zurilla and Nezu (2001, p. 212) defined problem-solving as "the self-directed cognitive-behavioral process by which a person attempts to identify or discover effective or adaptive solutions for specific problems encountered in everyday living." Understanding that people with an IDD/dual diagnosis have difficulties with adaptive skills, including some social skills and types of problem-solving, part of a therapeutic approach to prevent recidivism is assisting with skill development and support with problem-solving.

D'Zurilla et al. (2004) proposed a model of problem-solving that involves:
"(a) problem orientation, and
(b) problem-solving skills, also referred to as 'problem-solving proper or style.'"

Slide 33

Assisting the Justice System to Support Special Needs Offenders

If a person working in a corrections environment suspects a person has IDD, there are a number of interaction tips that can help build a positive rapport and increase the effectiveness of the interaction, treatment process or the person's ability to follow the rules.

Spence & Hughes (2003)

Slide 34

Assisting the Justice System to Support Special Needs Offenders

- When possible, limit distractions when communicating and interacting.
- Take extra time to explain expectations.
- Do not use slang or jargon.
- Be direct and straightforward.
- Speak clearly and use precise language.

Spence & Hughes (2003)

Many people with IDD have difficulty understanding abstract communication or concepts. Ideas and expressions of speech can be very difficult to understand.

Be very specific when giving directions. Explain clearly and, if possible, demonstrate what you would like them to do. When making a request, it may be helpful to offer a suggestion about how the person can complete the request. If you are confident that the person is able to read, write down the request. This may help them retain the information you are providing or the request you are making.

The use of visual cues can also be very effective to help with interpretation of verbal communication.

Slide 35

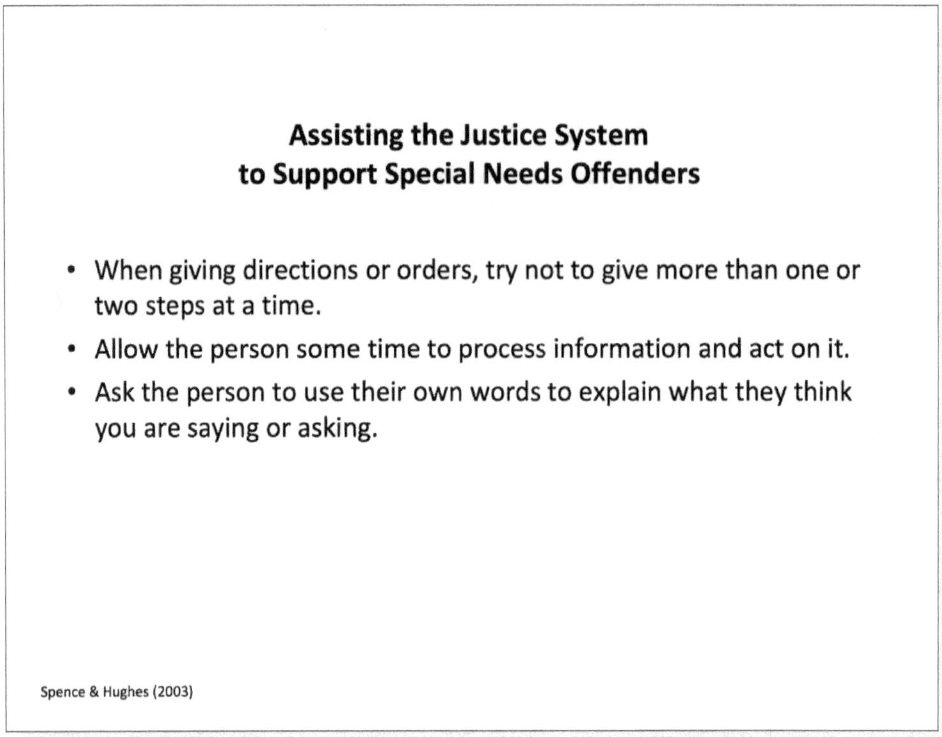

A person who has an IDD may have difficulty processing more than one or two pieces of information at a time. If this is the case, they may become overwhelmed by directions or orders that have multiple steps or instructions. Refusal to complete the steps doesn't necessarily mean refusal. The person could be overwhelmed, completing only one of the instructions or none at all. A person with an IDD may also need extra time to process information, determine what they are going to do and then initiate action.

Asking a person to interpret and tell you what you have said helps ensure they are not echoing your words, agreeing or disagreeing without understanding.

By asking them what they have understood, you are able to have a clearer understanding of what the person thinks you expect.

Slide 36

Assisting the Justice System to Support Special Needs Offenders

- Use open-ended questions as opposed to yes/no questions.
- Be aware of body language being consistent with verbal communication.
- Be sensitive to the impact psychotropic medication can have on a person's ability to process information. Side effects can cause fatigue, lower ability to concentrate and impact short-term memory, which affects interviews and interactions.

Spence & Hughes (2003)

Slide 37

Assisting the Justice System to Support Special Needs Offenders

- Many people with IDD are strongly motivated to do what they believe is expected of them.
- They learn to listen for certain words or inflections. They may even copy moods as they try to give "correct" answers.
- They want to be accepted by and to please others. Many have adapted by use of denial. They may affirm the last choice, agree or repeat the last word. For example:
  - *Q: "Do you understand what I have told you?" A: "Told you."*
  - *Q: "Do you want to take a break or keep going?" A. "Keep going."*

Spence & Hughes (2003)

Slide 38

Ultimately, our goals for supporting people with IDD/dual diagnosis when they come into contact with the justice system is to help them achieve the best possible outcome through treatment, rehabilitation and reintegration.

It's important to remember that the social services system is not at cross-purposes with the justice system. Each must take the opportunity to understand, advocate and educate, as appropriate, to the best possible outcome for the person involved.

References: Module XIII

Arboleda-Flórez, J. (2006). Forensic psychiatry: contemporary scope, challenges and controversies. *World Psychiatry*, June 2006, 5 (2) 87-91.

D'Zurilla, T. J., & Nezu, A. M. (2001). *Problem-solving therapies* (2nd ed.). New York: Guilford Press.

D'Zurilla, T. J., Nezu, A. M., & Maydeu-Olivares, A. (2004). Social problem-solving: Theory and assessment. In Chang, E. C., D'Zurilla, T. J., & Sanna, L. J. (Eds.), *Social Problem Solving: Theory, Research and Training* (pp. 11–27). Washington, DC: American Psychological Association.

Danzer, G. S., Wheeler, M. A., Alexander, A. A., & Wasser, T. D. (2019). Competency Restoration for Adult Defendants in Different Treatment Environments, *Journal of the American Academy of Psychiatry and the Law* Online February 2019, Volume 28, Issue 3, 1 Sep 2020 JAAPL.003819-19; https://doi.org/10.29158/JAAPL.003819-19.

Gardner, W. I. (1998). Initiating the case formulation process. In Griffiths, D. M., Gardner, W. I., & Nugent, J. (Eds.), *Behavioral Supports: Individual Centered Behavioral Interventions: A Multimodal Functional Approach* (pp. 17-66). Kingston, NY: NADD Press.

Griffiths, D., Taillon-Wasmond, P., & Smith, D. (Eds.), (2002). Offenders who have a developmental disability. In *Dual Diagnosis: An Introduction to Mental Health Needs of Persons with Developmental Disabilities.* Sudbury, ON: Habilitative Mental Health Resource Network.

Lunsky, P., Raina, Y., Jones, J. (2012). Relationship between prior legal involvement and current crisis for adults with intellectual disability. *Journal of Intellectual and Developmental Disability*, 37, 163-168.

Hauser, M. J., Olson, E., and Drogin, E.Y. (2014). Psychiatric disorders in people with intellectual disability (intellectual developmental disorder): forensic aspects. *Current Opinion in Psychiatry*, 117-121.

MODULE 13

Howlett, M. (2005). The Mental Health Commission of Canada – The Way Forward, 4.

Rickford, D. & Kimmett, E. (2005). *Troubled Inside: Responding to the Mental Health Needs of Men in Prison*. London, U.K.: Prison Trust.

Module XIV

The Importance
of Direct Support Professionals

Slide 2

Learning Objectives

- Recognize the role of Direct Support Professionals (DSPs) in providing quality supports to people with IDD/MI.
- Identify several workforce challenges of Direct Support Professionals.
- Recognize importance in building competency to ensure quality supports.

Slide 3

1. The role of the DSP
2. Workforce challenges
3. Including and empowering DSPs
4. Building competency
5. Supporting a competent workforce

Slide 4

Direct Support Professionals (DSPs) spend more time with the person with IDD/MI than any other professional. The competence of the DSP can make a big difference in the quality of life for people.

It is common for individuals with developmental or intellectual disabilities to experience psychiatric disorders also. People with IDD who experience mental illness (IDD/MI) often have complex needs. They may have difficulty with their behavior. They may have trouble communicating with staff and others. Describing and managing the symptoms of their mental illness may be very challenging for them. As a result, people with this dual diagnosis are at increased risk of being given unnecessary medication. They are more likely to have their rights restricted and to experience restraints. They may struggle to have meaningful relationships. They are at increased risk for abuse and neglect. They miss opportunities for community inclusion and participation.

Slide 5

The Role of the DSP in IDD/MI

- DSPs are often the ones charged with supporting skill building.
- They help the person engage in recommended therapies on a day-to-day basis.
- Using the word "professional" acknowledges the respected role of these persons in the community at large and makes the point that DSPs are valued caretakers.

Some people with IDD experience mental health challenges and/or difficulty with their behavior. People with a dual diagnosis (IDD/MI) are more likely to take multiple medications, including a psychotropic medication (NCID, 2016). They may miss opportunities for community inclusion and participation, employment and relationships without sufficient or effective supports.

Supporting a person effectively means taking all the challenges of behavior and mental health into account — clinical, environmental, quality of life. To be an effective member of a person's team, it is important that a direct support professional have knowledge in the following areas:

- principles of positive behavior support
- use and implications of medications
- the influence of mental health on behavior, symptoms
- risk factors for a crisis for intervention/prevention

Slide 6

Including DSPs in Planning

DSPs work closest with individuals and often determine the success and efficacy of interventions related to:

- Behavior planning
- Health and wellness
- Skill acquisition
- Employment and recreation
- Relationship building

Supporting for a person with IDD/MI means taking all the challenges of dual diagnosis into account — clinical, behavioral, quality of life. These concerns add a layer of complexity to the care one gives, which contributes to burnout. The need for supports is typically lifelong and begins at birth, greatly adding to the responsibility of family and other caregivers. These issues highlight the crucial need to provide support for DSPs and family caregivers.

Slide 7

Exercise

Consider the many ways DSPs have an impact in their roles at your program/agency.

How is this different for people with IDD/MI?

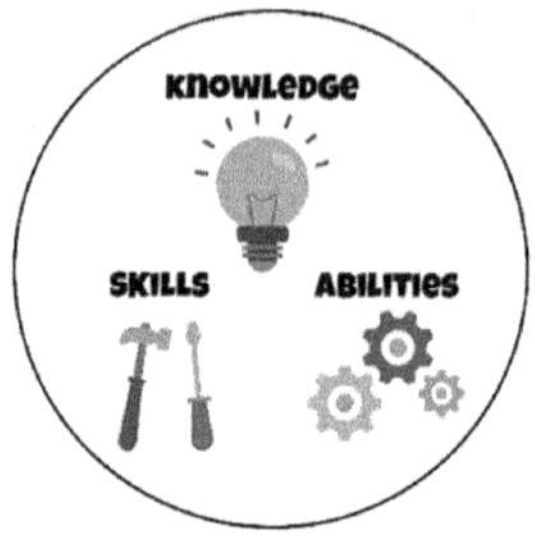

During this discussion, encourage participants to identify the values of DSPs who are reliable and competent. What knowledge, skills and abilities are essential to support someone with challenging behavior and mental health needs?

Below are some examples to generate discussion:

- Knowledge (PBS & MH/medication/crisis prevention)
- Communication (advocacy/with person/with other peers)
- Teamwork (sharing of ideas/professionalism)
- Observation and documentation (formal/informal)

Slide 8

Workforce Challenges

- DSPs generally are not certified or credentialed.
- Requirements for employment vary.
- DSPs have varying levels of education.
- Educational opportunities are often limited.
- DSPs generally work for low wages.
- DSPs' work experience is diverse.

This work requires an advanced level of skill and knowledge to do well. However, there is little available to guide DSPs and others in identifying the specific competencies a DSP should have. As a result, many DSPs are underqualified. Too often, they lack the support and training to do well. This lack of standards can make finding, hiring, training and retaining qualified DSPs difficult. As a result, many people with IDD/MI do not have adequate daily support.

Slide 9

Supervision Challenges

- Lack of support from managers.
- Limited resources.
- Staff turnover causes diversion from plan ("anyone can do it").
- Given directives without explanation.
- Not empowered to contribute.

DSPs are responsible for assisting individuals with IDD/MI with daily tasks; they work to implement care plans, to progress educational or career goals and to advance skill development and socialization. DSPs have varying educational backgrounds and are often underpaid and receive minimal training. Much time is devoted to required and mandatory training with little priority given to building capacity and professional development.

Slide 10

Training Challenges

- A lot is expected from staff who are often left out of the planning process.
- Required to implement, maintain, evaluate and assess plans they did not develop.
- Do not understand the cause of behavior or the goal of the plan, only given "strategy."
- Expected to use tools they are not familiar with.
- Passive role (instructed by "experts").

Supervisors of IDD/MI programs are often managing multiple issues, including personnel. Due to high turnover and the significant needs of individuals with people with IDD/MI, resources are often dedicated to acute and reactive issues with lesser time and consideration for team building and communication with those closer to the work.

Without the proper ongoing supervision and mentoring, direct support professionals are often in a "passive role" — receiving instructions and tasks related to a person's treatment or support plan, but the DSP is not valued as a contributing member of the team. This creates a disconnect between the DSP, who can provide timely, thorough, vital information on behalf of a person with IDD/MI, and the person's treatment goals.

Slide 11

Value of Including DSPs

- Staff often have most updated information.
- Opportunity for staff to take ownership in planning for the individuals they support.
- More likely to follow plans and strategies if involved in development.
- Increases staff efficacy in following plans or implementing strategies.

By including DSPs in the planning process and development of strategies, it acknowledges their role as a key informant/observer and increases the likelihood that they will demonstrate skills on the job.

Slide 12

Value of Including DSPs

- Greater consistency in support delivery.
- Staff learn to be more observant and more comfortable contributing information.
- More accurate and useful information will emerge.
- Individuals will associate staff with progress, and challenging behavior will decrease.

Often, clinicians, behaviorists, managers and other supervisors provide verbal or written directives to staff without an opportunity for team process or feedback. Including DSPs fosters empowerment and enables staff to understand their roles fully.

Slide 13

How Do We Empower Staff to Participate?

Activity: Using the ideas below, brainstorm ways to include DSPs in support planning.

- Ask DSPs for feedback, then listen.
- Change approach, welcome cooperation.
- Establish trusting relationships.
- Provide technical assistance and demonstrations.
- Show progress and include staff in modifications.
- Address requests in a timely manner.
- Be conscious of staff cultural diversity and concerns.

Slide 14

DSPs: Building Capacity

- Classroom and online trainings
- Team meetings
- On-the-job practice
- Mentoring and modeling
- Evidence-based skill standards
- DSP core competencies
- Credentialing programs

Classroom trainings are useful for initial coursework or information or learners who thrive in a group setting. It is also a helpful option to deliver content to introduce to all individuals at once. Virtual courses or webinars can support training or staff who have geographic, transportation, mobility or scheduling challenges that may not be accommodated by classroom training.

In-person trainings can also be done in small settings such as at team meetings with smaller, more focused objectives such as to review a treatment plan or a change in medication or provide updates. It is a good way to ensure consistency across support delivery and share important health or community information.

On-the-job training helps staff learn and practice skills in the setting where they will be used. It allows for timely feedback and an opportunity to clarify expectations.

Modeling helps staff receive and practice skills in the context where they will be used, along with barriers and real chances to adapt.

Mentoring allows the DSP to learn from a senior team member and gives that mentor a chance to highlight his/her knowledge. Having a more experienced and knowledgeable peer can help new DSPs adjust to their role and become more competent.

Competencies are an evidence-based set of knowledge, skills and abilities that reflect best practices.

Slide 15

NADD Direct Support Professional Certification

NADD has developed the NADD Competency-Based Direct Support Professional Certification Program to certify the competency of DSPs who support people with a dual diagnosis.

- Acknowledge the importance of the DSP in providing treatment and support to people with IDD/MI.
- Increase the capacity of DSPs to work with individuals with IDD/MI.

The goal of DSP certification through the NADD Competency-Based Certification Program is to improve the quality and effectiveness of services provided to individuals with a dual diagnosis through the development of competency-based standards for direct support professionals and through promoting their ongoing professional development.

More information at theNADD.org.

Slide 16

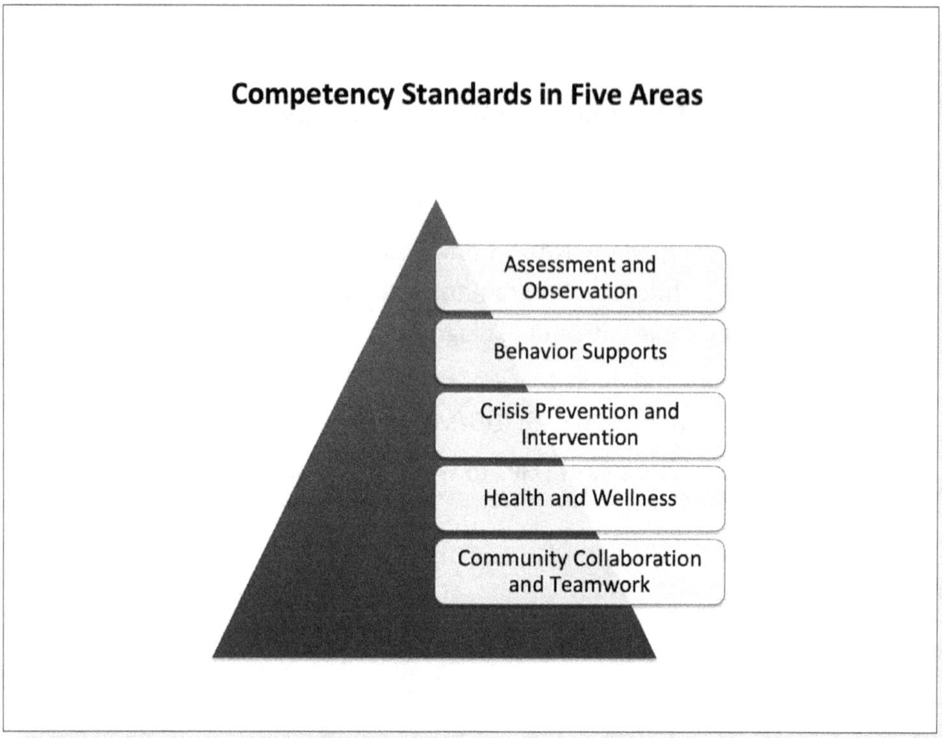

The skills and benchmarks in each competency standard include elements of critical thinking and communication, built upon a foundation in person-centered language and self-directed supports:

Assessment and Observation

- Knowledge and assessment of the observation process
- Use of assessment and observational tools
- Behavior assessment
- Documentation and communication related to assessment and observation

Behavior Support

- Knowledge and assessment of the causes and functions of challenging behavior
- Maintaining a supportive physical and social environment

- Responding to challenging behavior
- Teaching new behaviors and skills

Crisis Intervention and Prevention

- Knowledge and use of crisis prevention strategies
- Knowledge and use of crisis intervention strategies
- Documentation and communication related to crisis situations
- Managing stress and burnout

Health and Wellness

- Documentation and communication related to health and wellness
- Knowledge of health and wellness
- Use and implications of medication
- Illness management and recovery
- Knowledge of intellectual and developmental disabilities, mental health and co-occurring disorders

Community Collaboration and Teamwork

- Knowledge of service systems
- Building positive and cooperative relationships
- Promoting person-centered support, informed consent and advocacy
- Communication across systems

Slide 17

Core Competency

The Developmental Services Human Resources Strategy identified the core competencies of Direct Support Professionals, Direct Support Supervisors, Specialized Support Workers, Clinical Specialists, Managers and Directors.

The DSHR Strategy work also identified definitions and a process by which each competency can be measured and encouraged within each position.

Provincial Network on Developmental Services , Ontario, 2020

In 2010, the DS HR Strategy published a report and dictionary reflecting extensive work completed to recognize the core competencies required of superior performers in Ontario's Developmental Services Sector. Since that time, the core competencies have been implemented by DS agencies across the province and by colleges offering the DSW program.

Several assumptions underlie Hay Group's methodology for identifying the characteristics that distinguish the top performers in a particular job from average performers:

- Outstanding performers do their jobs differently and possess different competencies (i.e., characteristics, traits, motives) than average performers.
- The best way to identify the characteristics that predict superior performance is to study the behaviors of top performers.
- In every job, some people perform more effectively than others.

Slide 18

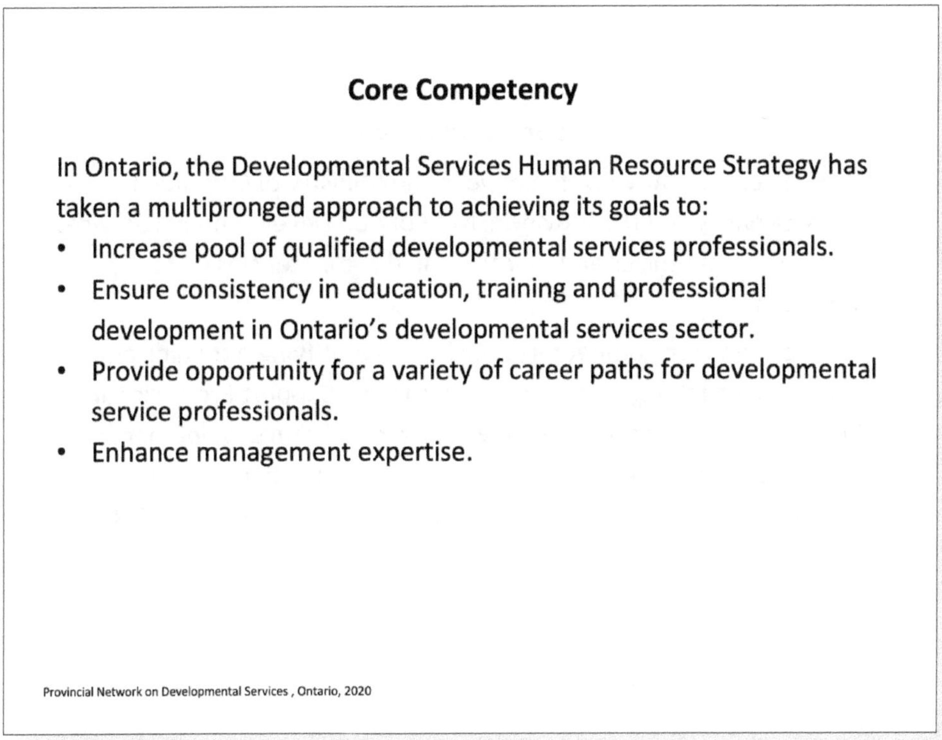

To achieve these goals, subcommittees of the DS HR Strategy participate in research, including gathering information from the sector and reviewing literature. Their work has been compiled into reports and documents to be shared with Ontario's DS sector, particularly those working in a human resources capacity.

A portion of the outcome from the work of the DS HR Strategy project was the identification of core competencies.

"Competencies are the underlying personal characteristics and behaviors of an individual that are important contributors to predicting outstanding performance in a job within a particular organization. They mark the difference between average job performance and outstanding performance. Furthermore, the competencies in a specific model are aligned with the organization's strategy and culture."

Slide 19

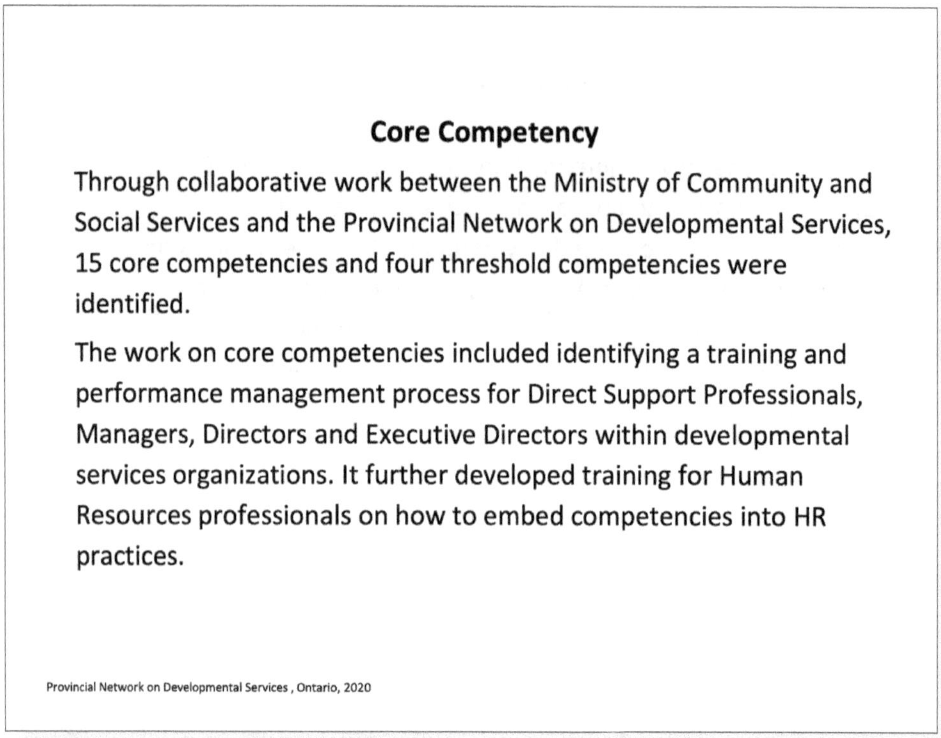

Threshold competencies are fundamental to all roles in the sector. It is recommended that they be used during recruitment as a way to identify "fit," since threshold competencies generally reflect the values in an organization. By comparison, the core competencies are also relevant in hiring as a reference for considering one's natural predisposition to develop a strength in the respective competencies. Once an individual is hired, the core competencies become a personal development and coaching focal point for developing one's behavioral strength in one's role.

Slide 20

Core Competencies

Advocating for Others	Collaboration
Creative Problem-Solving and Decision-Making	Developing Others
Fostering Independence in Others	Holding People Accountable
Initiative	Interpersonal Relationships and Respect
Leading Others	Managing Change
Relationship and Network Building	Resilience
Resource Management	Self-Development
Strategic Thinking	

The Hay Group, 2009

Work with the Hay Group facilitated the development of competency definitions to be supported by the "why it's important" statement. Together, they capture the essence of the competency, what is being measured and the way it helps support the employer's goals and values.

All of the competencies have four or more levels. There is a natural build in sophistication from one level to the next.

In all cases, several behavioral indicators are given that provide an example of the behaviors seen at that level and for that competency; they are intended to show what the level "looks like" and do not provide an exhaustive list.

Slide 21

Threshold Competencies

Flexibility	Self-Control
Service Orientation	Values and Ethics

The Hay Group, 2009

Together, the definition of the competency, why it's important, levels of demonstration within the competency and behavioral descriptors all capture the essence of the competency, what is being measured and the way it helps support the employer's and employee's goals and values.

For more information on the HR Strategy, Provincial DS Network and core competency project in Ontario, visit: http://www.ontariodevelopmentalservices.ca/resources/human-resources.

Slide 22

NADSP Code of Ethics

- Person-Centered Supports
- Promoting Physical and Emotional Well-Being
- Integrity and Responsibility
- Confidentiality
- Justice, Fairness, Equity
- Respect
- Relationships
- Self-Determination
- Advocacy

The NADSP Code of Ethics® developed by the NADSP is intended to serve as a straightforward and relevant guide for DSPs as they resolve the ethical dilemmas they face every day. It encourages them to achieve the highest ideals of the profession.

It is a requirement of DSPs who apply for NADD certification to follow the code of ethics; however, all staff should look to the values of this code as a guide to help make decisions when faced with competing demands or other dilemmas in their work.

Slide 23

Activity: David's dream is to go on a vacation to California to visit his brother. He is afraid to fly and barely has enough money to pay his current bills. After learning about this dream, his DSP should:

A. Focus on helping David recognize that he cannot possibly save enough for the trip.
B. Call David's brother and ask him to visit David's home instead. It's more practical and cost-effective.
C. Help David plan a more affordable vacation at a nearby resort.
D. Encourage David to develop a plan to reach his dream by assisting him with budgeting money and addressing his flying anxiety through desensitization.

While all of the answers may seem like supportive options, the correct answer is D because it is most consistent with the NADSP Code of Ethics.® While A through C may not be harmful, they are not person-centered, nor do they demonstrate allegiance to David.

Allow the participants an opportunity to discuss this scenario as necessary with the understanding that sometimes the best answer is not the only response but is that which is most in parallel with the values on the previous slide. While we can and may explore other options and strategies either simultaneously and eventually, "D" is most in parallel with the values set forth in NADSP Code of Ethics.®

Slide 24

Beyond Training

- Training is not complete until staff can demonstrate the skill on the job.
- Develop methods and documents to evaluate and demonstrate competency.
- Consider how to apply the NADSP Code of Ethics® when faced with competing demands and expectations.

Slide 25

Effective Team Process

- Design team meetings to prioritize and solve problems; use competency areas as the roadmap to generate solutions.
- Identify how to modify plans in response to the changing behavioral and psychiatric needs of the persons served.
- Prepare individuals and information for appointments with health professionals.
- Set expectation of DSP contribution and feedback.

Due to high turnover and the significant needs of individuals with IDD/MI, resources are often dedicated to reactive issues with lesser time and consideration for team-building and communication with those closer to the work. Best practice in IDD/MI includes a team process with the DSP in a valuable role. Create opportunities during team meetings, supervisions, informal mentoring and other interactions for clinicians, behaviorists, direct staff, individuals and families to interface and communicate.

Slide 26

Building Competency: Outcomes

- DSPs feel valued and take pride in the direct support work provided to individuals who have IDD/MI.
- DSPs are recognized for the skills, knowledge and values they have acquired in the field of dual diagnosis.
- By utilizing competency standards as guidelines, staff are empowered and valued.
- Greater consistency and efficacy in support delivery for people with mental and behavioral health needs.

Supporting DSPs in their career provides meaning to their work and provides the opportunity to recognize excellence in this important work.

Furthermore, we want to highlight ongoing ways to build capacity as individuals, as teams, as an agency, as a state and as a field to ensure we are always demonstrating competency and best practice in IDD/MI.

References: Module XIV

The Centers for Medicaid & Medicare Services (CMS) Road Map of Core Competencies for the Direct Service Workforce (2011). Prepared by the University of Minnesota Research and Training Center on Community Living. https://ici.umn.edu/products/docs/DSW_Competencies_Phases_1_and_2.pdf.

Cheplic, M. (2018). Behavioral Support and the NADD Credential. Direct Support Workforce Insider. The Boggs Center on Developmental Disabilities.

Developmental Services Human Resources Strategy, Provincial Network on Developmental Services, Ontario, 2021. Developed in collaboration with The Hay Group, Ltd., 2011. Available at http://www.ontariodevelopmentalservices.ca/resources/core-competencies. Retrieved February 2, 2021.

National Core Indicators Adult Consumer Survey 2015-16 Final Report (2017). National Association of State Directors of Developmental Disabilities Services and the Human Services Research Institute. www.nationalcoreindicators.org.

Consumer Outcomes Final Report 2010-2011 NCI Adult Consumer Survey Data, August 2012. Alexandria, VA: National Core Indicators.

McGilvery, S., & Sweetland, D. (2011). *Intellectual Disability and Mental Health: A Training Manual in Dual Diagnosis.* Kingston, NY: NADD Press.

Moore, D., and Cheplic, M. (2018). Hiring and retaining competent direct support professionals. *The NADD Bulletin*. Vol. 21 Issue 1.

NADD (2014). The NADD competency-based direct-support professional certification program. http://acp.thenadd.org/dsp.htm. Retrieved October 2020.

The National Alliance for Direct Support Professionals (*NADSP*) Code of Ethics, https://www.nadsp.org/wp-content/uploads/2018/07/CodeOfEthicsBrochure.pdf.

National Association of State Mental Health Program Directors (2017).

MODULE 14

The Vital Role of Specialized Approaches: Persons with Intellectual and Developmental Disabilities in the Mental Health System.

Module XV

Collaborating Across Systems

Slide 2

Inter-Systems Collaboration

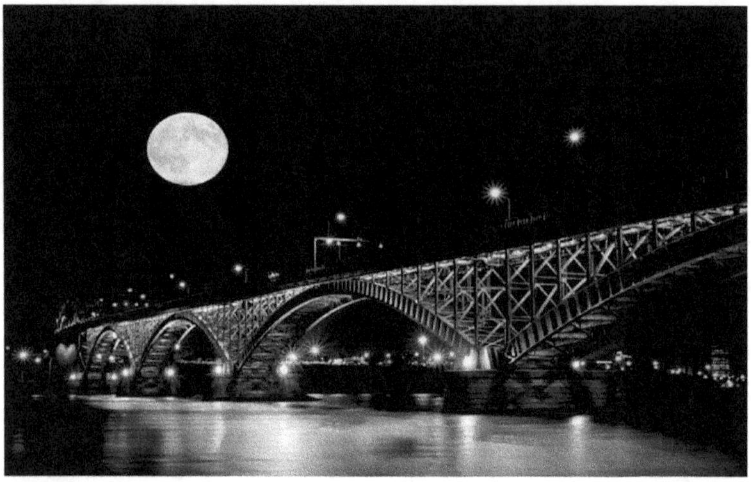

Peace Bridge, Niagara Falls USA/Canada

Slide 3

Learning Objectives

- Discuss how limited collaboration between mental health and IDD systems can result in barriers to service delivery.
- Recognize that assessment of individual need is at the center of effective person-centered service planning for individuals with MI/IDD.
- Identify the four planning and practice elements essential to working together and the factors that make each of these achievable.

Slide 4

Collaborating Across Systems

- Barriers to service delivery
- Principles in service planning
- Community collaboration and teamwork
- A framework to promote cross-system collaboration
- Service planning recommendations

Effective services do not occur in a vacuum but rather as a result of deliberate planning by a variety of stakeholders. At a national, state or county level, there is usually a process of planning that is important and a prerequisite to future implementation.

Although the MH and IDD service systems are the two significant bureaucratic structures, there are usually other systems that need to be addressed in terms of inter-systems collaboration. The other systems include for example: education, health, substance abuse, emergency response, criminal justice, among others.

In this module, we will explore the planning process and provide ideas about how the mechanism of planning can be accomplished.

Slide 5

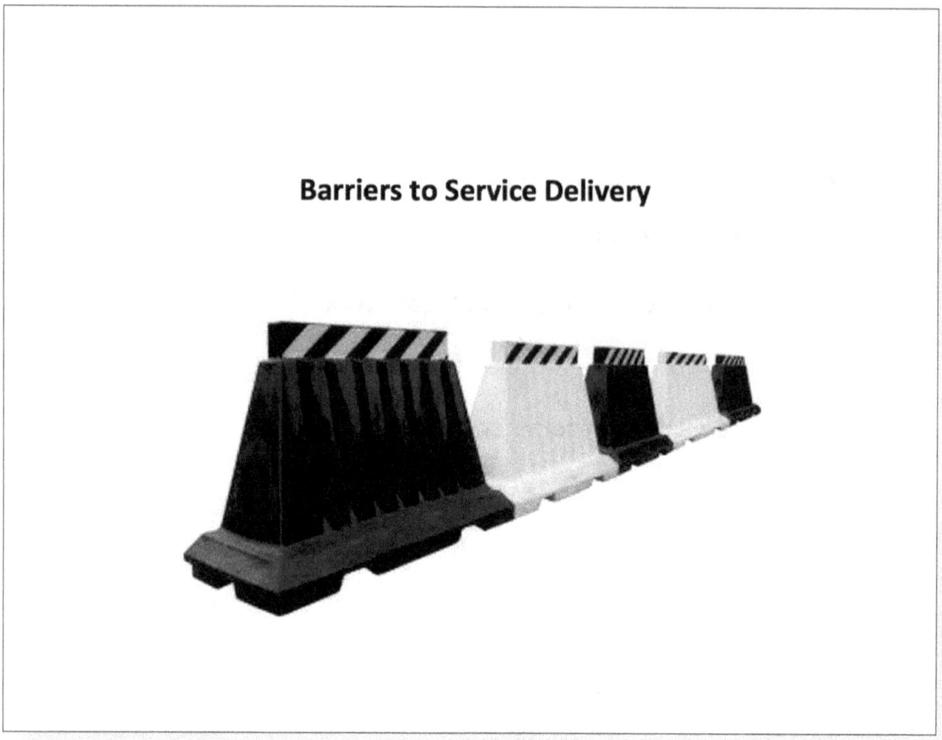

Systems and their related services are often fragmented. Each system is its own silo. People with IDD who have co-occurring mental health disorders frequently are not understood and do not have their needs met (SAMHSA, 2006).

Slide 6

Dual Diagnosis Policy Barriers

The Typical Picture:

Individuals with MI and IDD are among the most challenging persons served by both MH and IDD service delivery systems.

Moseley, 2004

Historically, people with a dual diagnosis often fall through cracks of the service delivery system, as neither the MH nor IDD service delivery system has wanted to take responsibility for their care and treatment (Fletcher, 1993 dissertation).

The lack of inter-system planning has resulted in a splintered system of care and has created a quagmire for both the MH and the IDD service delivery systems.

The lack of behavioral health and primary care providers with the specialized training to diagnose and treat this population results in preventable and expensive health care and treatment, repeated hospitalizations, problematic drug interactions and the overuse of psychotropic medications (NADD, 2018).

Slide 7

Discussion:

Think about your experience.

How do systems barriers or gaps contribute to unmet needs of people with IDD/MI?

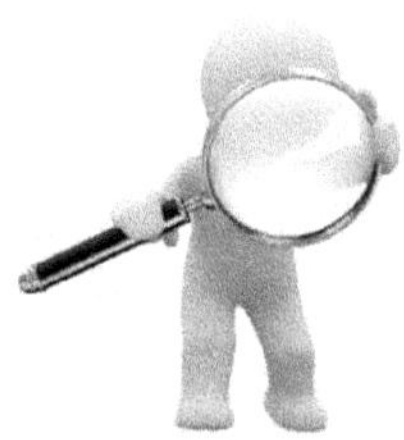

Examples may include access to health and health care, emergency preparedness response and public health and housing.

Slide 8

The Typical Picture:

- Failure to plan services
- Failure to fund flexible services
- Failure to obtain technical assistance

Mosely, 2004

The failure to plan for services for individuals who have IDD and MI has resulted in inadequate care and treatment for this group of people. We live in a "silo" structure of service delivery. The IDD system lives in its own silo, while the MH system lives in another (SAMHSA, 2006). Each has its own criteria of eligibility and funding streams, as well as policies and regulations. Problems include difficulty negotiating the separate systems (Fletcher, 1993).

The lack of strategic planning has led to challenges faced by states and communities. We have significant systems barriers highlighted by eligibility and access barriers, as well as financial challenges (SAMHSA, 2006).

As a result of the failure to strategically plan for appropriate cross-system services, people with a dual diagnosis have not received the services they need. As pointed out, "In spite of many innovative developments in service delivery for people with disabilities, success for people with a dual diagnosis has lagged behind that for other groups" (Fletcher, Beasley & Jacobson, 1999).

Mental health services may be available, but access is frequently difficult for people who have IDD and mental health problems (Mosley, 2010).

There is limited use of medical waivers by states to help address the service needs of persons with co-occurring disorders (SAMHSA, 2006).

Slide 9

The Typical Picture:

- MH providers perceive that they do not have the skills to serve adults or children with a dual diagnosis.
- IDD providers do not understand the services the MH sector offers.
- MH providers do not understand the services the IDD sector offers.

To some extent, policy barriers can be rooted in a lack of understanding of how one system can collaborate with another. Individuals with IDD co-occurring with mental illness are typically supported through different state agencies (Mosley, 2004). Structural differences between the IDD system on the one hand and the mental health system on the other have resulted in misconceptions and the general lack of understanding of how the two systems can work in a collaborative way.

There is a lack of adequate training for professionals to recognize the possibility of a co-occurring mental health disorder in a person who has IDD (SAMHSA, 2006).

There is a near absence of inter-systems professional training, and this has led to clinical myths and mistrust.

Slide 10

MH System

- Short-term episodic treatment
- Focus on psychiatric needs
- Recovery model
- Local authority
- Medication treatment
- Consumer/client /patient

IDD System

- Services/supports over lifetime
- Emphasis on direct support
- Self-determination
- State authority
- Behavioral support (PBS)
- Self-advocate/consumer

← **Little Collaboration** →

Each service delivery system has its own philosophy of care and treatment approaches. Even the language used in each system can be different than language used in the other system. The professional staff find it difficult to understand and grasp each other's perspective.

Slide 11

Institutions Provided Care in These Disciplines:

- OT
- PT
- Speech
- Psychology
- Medical
- Dental
- Other

Individuals historically served in an institutional system had services provided from multiple disciplines. These services may not have been provided in a well-coordinated interdisciplinary model, but nevertheless an array of services may have been available (Kelly, 2016).

Slide 12

From Institutionalization to Home and Community: Complexities Challenging Community Support Systems

Complex Support Profile/Issues	Challenges
Individual with relatively minor support needs for typical daily living needs but with diagnosis of borderline personality disorder	• Frequent staffing changes throughout the day more challenging, but may be necessary • Professional oversight of interventions as often as needed • Professional help for support staff to sustain the challenges daily and consistently implement needed intervention strategies
Individuals with anticipated needs for crisis services	• Quick access to crisis services by professionals familiar with the individual and his/her needs
Individual with a dual diagnosis who needs medication, behavioral strategies and instructions for family/staff support	• Coordination of medication changes/needs with implementation of behavioral strategies • Clear guidelines on which professional to seek when problems occur • Consistency in instructions to family/staff across professionals
Individual with significant medical issue and co-occurring behavioral health need	• Coordination and prioritization of needed medical interventions when behavioral issues may impact cooperation • Coordination of needed medication changes and impact on behavioral presentation and strategies

As people moved from institutions to home and community living, planning for needed supports did not adequately consider the complexities of needs. This lack of planning resulted in inadequate cross-systems collaborations. Also, there was not adequate funding to address the multiple cross-systems needs for people with complex challenges (Kelly, 2016).

Slide 13

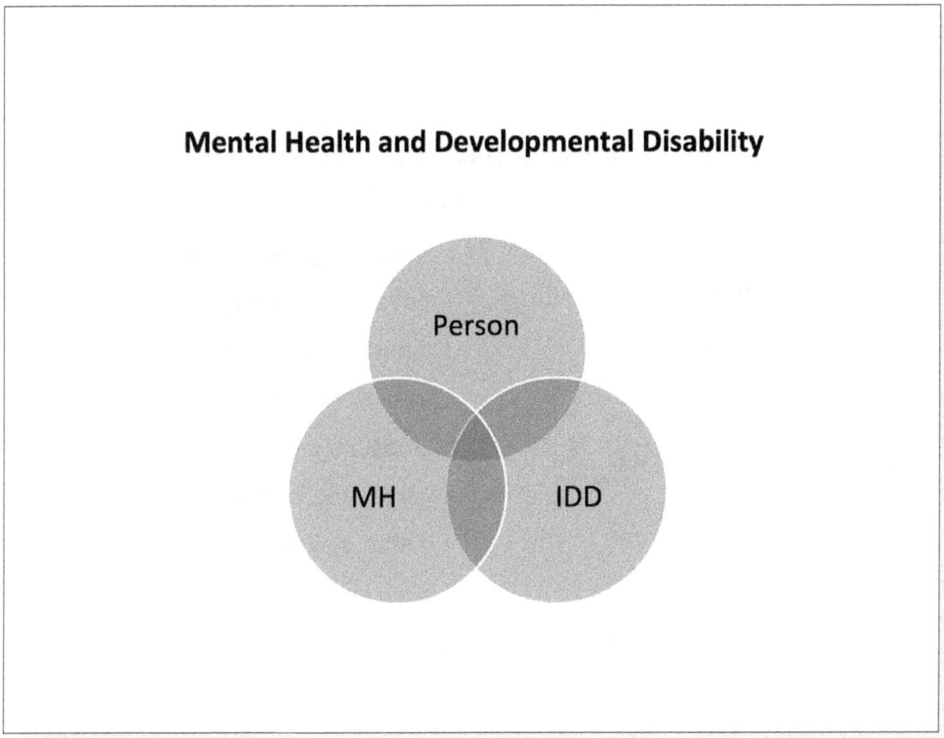

Individuals with a dual diagnosis (IDD/MI) may interface with minimally two systems, one addressing the developmental disability needs and one addressing the mental health needs (Brockman et al., 2009).

The populations of people with co-occurring needs are very heterogeneous, and their support needs change over their lifetimes. Individuals with IDD and co-occurring MI require a flexible array of services to help them effectively reside in the community (NADD, 2018).

Slide 14

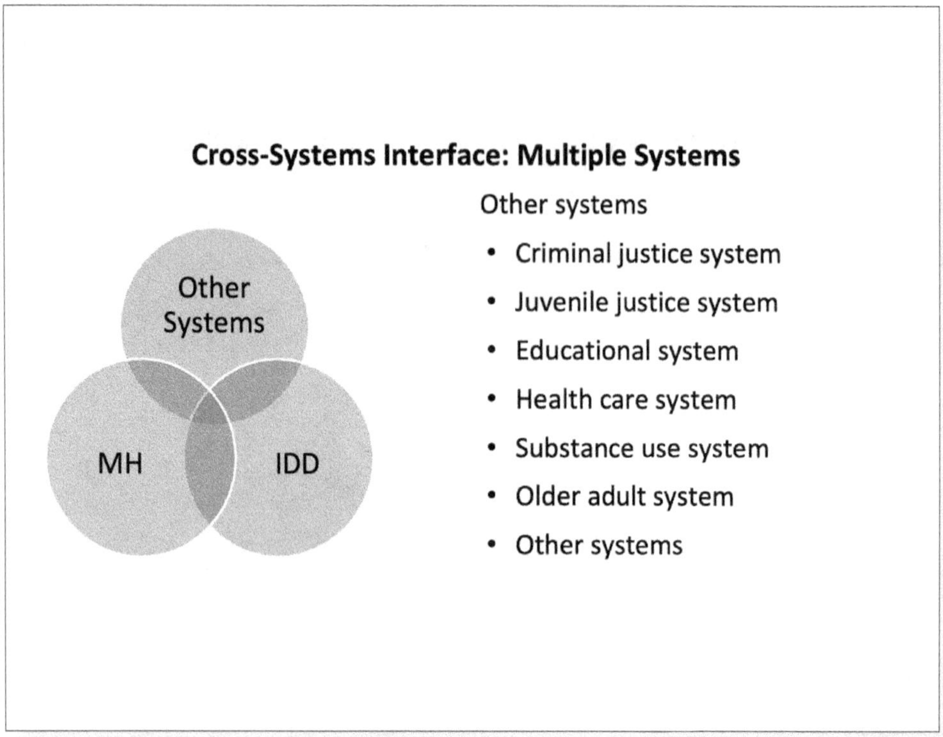

There is often the need to involve multiple systems to address the complex needs of individuals. Although the IDD and MH systems may be primary for many people with a dual diagnosis, other systems need to be brought to the planning table to address the fact of multiple systems for people with complex and challenging needs.

Service systems include education, health care, DD/IDD services, mental health services, inpatient referral process, the justice system, foster care, youth services, community disability services, transportation and employment. This includes housing, transportation, employment support, case management and education. It also includes other types of systems, such as criminal justice diversion programs or community mental health clinics.

Slide 15

Over the last 40 years, both the mental health and the developmental disabilities service systems have changed dramatically. Services that once were provided almost exclusively in institutional settings now are part of a broad, community-based service delivery system, and individuals who once would have spent their lives in state hospitals or schools now live independently or in small group homes in community settings. For both service systems, self-determination and community integration have become critical — and attainable — goals (NASMHPD, 2004).

Slide 16

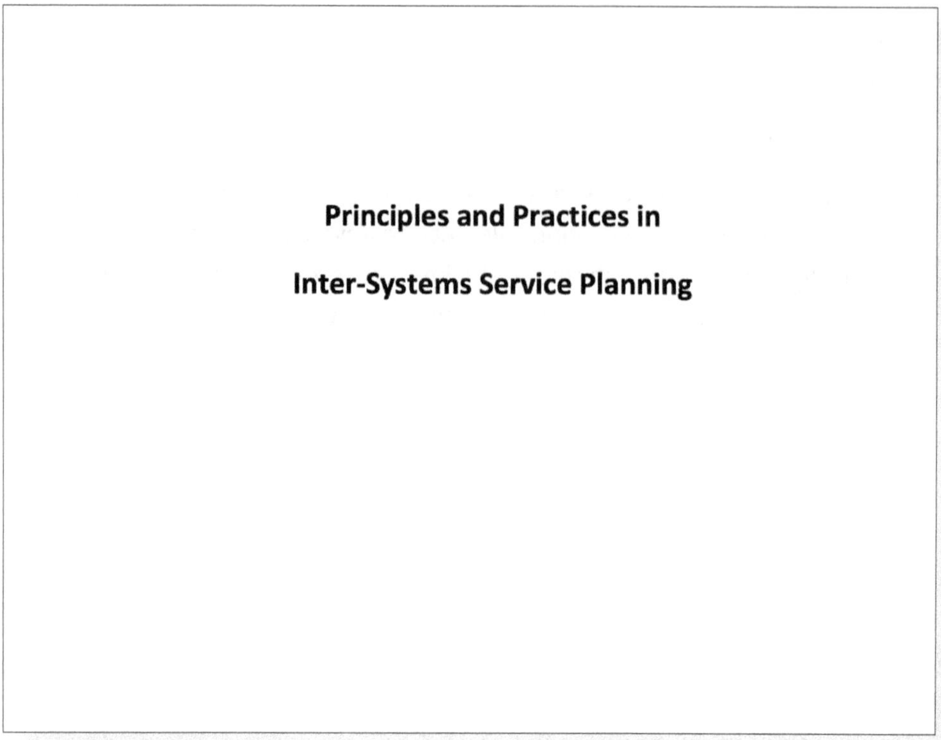

It is important that the systems' stakeholders agree on principles in service planning. The service principles lay out the foundation upon which cross-systems practices can occur.

Slide 17

Dual Diagnosis Planning Principles

- Co-occurring disorders should be treated as multiple primary disorders, in which each disorder receives specific and appropriate services.
- Collaboration of appropriate services and supports must occur as needs are identified.
- Services provided to the individual are consistent with what the person wants and what supports are needed.

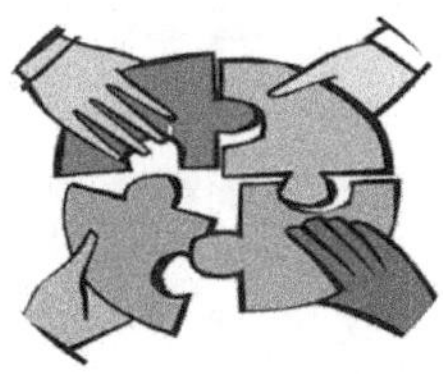

Fletcher, Beasley & Jacobson, 1999

The issue of what is the primary vs. the secondary diagnosis has served as an obstacle to service planning and practice. It is important to get beyond this issue in service planning. If a person is receiving treatment services for a mental health disorder, the psychiatric diagnosis is considered primary. If that same person is receiving residential services from an IDD provider, then a developmental disability diagnosis is considered primary for that provider.

Slide 18

Dual Diagnosis Planning Principles

- Services are determined on the basis of comprehensive assessment of the *needs* of each individual.
- Services are based on individual needs and not solely on either MH or IDD diagnosis.
- Emphasize early identification and intervention.

Fletcher, Beasley & Jacobson, 1999

All services need to be based on an assessment of the needs of the person. This assessment needs to consider areas such as mental health issues, developmental needs, health needs, family, etc.

Slide 19

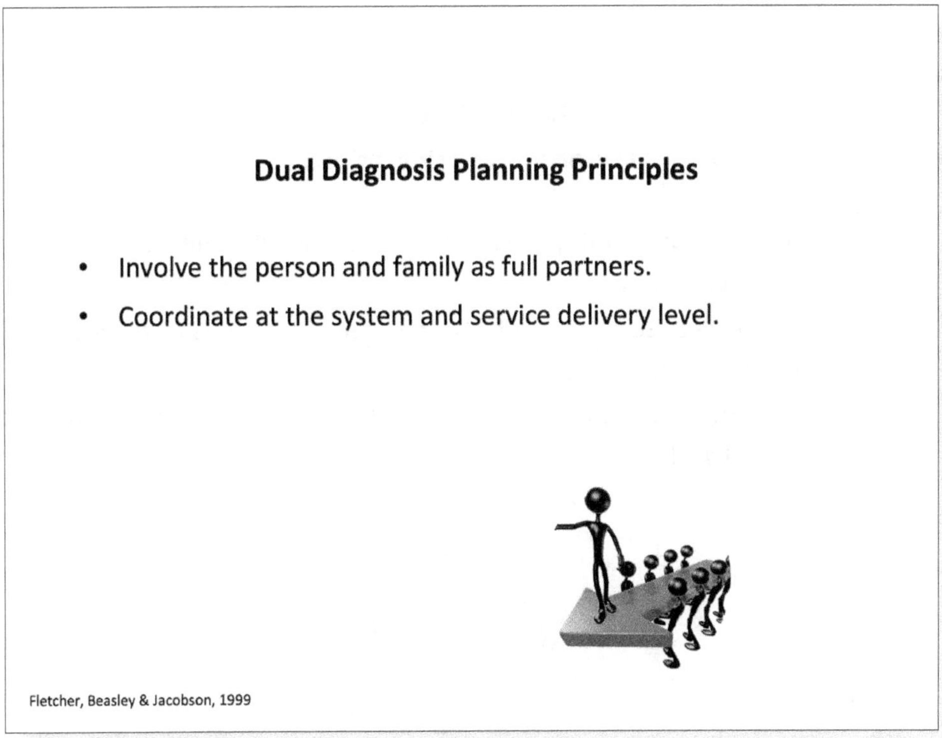

The individual and his/her family need to be an integral part of the planning process. Also, the person and family should be empowered to contribute to treatment decisions that are based on a person-centered approach.

Cross-systems planning and practice should occur at the systems level (macro) as well as at the service delivery level (micro). Systemic inter-systems planning can take place at the county, regional or state level (macro). The service delivery level involves individual planning at the local level (micro).

Slide 20

Service Systems
Important Considerations

- Support access to state and local services, benefits and community-based resources.
- Recognize cultural, accessibility and linguistic barriers to service access and take steps to improve the situation.
- Advocate for a community inclusive of all citizens, including those with IDD/MI.

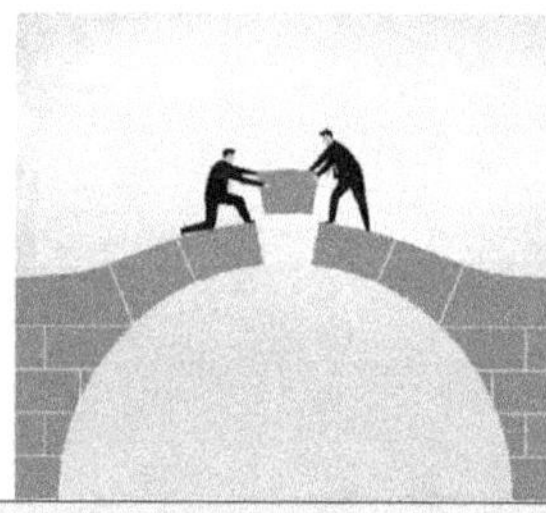

NADD-DSP

Most of the time, the first suggestions that come from professionals are things that have been done before or are easy to do.

Support individuals in understanding conflicts between systems and sorting through information in order to decide how to approach these issues. Sometimes systems or services have different funding sources, they are housed in different buildings or require separate referrals/ authorization to access. This can be challenging to navigate for individuals, family and staff.

Other times, there isn't capacity to support someone with multiple needs, such as IDD/MI, within one system and we need to work to encourage collaboration in the community on his/her behalf.

Diversity issues are inadequately managed in services, failing to represent the people we support. When the system or the community is only capable of accommodating people to a certain extent, that isn't true inclusion.

Slide 21

Facilitating Positive and Cooperative Relationships

- Navigate recommendations between systems (e.g., psychiatrists and other health professionals, employment, residential settings).
- Build positive and cooperative relationships with other health and mental health professionals.
- Work positively with multiple systems as a collaborative and cooperative member of the team.
- Maintain professional and empathetic communication and partnership with family members and friends of the individual.
- Advocate with allegiance to the individual served.

NADD, n.d.

We need to maintain positive cooperative relationships with other agencies for the benefit of individuals' well-being.

This level of professionalism maintains open communication, which can help in devising treatment modalities, as well as planning next steps.

It includes effective problem-solving in a team setting for the benefit of the person supported.

A DSP or clinician is often in the position to make contact with and facilitate supports across multiple systems and acts as the liaison between individuals and other professionals providing services. As the main point of contact, that staff person is responsible for providing accurate information, communicating the needs of individuals and ensuring a collaborative approach to treatment.

Slide 22

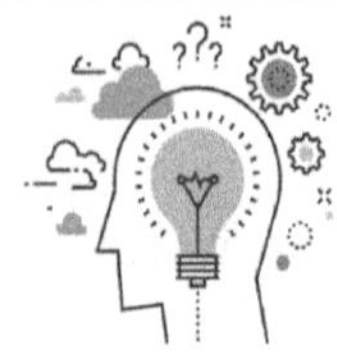

Discussion

During a meeting with Conner, a young adult with autism and anxiety disorder, his father is monopolizing the conversation and answering for his son.

Topics including choosing a college, auditioning for the community theater and an overnight camping trip. Dad is worried about Conner's ability to manage his diagnosis away from home or take the correct bus to the theater.

- How do we honor Connor's choice and respect the family?
- What other systems may be a resource?

Consider the needs of the audience when facilitating this activity: Discuss how your approach may change if the young man is 16 years old vs. 21 years old?

Adjust/add other demographic information as needed for learners.

Encourage participants to review the guidelines on the previous slide. Also, consider how we can be respectful of the young man's father and his concerns. How can the team explore the risks and opportunities by making a list of questions of additional resources? Are there goals, behaviors, symptoms or other challenges we need to manage before these possibilities can be considered as realities?

Who/how can we connect and collaborate in the community?

Slide 23

Effective Planning and Practice Elements

1. Leadership
2. Effective staff
3. Effective treatment
4. Staff training

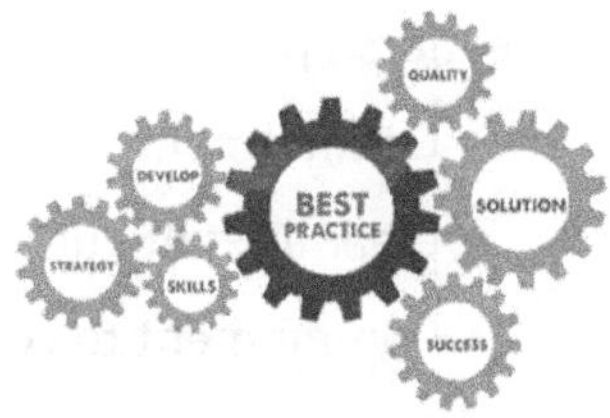

Adapted from Moseley, 2010

Each of these four practice elements is relevant to advance inter-systems collaboration. The elements taken together are designed to have a synergistic effect on promoting inter-system collaboration.

Slide 24

Effective Planning and Practice Elements

1. Leadership
    - Commitment
    - Clear lines of authority
    - Commitment to collaboration
    - Focus on the individual

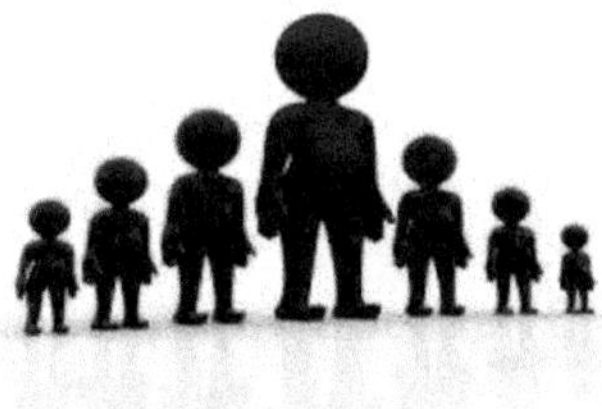

Adapted from Moseley, 2010

Leadership's embrace of inter-systems collaboration is essential. Without leadership to support advancing inter-systems collaboration, little can be accomplished from a systemic perspective. Identifying a "champion of the mission" from a leadership position would facilitate the process and lead to a more likely positive outcome.

Slide 25

Effective Planning and Practice Elements

2. Effective Staff

- The right person
- The right match
- Build trust, dependability
- Focus on the inter-system
- Collaboration system
- IDD/MH interface

Adapted from Moseley, 2010

It is important that the "right" staff be at the inter-systems collaboration table. Systems planning requires decision makers who can effectively represent their constituency or system in a manner that seeks to promote inter-system collaboration.

Slide 26

Effective Planning and Practice Elements

3. Effective Treatment
   - Appropriate psychiatric diagnosis
   - Effective medication treatment if needed
   - Positive behavioral supports
   - Effective treatment strategies such as DBT, CBT

Adapted from Moseley, 2010

Treatment follows diagnosis. Therefore, identifying the appropriate diagnosis is crucial. The DM-ID (Fletcher et al., 2007) can assist in the diagnostic process. Once a diagnosis has been established, there may be a need for medication. Medication treatment should be aligned with a psychiatric diagnosis. A holistic approach to care and treatment essentially requires both a mental health and a developmental disability approach. Positive behavioral supports should be used along with mental health treatment. Psychotherapy such as DBT and CBT have been growing substantially as they are adopted and applied to people with a dual diagnosis.

Slide 27

Effective Planning and Practice Elements

4. Staff training
   - DSP
   - Clinicians
   - Service coordinators

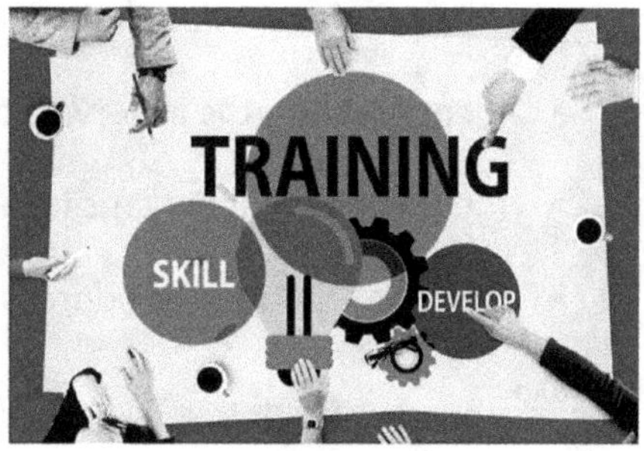

Adapted from Moseley, 2010

Staff training at all levels is a prerequisite to effective planning and practice. At all levels, staff needs knowledge, practice, skill and competency. For example, DSPs need to learn how to observe behaviors that might be indicative of a mental health disorder. Clinicians need to appropriately identify specific psychiatric disorders in persons with limited language skills. Additionally, service coordinators, supervisors and administrators need to know how to negotiate the complexities of various systems.

Slide 28

Purpose/Function of a Dual Diagnosis Committee

- Gather relevant data/information
- Identify strengths in service delivery systems
- Identify challenges/gaps in service delivery system
- Develop solutions to address challenges and gaps

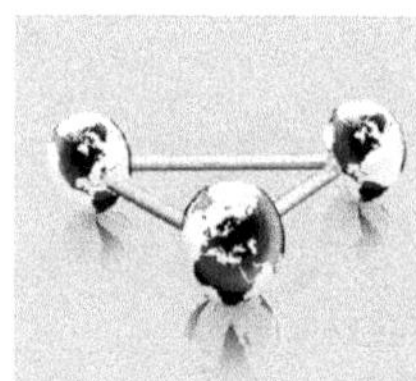

Developing a local, regional or statewide task force can be very important and useful in the attempt to improve service delivery. The task force can gather information and data to analyze relative strengths and weaknesses in the service delivery system for people with a dual diagnosis. Once there is a clear picture of where service pressures, challenges and gaps exist, a network can build strategies to address them, building on the identified strengths.

Slide 29

Stakeholders from other than MH & IDD systems could be included as appropriate. These include but are not limited to representatives from:

- Substance abuse
- Justice
- Health department
- Social services
- Parents
- Consumers
- Advocacy organizations
- Special education
- Early intervention
- Child welfare
- Coordinated children's services
- Service providers
- Senior services

The dual diagnosis task force needs to include decision-making representation from the MH and IDD systems. The composition of the committee should also include representatives from service providers, family representation and advocacy organizations.

The working group could include other constituents either on an ongoing or as-needed basis. The stakeholders would include, for example, representation from the criminal justice system, special education and substance abuse.

There is a need for comprehensive service components to be available, accessible and appropriate for each individual. This involves an array of service components that need to be coordinated.

Slide 30

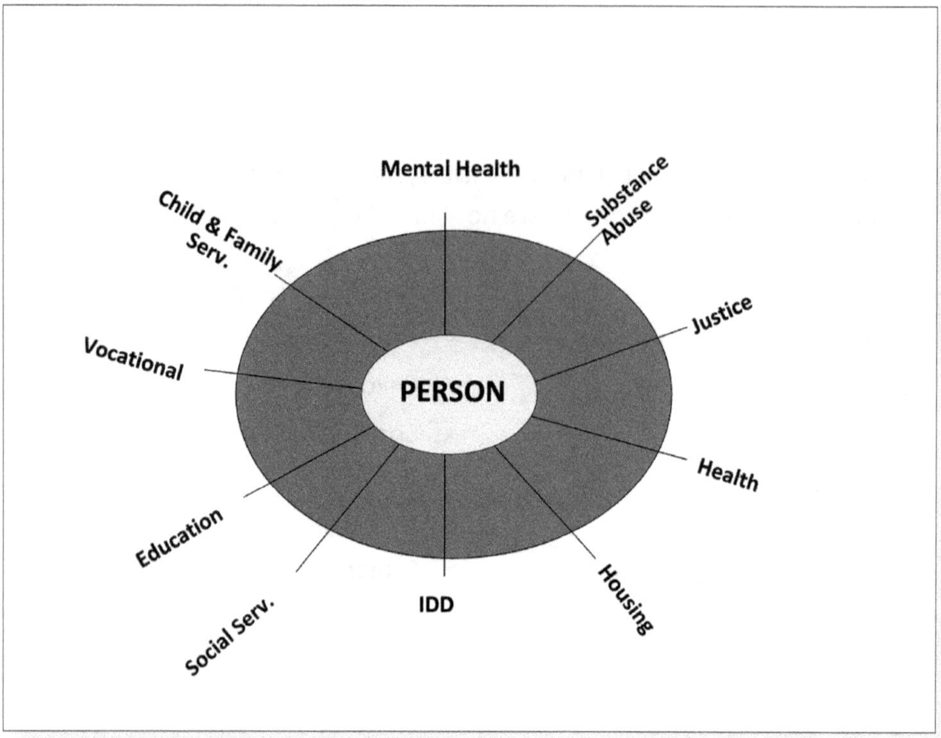

A number of systems need to be involved when it comes to supports, care and treatment for persons with a dual diagnosis. With the person in the middle, person-centered planning can take place. This would involve an analysis of what the individual wants along with what the individual needs.

Slide 31

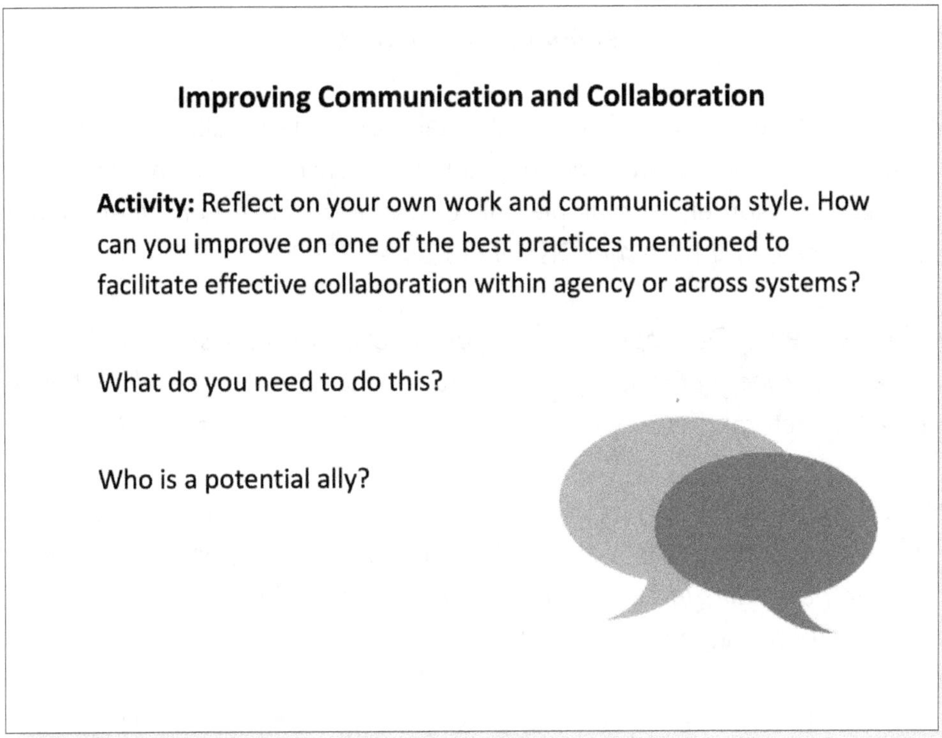

Some questions for considerations to target improvement on a micro and macro level:

- Do you come prepared to meetings, ready to advocate with recommendations that reflect the person's needs?
- Do you need to learn more about how another service system works? Or how your job role fits into the larger structure of the person's team or organization?

MODULE 15

References: Module XV

Brockman-Frazee, L., Baker-Ericzén, M., Stahmer, A., Mandell, D., Haine, R., & Hough, R. (2009). Involvement of youth with autism spectrum disorders or intellectual disorders in multiple public service systems. *Journal of Mental Health Research in Intellectual Disabilities*, 2 (3), 201-219.

Fletcher, R. (1993). *Developing a Policy for the Dually Diagnosed: A Policy Management Model for Providing Mental Health Services to the Mentally Ill-Mentally Retarded.* (Doctoral dissertation). New York: The City University of New York.

Fletcher, R., Beasley, J., & Jacobson, J. (1999). Support service systems for people with dual diagnosis in the USA. In Bouras, N. (Ed.), *Psychiatric and Behavioural Disorders in Developmental Disabilities and Mental Retardation.* Cambridge: Cambridge University Press.

Fletcher, R., Loschen, E., Stavrakaki, C., & First, M. (Eds.). (2007). *Diagnostic Manual – Intellectual Disability: A Textbook of Diagnosis of Mental Disorders in Persons with Intellectual Disability.* Kingston, NY: NADD Press.

Kelly, B. B. (2016). *Breaking Down Silos: Innovation in Dual Diagnosis Systems.* Kingston, NY: NADD Press.

McGilvery, S., & Sweetland, D. (2011). *Intellectual Disability and Mental Health: A Training Manual in Dual Diagnosis.* Kingston, NY: NADD Press.

Moseley, C. (2004). *Picking Up the Pieces of Our Own Mistakes: Supporting People with Co-Occurring Conditions.* Washington, DC: National Association of State Directors of Developmental Disabilities Services.

Moseley, C. (2010). Population based strategies for supporting people with co-occurring mental illness and intellectual/developmental disabilities. Olmstead Policy Academy.

SAMHSA (2006). Matrix model. SAMHSA's national registry of evidence-based programs and practices. Washington, DC.

NADD (2014). The NADD competency-based direct-support professional certification program. http://acp.thenadd.org/dsp.htm. Retrieved February, 2014.

NADD (2018). Including Individuals with Intellectual/Developmental Disabilities and Co-Occurring Mental Illness: Challenges That Must Be Addressed in Health Care Reform.

NASMHPD (2004). Serving Individuals with Co-Occurring Developmental Disabilities and Mental Illnesses: Systems Barriers and Strategies for Reform.

Appendix: Training Checklist

APPENDIX

Introduction
Cultivating Training Mastery Checklist

General Trainer Considerations and Practices

☐ Cultivate self-awareness. Develop an understanding of your culture (the shared, learned, symbolic system of values, beliefs and attitudes that shape and influence perception and behavior) and how these factors influence your worldview.

☐ Cultivate emotional intelligence. This is defined by Lee Gardenswartz, Jorge Cherbosque and Anita Rowe from the Emotional Intelligence and Diversity Institute (https://www.eidi-results.org/): "Emotional Intelligence is the ability to feel, understand, manage, articulate, and effectively apply the power of emotions as a source of human energy."

☐ Be a continuous learner and keep up to date with the current research on adult learning and the current best practices in the field of study you are training.

☐ Have a system in place (like this checklist) to ensure that the only uncertainty going into the training is what the audience or environment may produce.

☐ Develop your knowledge and experience relating to the material you are training. Be prepared to talk in depth and with familiarity about the content you are teaching.

Preparation Before the Training

☐ Understand the needs, characteristics and makeup of the audience.

- ☐ Understand the training goals of the organization or individual hiring you to train.
- ☐ Incorporate effective, emotionally compelling stories and relevant examples throughout your session.
- ☐ Create a clear outline or agenda for each day that spells out the breaks, lunch and ending times.
- ☐ Plan to start and end each day with an exercise that brings people together.
- ☐ Link learning objectives to the organization's (or individual's) identified training needs and goals.
- ☐ Ensure every topical area leads to the next. (It must all be connected and coherent.)
- ☐ Incorporate *as many interactive exercises as you can manage effectively*, grouping people differently with each exercise and being cognizant of the hierarchical relationships in the room. Make sure the exercises are concretely linked to the learning objectives.
- ☐ Ensure training methods attract the engagement of all types of learners and are inclusive of different learning styles.
- ☐ Make sure the examples, images and vignettes are relevant and that your language is culturally appropriate for each unique group.
- ☐ Have the chairs and tables organized for maximum group work.
- ☐ Ensure the lighting is as soft and inviting as the space will allow.
- ☐ Try to manage the room temperature effectively.
- ☐ Have good treats and beverages available throughout the session.

☐ Incorporate frequent breaks into the schedule.

☐ Provide a gift or tool to the group (if possible), such as a notebook to record observations or some other item that will remind the participants of the training in the future.

☐ If you have handouts, ensure they are attractive and professional.

☐ Develop a backup plan for presenting your training should technology not work correctly.

☐ If you are not bringing these materials yourself, make sure you have arranged for all the audio-visual equipment (computer, projector, adapter, flash drive with your presentation, microphone, etc.), meeting supplies (flip chart, Post-its, pens, Sharpies, ice-breaker materials, etc.) and training materials (handouts, workbooks, etc.) to be waiting for you when you arrive.

☐ Once the training is designed and planned, create a script or outline for yourself.

☐ Involve people in the process of learning and sharing so the collective experience of the group enhances the learning for everyone involved.

☐ Keep people moving around and interacting as much as you can.

☐ Prepare your evaluation tool for end-of-day feedback from participants. If you are training on behalf of NADD, there will be an evaluation tool to administer. If not, you can create your own or use the evaluation tool included in the appendix of this book.

During the Training

☐ Arrive at the training location very early. This will give you time to make sure everything is working and the environment is as exactly as you had planned (AV and safe electrical cord placement, lighting, temperature, training materials placed where you want them, general room setup, etc.).

- ☐ To set the tone and create an informal and welcoming environment, greet and spend time with participants as they arrive. Ask them about themselves and what excites them about their work. Modeling this as people enter the room provides a natural segue for you to ask people to share their own experience throughout the day.
- ☐ Practice active listening and respecting the perspectives of others.
- ☐ When you first address the group, tell them about yourself, ideally including a relevant short story and elements of your background that relate to the material you are training.
- ☐ Co-create a set of ground rules to make expectations clear regarding things like being on time, respecting other opinions, texting, taking phone calls or doing other work while in the training.
- ☐ Model the established ground rules.
- ☐ Utilize body language consciously (gesture with hands and arms, move around the space effectively, visually connect with all participants, etc.).
- ☐ Personally connect in some way with each person in the room, so everyone feels seen, heard and valued.
- ☐ Always scan the room for engagement. Ask for feedback if you sense things are not working well. Change your approach if how you are teaching a segment is not being received as you had hoped.
- ☐ Let the group know ahead of time that you will seek their feedback at the end of each day so you can learn from their experience and improve your capacity as a trainer.
- ☐ Create a "parking lot" or place where you can capture questions and issues that need to be addressed.

- ☐ Near the end of the day, circle back to discuss the "parking lot" items.
- ☐ Before you end the session and invite people to complete their evaluations, thank them for their engagement, for dedicating the time to increase their skills and for the learning you gained by working with them.
- ☐ Give participants specific information on how they can contact you or NADD for additional resources or learning opportunities.
- ☐ At the end of the day, seek the participants' feedback and allow enough time for people to complete the evaluation before they leave the room.

After the Training

- ☐ Collect the evaluations.
- ☐ Return the room to its original condition. You may want to ask for volunteers to help you.
- ☐ Take all feedback and consider each comment for the lessons so you may learn from them and incorporate them into your next training. If there are trends, those are worthy of deep consideration and learning. Isolated comments may not be particularly helpful.
- ☐ If you are doing a multi-day training, start each subsequent day with a very general summary of the trends of the feedback (not individual comments) and how you are addressing the insights.

Digital Training

- ☐ If possible, conduct the training on a digital platform that allows for video participation and breakout sessions.
- ☐ Utilize emotionally compelling stories, videos and pictures, which are even

more important when training remotely.

- ☐ To keep participants focused, break the training modules into small increments of about 20 minutes, with engaging activities between the 20-minute increments.

- ☐ To ensure participant learning, break up the trainings over multiple days, with no more than four full hours in a day, including breaks.

- ☐ Be trained and proficient with the digital platform you are using. (This is critical.)

- ☐ Before the day of your training, practice all aspects and phases of your training to make sure they work effectively (group video engagement, breakout sessions, screen share, etc.).

- ☐ Be sure you present a professional and calming presence. Don't wear bright colors or extreme patterns. Wearing a pastel color with a gentle neutral background is important.

- ☐ Be aware of your vocal tone and where your eyes are focused. Be a welcoming presence to those watching and listening.

- ☐ Add to your opening session a tutorial on the details of the digital platform so participants know how to use the chat function, how to raise their hand to speak, why it is important to remain muted unless speaking, etc.

- ☐ To maintain a professional atmosphere, incorporate into the tutorial a description of digital etiquette, including how to: position their camera, use the microphone, create the best lighting, ensure their environment is free of distractions, etc.

- ☐ Convert your evaluation process into an automated survey format and allow for completion after each day of training, so you can learn from participant feedback before you next train.

Appendix: Pre- and Post-Tests

Module I: Understanding Dual Diagnosis Basics

APPENDIX

1. Which of the following is the most accurate description of a dual diagnosis?
   (a) Coexistence of two disabilities: intellectual/developmental disability (IDD) and mental illness (MI)
   (b) Coexistence of two or more mental health diagnoses
   (c) Coexistence of a mental health disorder and complex behavioral support needs
   (d) Coexistence of two or more distinct "personalities"

2. True or false: In 2013, the *DSM-5* updated terminology from "mental retardation" to "intellectual disability" or "intellectual developmental disorder."
   True

3. True or false: Adaptive functioning refers to a person's capacity to gain personal independence, based on the person's ability to learn and apply conceptual, social and practical skills in their everyday life.
   True

4. People who have an intellectual/developmental disability often have impairments of general mental abilities that impact adaptive function, which determine how well an individual copes with everyday tasks in the:
   (a) Conceptual domain, the social domain and the practical domain
   (b) Conceptual domain, the practical domain and the vocational domain
   (c) Practical domain, the conceptual domain and the recreational domain
   (d) Conceptual domain, the social domain and the virtual domain

5. Intellectual/developmental disabilities can be categorized as:
   (a) Mild, moderate, profound and extreme
   (b) Invisible, moderate, severe and profound
   (c) Moderate, profound, debilitating and severe
   (d) Mild, moderate, severe and profound

6. For people who have intellectual/developmental disabilities, mental health disorders can be caused by:
   (a) Brain abnormalities
   (b) Bio-psycho-social influences
   (c) Vulnerabilities from environmental factors
   (d) All of the above

7. True or false: It is likely that about 25% of people who have an intellectual/developmental disability will develop a mental health problem at some point in their lives.
   False

8. Psychological vulnerability factors for developing mental health challenges for people who have intellectual/developmental disabilities do *not* include:
   (a) Rejection/deprivation/abuse
   (b) Life events/separations/losses
   (c) Poor self-acceptance/low self-esteem
   (d) Autism spectrum disorder and other neurodevelopmental challenges

9. What might assist a person with IDD through some of their learning issues?
   (a) Strategies to gain attention: using the person's name frequently
   (b) Positive support strategies
   (c) Errorless learning strategies (setting the person up for success)
   (d) All of the above
   (e) (a) and (b) only

10. True or false: People who have a dual diagnosis experience similar employment rates and make as much money as those who have an intellectual/developmental disability only.
    False

Module II: The Genetics of IDD: Syndromes and Phenotypes

1. Among the causes of intellectual/developmental disabilities are:
   (a) Chromosomal abnormalities
   (b) No known causes
   (c) Exposure to toxins
   (d) All of the above

2. True or false: Deletions and duplications of chromosomes along a DNA strand are quite common and collectively account for a significant minority of genetic causes of intellectual disability.
   False

3. The specific and characteristic repertoire exhibited by people with a genetic disorder best describes:
   (a) Genetic phenotype
   (b) Behavioral phenotype
   (c) Chromosomal abnormality
   (d) The behavior of black holes approaching a vacuum

4. There are many benefits of genetic testing, but this is *not* considered one of them:
   (a) Identification of a specific syndrome that may have associated medical vulnerabilities and behavioral phenotypes or specific behavioral patterns
   (b) Early diagnosis assists with early identification of strengths
   (c) Identification of which parent has contributed the chromosomes causing the abnormality
   (d) Preventative health care for medical vulnerabilities

5. True or False: Recent studies indicate there are epigenetic changes associated with FASD.
   True

6. Of the following, which are considered to be medical vulnerabilities associated with Down syndrome:
   (a) Congenital heart defects
   (b) Respiratory and hearing problems
   (c) Thyroid conditions
   (d) Childhood leukemia
   (e) All of the above
   (f) None of the above

7. Fragile X syndrome is a genetic condition that causes a range of developmental problems. Which of the following is *not* associated with Fragile X?
   (a) Can affect males and females equally
   (b) Can result in a predisposition to anxiety and hyperactive behavior
   (c) About one-third of people who have Fragile X also have features of autism spectrum disorder, such as impairments with communication and social interactions
   (d) Fragile X syndrome does not always cause intellectual disability, but most people who have Fragile X have a mild or moderate intellectual disability

8. People with autism spectrum disorder tend to have difficulty with:
   (a) Social disinhibition
   (b) Weight control
   (c) Communication/language
   (d) Impulsiveness

9. The behavioral phenotype of Angelman syndrome is characterized by each of the following *except*:
   (a) A happy demeanor with prominent "smiling"
   (b) Repeated self-injury
   (c) General exuberance associated with hypermotive behavior
   (d) Reduced behavioral adaptive skills
   (e) A full range of emotions (prominent smiling is potentially a motor reaction to physical or mental stimuli)

10. True or false: Treatment of ASD usually focuses around early intervention with proper medical care, education/behavior therapy, language and speech therapy, occupational therapy and physical therapy.
    True

Module III: Comprehensive Assessment Practices

1. Which model is the most clinically useful in identifying the nature of challenging behavior in persons with IDD?
   (a) Medical Model
   (b) Communication Model
   (c) Behavior Model
   (d) Integrative Model

2. Possible functions of challenging behavior in people with IDD/MI can include:
   (a) To gain attention from others
   (b) To escape or avoid demands
   (c) To obtain tangible items or opportunities
   (d) All of the above

3. Best practice in assessment and diagnosis for people with IDD/MI refers to:
   (a) The Bio-psycho-social model
   (b) Behavior analysis
   (c) Mental health assessments
   (d) An annual physical completed by a health professional

4. One of the first steps to completing a functional assessment is:
   (a) Describing the target behavior; assigning an operational definition
   (b) Understanding the behavior from the perspective of the person who directly observes it and the problem it causes for other people
   (c) Identifying the patterns of triggers to help figure out how a behavior is maintained
   (d) Assessing the effectiveness of different approaches on the target behavior

5. Which of the following is the most suggestive indicator that a behavior

pattern may be the result of a mental illness:
(a) The behavior is exhibited only at home
(b) The behavior occurs in all environments; it is not observed just in specific settings
(c) The behavior never occurs when the person's favorite direct support professional is supporting him/her
(d) The person appears to be able to start and stop the behavior at will

6. The bio-psycho-social model __________________________
   (a) Does not require the review of existing data or background information to contribute to the assessment process
   (b) Recognizes that mental health is defined only by the relative absence of psychological distress
   (c) Incorporates the effects of biomedical and psychological factors and how these influences interrelate
   (d) Recognizes that the clinical interview can be completed by reviewing the documented history and reports compiled about the person

7. Which of the following statements is accurate?
   (a) Medical problems in people with IDD are easily recognized
   (b) Dental problems in people with IDD are easily recognized
   (c) Rapid onset in a change in behavior patterns is likely because behavioral problems are directly associated with having the condition of IDD
   (d) Causes of self-injurious behavior in people with IDD can be related to an underlying medical condition

8. True or false: In addition to the client's health history (medical, psychological, substance use), clinicians should obtain the health history of family members.
   True

9. True or false: People with IDD experience the full range of psychiatric disorders as compared to the general population.
   True

APPENDIX

10. Medical conditions:
    (a) Can be present when behavioral problems are exhibited
    (b) Are often underdiagnosed
    (c) Can be masked as behavioral problems
    (d) All of the above

Module IV: Mental Status Exam

1. True or false: The Mental Status Exam (MSE) is intended to be part of a comprehensive assessment of a person's overall condition at the time the exam is administered.
   True

2. The higher-level functions of the brain involved in gaining knowledge and comprehension are referred to as:
   (a) Theory of mind
   (b) Stream-of-consciousness thought
   (c) Cognitive functions
   (d) Functional analysis

3. Which one is *not* a common challenge encountered when completing a proper diagnosis for a person who has an intellectual/developmental disability and a mental health problem?
   (a) Intellectual distortion
   (b) Baseline exaggeration
   (c) Lack of independent identity
   (d) Psycho-social masking

4. True or false: When completing a Mental Status Exam (MSE), the clinician does not need to have an understanding of the person's baseline behavior since the MSE only provides a quick snapshot of the mental status at the time of the assessment.
   False

5. Assessment of mood and affect involves assessing and:
   (a) Describing the predominant mood and its impact on others
   (b) Describing how the person responds to intentional changes in affect of the clinician
   (c) Describing the predominant mood of the person and the person's outward expression of internal emotions
   (d) Describing the general atmosphere of the assessment environment to

interpret the impact on the assessment process

6. Fill in the blank: ___________ can be a significant problem for making a good diagnosis as care providers may see only the escalation of the problem behavior rather than note it along with other symptoms of a psychiatric disorder.
   (a) Effective field theory
   (b) Hashimoto's disease
   (c) Baseline exaggeration
   (d) Paparazzi effect

7. True or false: People with IDD may have preexisting challenges with hyperactivity, challenges with gait, coordination and verbal communication that need to be understood by the clinician when conducting the MSE.
   True

8. When assessing thought process and content as part of the MSE, which of the following is not a consideration?
   (a) Obsessions
   (b) Self-talk
   (c) Telekinesis
   (d) Phobias

9. When assessing cognitive function in a person who has an intellectual/developmental disability, a clinician would *not* consider:
   (a) Attention and concentration
   (b) Developmental level
   (c) Memory
   (d) Daily living skills

10. True or false: Judgment and insight cannot be assessed for a person with an intellectual/developmental disability.
    False

Module V: Overview of the Diagnostic Manual for Persons with Intellectual Disability (DM-ID-2)

APPENDIX

1. The DM-ID-2 was developed in part because of which of the following:
   (a) The DSM-5 relies on self-reporting of signs and symptoms, which is difficult to ascertain in individuals with IDD
   (b) Diagnostic categories are different for people with IDD
   (c) The *DSM-5* is a reliable tool for diagnosing individuals with IDD
   (d) The greater the IDD, the more reliable was the *DSM-5*

2. The DM-ID-2 diagnostic system ________________
   (a) Focuses on comparing the DSM and the International Classification System (ICD)
   (b) Focuses on the International Classification System (ICD)
   (c) Compares the DSM-5 and the DM-ID-2 diagnostic criteria
   (d) All of the above

3. Psychiatric diagnosis tends to ________________
   (a) Vary greatly from person to person
   (b) Require biological markers
   (c) Differ only by age
   (d) Not apply to children

4. Which of the following is *not* something clinicians should do when speaking to an individual with IDD:
   (a) Speak in a monotone voice
   (b) Ask one simple question at a time
   (c) Wait for the answers before proceeding
   (d) Use visuals

5. True or false: In the assessment process, information on individuals with IDD should be provided only by clinicians and staff.
   False

6. True or false: Behavioral phenotype denotes a set of behaviors that are genetically determined and are associated with a particular genetic disorder.
   True

7. True or false: The DM-ID-2 is an acronym to describe people with IDD.
   False

8. Which of the following is not an adaptation used in the DM-ID-2?
   (a) Modification of symptom duration
   (b) Changes in symptom count
   (c) Addition on symptom equivalents
   (d) Use of medications

9. A ______________ perspective is emphasized throughout the DM-ID-2 to assist the clinician in recognizing psychiatric disorders.
   (a) Developmental
   (b) Depressive
   (c) Reactive
   (d) Childhood

10. An accurate DM-ID-2 diagnosis can lead to all of the following *except*:
   (a) Effective treatment
   (b) An increase in the level of IQ
   (c) Better quality of life
   (d) Improved outcomes

Module VI: Signs and Symptoms of Mental Illness

1. What is the difference between anxiety people commonly feel in everyday life and having an anxiety disorder?
(a) Whether people see a therapist
(b) There is no difference
(c) Whether the anxiety interferes with quality of life
(d) If the person takes medication

2. Which factor(s) can complicate diagnosis of mental health disorders in people with IDD?
(a) People with IDD may have narrow communication that can limit their ability to describe their symptoms
(b) People with IDD may experience symptoms of mental health disorders differently
(c) The symptoms a person is experiencing may be connected to a known IDD diagnosis, when there may actually be another condition
(d) All of the above

3. True or false: Depression is not diagnosed as quickly for people with IDD as for the general population as onset tends to be more insidious and changes in baseline are not as apparent.
True

4. ________________ refers to the process of attributing all an individual's symptoms to a known condition.
(a) Assessment
(b) Diagnostic overshadowing
(c) Polypharmacy
(d) Screening

5. True or false: A person with bipolar disorder will show cycling moods (periods of mania and periods of depression) over the course of days or hours.
False

6. This disorder involves excessive anxiety or worry occurring more days than not for at least six months, about a number of events or activities:
   (a) Phobia
   (b) Generalized anxiety disorder
   (c) Panic disorder
   (d) Obsessive-compulsive disorder

7. ________________ cause difficulty perceiving and relating to situations and people, including oneself.
   (a) Personality disorders
   (b) Mood disorders
   (c) Phobias
   (d) Compulsions

8. Psychosis may present in someone with IDD with which of the following symptoms?
   (a) Delusions
   (b) Hallucinations
   (c) Disorganized speech
   (d) All of the above

9. Which is an example of a wellness strategy to help manage anxiety?
   (a) Avoiding work when feeling nervous
   (b) Skipping a party where you don't know many people
   (c) Staying awake all night and worrying about a test the next day
   (d) Attending weekly yoga classes with a friend

10. Which is the greatest indicator that behaviors may indicate an underlying mental health condition?
   (a) The behavior never occurs when the person is at work
   (b) The behavior occurs less frequently if the person eats breakfast
   (c) The behavior occurs in all environments/across settings
   (d) The behavior is only observed at home

Module VII: Positive Support Strategies and Wellness

APPENDIX

1. Which of the following is an example of positive behavior support (PBS)?
   (a) Overcorrection following property destruction
   (b) Teaching conversation skills
   (c) Toothbrushing goals
   (d) Using the Whately Principle to craft a reward scheme that will generalize

2. Which is a reason that inappropriate behavior is difficult to change?
   (a) It probably works for the person based on their history
   (b) It makes sense to the person
   (c) Both are true
   (d) Neither is true

3. Which of the following is not something PBS considers?
   (a) Quality of life
   (b) Effective consequence strategies
   (c) Learning history
   (d) Skill-building

4. When starting a conversation, it is a good idea to:
   (a) Start with limit-setting statements
   (b) Remind the person you are in charge
   (c) All of the above
   (d) None of the above

5. How might one effectively adapt an environment that causes problems for a person?
   (a) Tell the person to ignore whatever is bothering them
   (b) Change the troubling feature, such as choosing a more pleasant tone for an alarm
   (c) There is no effective way to change an environment
   (d) Use Hastur's Behavioral Model as an analysis method

6. What is the purpose of relaxation?
   (a) Supporting a person to be calmer
   (b) Supporting a person to handle stress better
   (c) It is a simple way to improve quality of life
   (d) All of the above

7. Which is an example of Feil's Validation Strategy?
   (a) Asking what a person's favorite beverage is if they are upset over losing their drink
   (b) Reminding the person that their roommates haven't ever stolen things
   (c) Correcting misperceptions
   (d) All of the above

8. Wellness interventions are:
   (a) A good starting point for interventions
   (b) Unlikely to make things worse
   (c) Both (a) and (b) are true
   (d) Neither (a) nor (b) is true

9. Which of the following is not a wellness intervention?
   (a) Improving relaxation
   (b) Promoting reading
   (c) Natural consequences
   (d) Nature walks

10. PRN stands for:
    (a) Per Resources Nullification
    (b) Pro Re Nata
    (c) Pax Riley Non
    (d) Pickman Rand Nephren

Module VIII: Crisis Prevention and Intervention: Reducing Risk

1. ________________ refers to strategies and responses used once signs of crisis are already present.
   (a) Behavior modification
   (b) Crisis intervention
   (c) Crisis prevention
   (d) Informed consent

2. True or false: Most crises can be prevented or interrupted before harm occurs.
   True

3. A crisis plan should:
   (a) Outline what constitutes a crisis for the person and which actions to take to prevent and respond to crises
   (b) Include a list of PRN medications to keep administering until the person is calm
   (c) Only be used if 911 or other emergency services are called
   (d) Require authorization from a psychiatrist

4. ________________ are lifestyle measures (such as relationships, routine and wellness) that minimize the impact of a crisis or prevent a behavior from escalating.
   (a) Symptoms
   (b) Protective factors
   (c) Risk factors
   (d) Triggers

5. Factors that can precipitate a crisis include:
   (a) Grief and loss
   (b) Medication changes or side effects
   (c) Unemployment

(d) All of the above
(e) Only (a) and (b)

6. Crises can be prevented:
   (a) By keeping people isolated from the community and each other
   (b) After the first time a person goes to the emergency department
   (c) By addressing environmental, biological, psychological and social factors that contribute to behavior
   (d) With enough medication

7. What are some challenges with the current crisis system for people with IDD?
   (a) There is a lack of psychiatric services for both adults and children with IDD
   (b) Lack of available community programs leads to overutilization of emergency resources
   (c) People with IDD are at risk of losing homes or jobs following inpatient admission
   (d) All of the above

8. True or false: Risk assessment used to evaluate a crisis for the general population is not an applicable tool for people with IDD.
   False

9. During the __________________ phase of crisis intervention, helpful responses include supportive verbal techniques, maintaining safety, providing distraction and validation.
   (a) Baseline
   (b) Prevention
   (c) Escalation
   (d) Resolution

10. __________________ is based on the idea that negative outcomes result from faulty systems, rather than ineffective people.
   (a) Collaboration
   (b) Triage
   (c) Training
   (d) Inclusion

Module IX:
Adapting Therapy Practices

1. Which of the following is *not* an adaptation to therapy with people with IDD:
   (a) Frequency of sessions
   (b) Duration of therapy over time
   (c) Therapist needs to be supportive
   (d) Longer individual session time

2. Which of the following therapeutic modules can apply to individuals with IDD:
   (a) Group therapy
   (b) Support therapy
   (c) Dialectical behavior therapy
   (d) All of the above

3. The therapist can use the following strategies to modify the complexity of therapy:
   (a) The use of repetition for the person to internalize the material discussed in therapy
   (b) Breaking down interventions into smaller pieces to ensure understanding before moving on to the next topic of discussion
   (c) The use of reflection to ensure understanding of the materials discussed
   (d) All of the above

4. Finish this sentence with the most appropriate response: Group therapy for people with IDD who have experienced trauma ____________________.
   (a) Helps people foster meaningful relationships and establish a sense of trust, and helps decrease feelings of inadequacy and loneliness
   (b) Is not beneficial, as people with IDD cannot benefit from insight-oriented group therapy
   (c) Adapts a standard, uniform technique and engages significant others in the therapeutic process
   (d) All of the above

5. Cognitive Behavior Therapy (CBT) is effective in helping improve a person's overall functioning through:
   (a) Psychoanalytic psychotherapy
   (b) Applied behavior analysis
   (c) Supportive therapy
   (d) Skill development and more adaptive cognitive appraisals of events that trigger intense responses

6. Identify the true statement below:
   (a) EMDR is a recommended treatment for people with IDD who have experienced trauma
   (b) CBT has not yielded positive results among people with IDD
   (c) The general underdiagnosis of PTSD among people who have an IDD does not lead to a large portion of those with PTSD never receiving treatment
   (d) Positive identity development is not an effective trauma-informed intervention

7. The reason communication with collaterals as an adaptation is valuable is because of all *except* the following:
   (a) A therapist should not work in isolation, but be part of the holistic treatment/ habilitation/care planning team
   (b) If the individual is living with natural family, employing a family-systems approach can be incorporated as an adjunct to individual therapy
   (c) Other caregivers can provide important collateral information
   (d) Therapists can validate the feelings of the client

8. True or false: The therapist should never communicate with collaterals.
   False

9. Guiding principles for instilling hope include the following *except*:
   (a) Using positive language
   (b) Staying focused on strengths
   (c) Not raising expectations
   (d) Celebrating accomplishments

10. Complete the question with the most appropriate response: A person with IDD may seek therapy ___________________.
    (a) For reasons as varied as the reasons people without IDD seek therapy
    (b) People with IDD do not have the same problems as people without IDD
    (c) When they have memory retention and self-awareness to participate in traditional models of therapy
    (d) Only when their support staff have thoroughly assessed the nature of their maladaptive behavior

Module X: Trauma-Informed Supports

1. When Xavier was a teenager, he was abused by a staff member at his school program. He is afraid of men who wear neckties and eyeglasses. What is a trauma-informed intervention to support Xavier?
   (a) Limit his DSPs and social relationships to women only
   (b) Identify what makes Xavier feel safe and provide it when he encounters a trigger
   (c) Take him to places and events where only family members are present
   (d) Give Xavier a PRN of an antianxiety medication when he goes out

2. ________________ trauma refers to the type of trauma experienced by hearing about abuse or encounters that happened to other people.
   (a) Vicarious
   (b) Direct
   (c) Complex
   (d) Chronic

3. Whether or not trauma leads to longer-term issues, such as a disorder, depends on:
   (a) The type of developmental disability a person has
   (b) Duration, intensity and intentionality of trauma
   (c) Whether the person has verbal language
   (d) If the person takes medication following the event

4. Possible trauma events for individuals with IDD include:
   (a) Uncertainty of safety and basic needs being met
   (b) Witnessing violence
   (c) Loss of home or job or support services
   (d) All of the above

5. True or false: Everyone will be exposed to events in their lifetime that put them at risk of post-traumatic stress disorder.
   True

6. ____________________ means understanding how trauma affects a person and knowing effective strategies to help them achieve safety and wellness
   (a) Trauma-informed
   (b) Avoidance behavior
   (c) "Fight or flight"
   (d) Positive identity development

7. Trauma is processed and stored in the ____________________ system of the body
   (a) Nervous
   (b) Circulatory
   (c) Limbic
   (d) Digestive

8. Three keys to recovery in a trauma-informed support are:
   (a) Therapy, medication and behavior modification
   (b) Safety, connection and empowerment
   (c) Redirection, refocusing and reframing
   (d) Compliance, consequences and counseling

9. Behaviors that may stem from a history of trauma include:
   (a) Eating nonedible items
   (b) Entering others' personal space
   (c) Refusing medications
   (d) All of the above

10. True or false: Once a person's identity is established, it cannot be improved or changed.
    False

APPENDIX

Module XI:
Childhood and Adolescence

1. Functioning and behavior are influenced by:
   (a) The Eltdown gland
   (b) Stages of development
   (c) A static pathway all young people follow
   (d) None of the above

2. Cultural perspectives of the family must:
   (a) Always be taken into account
   (b) Sometimes be taken into account
   (c) Never be taken into account
   (d) Be considered only when they clash with treatment goals

3. One of the first people to study the development of a personal identity was:
   (a) Randolph Carter
   (b) Tara Maclay
   (c) B.F. Skinner
   (d) Erik Erikson

4. A sense of identity includes:
   (a) Gender identity
   (b) Sense of purpose
   (c) Knowledge of character traits
   (d) All of the above

5. Which of the following is *not* true about most cases of bullying?
   (a) It's done by someone with more power or social support to someone with less power or social support
   (b) It often includes the abuser blaming the target for the abuse
   (c) It often leads to vengeance spells
   (d) In most bullying situations, the target cannot stop the bullying by their own actions

6. Cyberbullying is:
   (a) Becoming less common quickly due to efforts by social media companies
   (b) Difficult to prosecute due to the court case *Gibbous vs. Pnakotic*
   (c) Likely to cause real-world problems for targets
   (d) Not a big worry because it is all online anyway

7. Which of the following is *not* a common adolescent problem?
   (a) Senescence
   (b) Eating disorders
   (c) Depression
   (d) Substance abuse

8. Which of the following is an eating disorder?
   (a) Anorexia nervosa
   (b) Bulimia
   (c) Both (a) and (b)
   (d) Neither (a) or (b)

9. Substance dependence is an extra concern for youth with IDD due to:
   (a) Lack of understanding of long-term consequences
   (b) Greater access to street drugs than typical youth
   (c) Higher risk of physical dependence than typical youth
   (d) All of the above

10. What is the best way to help a young person with IDD be safe in the community?
    (a) Use Hazred's decision matrix
    (b) Teach the young person who and what can be dangerous
    (c) Follow the same routines always, as that builds comfort
    (d) Look for the appearance of safety

Module XII: Wellness and Aging

1. True or false: Older people with IDD generally have poorer health, greater need for support and experience greater health-related functional decline than do older people without IDD.
   True

2. Life expectancy for people with Down syndrome has __________________ in recent decades.
   (a) Remained the same
   (b) Increased dramatically
   (c) Decreased dramatically
   (d) Decreased slightly

3. True or false: Older adults are not able to learn new material or remember new things as they age.
   False

4. Some factors that might affect aging in people with IDD include:
   (a) Genetics
   (b) Lifestyle
   (c) Health
   (d) All of the above

5. __________________ is a technique or modification to our behavior or environment that we use to compensate for a deficit, weakness, injury or perceived inadequacy in a specific area or skill.
   (a) Sensory changes
   (b) Compensatory strategy
   (c) Dementia
   (d) Memory

6. Which of the following sensory changes can be associated with aging?
   (a) Decreased social isolation
   (b) Increased attention span

(c) *Increase in falls*
(d) None of the above

7. Some helpful interventions to create a supportive environment and increase comfort include:
(a) Minimize the time aging people spend in the community
(b) Provide proper lighting, reduce background noise and minimize clutter, such as rugs
(c) Introduce new food and people to the environment
(d) Encourage older people to retire

8. Which of the following is *not* a negative social aspect of aging?
(a) Cognitive decline
(b) Grief and loss
(c) Travel
(d) Accepting mortality

9. ________________ is a legal document in which a person specifies what actions should be taken for their health if they are no longer able to make decisions for themselves because of illness or incapacity.
(a) An advance healthcare directive
(b) Wellness plan
(c) Primary care toolkit
(d) A compensatory strategy

10. Wellness recommendations identified as those with the greatest potential for changing or improving healthy aging include:
(a) Promoting health and preventing illness/injury
(b) Optimizing mental and physical health
(c) Managing chronic conditions
(d) All of the above

Module XIII: Justice System Considerations

1. True or false: In the early part of the twentieth century, it was an accepted theory that people who have an intellectual/developmental disability were inherently criminal in their nature.
   True

2. This is *not* a reason there are challenges in capturing accurate prevalence rates of people who have an intellectual/developmental disability who interact with the justice system:
   (a) Underreporting to police services
   (b) Stats tend to represent the arrest and conviction rate as opposed to the true offending prevalence
   (c) People with IDD rarely get arrested
   (d) Research more often focuses on the rates of recidivism as opposed to the rates of offending

3. Counterfeit criminality is:
   (a) The concept that criminal behavior is performed for reasons other than criminality or criminal gain
   (b) The concept that a person with IDD can appear innocent even if they are guilty of committing a crime
   (c) When someone is falsely accused of a crime
   (d) The same as bait-and-switch, which is unethical but not always illegal

4. Which of the following is *not* considered an effective means to support people who have IDD in avoiding criminal behavior?
   (a) Assist people in developing friendships and learning about different types of social interactions
   (b) Ensure people are aware of the laws in their state/province so they can avoid breaking the law
   (c) Ensure people have an opportunity to advocate for themselves in ways they want

(d) Provide an opportunity for people to practice social skills in a variety of situations and environments

5. True or false: A person who has IDD frequently has specific vulnerabilities that can lead to initial involvement with the justice system and faces challenges that can often make it difficult to end that involvement or avoid future involvement.
   True

6. When people who have an IDD become involved with the justice system, they frequently experience prejudice, lack of understanding and fear. They often experience difficulties with:
   (a) Not being recognized as having a disability
   (b) Being victimized at high rates
   (c) Being denied opportunities for reparation
   (d) All of the above
   (e) (a) and (c) only

7. Fill in the blank: Fitness to stand trial, or __________, refers to the ability of a person accused to participate in their own defense.
   Competence

8. Forensic psychiatry relates to:
   (a) Understanding the behavior and motivation of people who commit homicide
   (b) Assessment and treatment of dangerous psychopaths
   (c) The assessment, treatment and rehabilitation of people with serious mental illness who have come in contact with the law as a result of committing a crime
   (d) The gathering and analysis of all crime-related psychological and psychiatric evidence in order to come to a conclusion about a suspect

9. True or false: A diagnosis of IDD and a mental illness means a person will be found unfit to stand trial.
   False

10. Which of the following is *not* an ethical consideration that should be discussed before caregivers and service providers develop crisis plans that include calling police services:
    (a) Is it the responsibility of the provider to manage aggressive behavior?
    (b) Should a person who has IDD be charged for aggression to caregivers or providers?
    (c) What is the goal of the intervention?
    (d) What is the caregiver's or service provider's expectation of police services?
    (e) None of the above

Module XIV: The Importance of Direct Support Professionals

1. In general, ________________ spend more time with the person with IDD/MI than any other team member and can make a big difference in the quality of life for people.
   (a) Behavior specialists
   (b) Psychiatrists
   (c) Direct support professionals
   (d) Pharmacists

2. Luke wants to try out for the community theater since he was in his high school play and he misses performing. His mom doesn't want him to go to auditions because Luke has depression and she is concerned that rejection will trigger a mental health crisis. How can Luke's Direct Support Professional best support Luke?
   (a) Talk with Luke about different options and prepare him for possible outcomes
   (b) Call to schedule a psychiatrist's appointment in anticipation of increased need for medication
   (c) Partner with Luke's mom to find a more realistic goal for him
   (d) Offer Luke a preferred activity if he skips the audition

3. True or false: When we include Direct Support Professionals in planning for persons with IDD/MI, more accurate and useful information will emerge.
   True

4. Identify a workforce challenge(s) in the field of IDD/MI:
   (a) Most Direct Support Professionals are not certified or credentialed
   (b) Requirements for employment vary according to agency or employer
   (c) Direct Support Professionals generally work for low wages
   (d) All of the above

5. The NADSP Code of Ethics®:
   (a) Is intended to serve as a straightforward and relevant guide for Direct
   (b) Support Professionals to help resolve the ethical dilemmas they face every day
   (c) Encourages Direct Support Professionals to achieve the highest ideals of the profession
   (d) Includes the principles of confidentiality, respect, self-determination and advocacy
   (e) All of the above

6. Which of the following is *not* a challenge many Direct Support Professionals face in their work?
   (a) A lot is expected from Direct Support Professionals who are often left out of the planning process
   (b) Direct Support Professionals are unwilling to participate in training
   (c) Direct Support Professionals are often required to implement, maintain, evaluate and assess plans they did not develop
   (d) Some Direct Support Professionals are expected to use tools with which they are not familiar

7. ____________________ helps staff learn and practice skills in the setting where they will be used.
   (a) Classroom training
   (b) Virtual courses
   (c) On-the-job training
   (d) Certification

8. The goal of programs such as the NADD Direct Support Professional Certification and the Ontario Developmental Services Human Resource Strategy is to build capacity among workforce professionals through a set of standards called:
   (a) Core competencies
   (b) Requirements
   (c) Expectations
   (d) Learning skills

9. True or false: Training is not complete until a Direct Support Professional can demonstrate the skill on the job.
   True

10. An outcome(s) of Direct Support Professionals who demonstrate competency in IDD/MI include:
    (a) Greater consistency and efficacy in support delivery for people with mental and behavioral health needs
    (b) More turnover and lower wages for Direct Support Professionals who work in the field of IDD/MI
    (c) Direct Support Professionals are less empowered to provide feedback and contribute to planning
    (d) Direct Support Professionals who require more supervision

APPENDIX

Module XV: Collaborating Across Systems

1. Lack of strategic planning has led to a "silo system" that:
   (a) Provides a plan to use state agencies as support
   (b) Confines people with a dual diagnosis to small areas
   (c) Ensures that people can escape the hustle and bustle of the city
   (d) Results in access barriers to required services

2. The MH and IDD systems:
   (a) Often do not collaborate, fostering divide between them
   (b) May work together if the person pursues
   (c) Will collaborate if the person requires treatment
   (d) Always actively collaborate for betterment

3. Services for people with a dual diagnosis need to be:
   (a) Based primarily on a comprehensive assessment
   (b) Based primarily on the mental health concerns
   (c) Based primarily on what services are available
   (d) Based primarily on the level of ID

4. True or false: Dual diagnosis planning principles are based only on MH or IDD diagnoses.
   False

5. A holistic approach to care and treatment requires:
   (a) Neither a mental health nor a developmental disabilities approach
   (b) A focus on a mental health approach
   (c) A focus primarily on developmental disabilities
   (d) Both a focus on mental health and developmental disabilities

6. Intersystem collaboration means:
   (a) Interacting with your agency colleagues
   (b) Interacting with the person being served

(c) Interacting with staff from other systems
(d) Interacting with the individual and their family

7. The goal of community collaboration is to:
    (a) Improve access to and availability of human services
    (b) Raise awareness for individuals within a community
    (c) Build a more effective system for individuals
    (d) All of the above

8. Co-occurring disorders should be treated:
    (a) By the severity of the disorder, with the more severe being treated first
    (b) There is no such thing as co-existing disorders
    (c) As multiple primary disorders, with each requiring active treatment and supports
    (d) By the severity of the disorder, with the milder disorders being dealt with first

9. People with a dual diagnosis generally:
    (a) Experience difficulty fitting into both systems
    (b) Can never fit into either system
    (c) Easily fit into the MH system
    (d) Easily fit into the IDD system

10. The purpose of a Dual Diagnosis Committee includes:
    (a) Using the courts to catalyze change
    (b) Protecting persons with a disability abroad
    (c) Gathering relevant information to analyze strengths/weaknesses
    (d) Building an international headquarters for people with a dual diagnosis

Index

INDEX

INDEX

INDEX

INDEX

INDEX

I N D E X

INDEX

www.ingramcontent.com/pod-product-compliance
Lightning Source LLC
LaVergne TN
LVHW081959200926
848481LV00010B/2773

* 9 7 9 8 9 8 5 3 3 6 6 2 7 *